Introduction to
Public Health
Program Planning

D1560658

Joanna Hayden, PhD, CHES

Professor Emeritus, Department of Public Health,
William Paterson University

JONES & BARTLETT
LEARNING

World Headquarters
Jones & Bartlett Learning
5 Wall Street
Burlington, MA 01803
978-443-5000
info@jblearning.com
www.jblearning.com

Jones & Bartlett Learning books and products are available through most bookstores and online booksellers. To contact Jones & Bartlett Learning directly, call 800-832-0034, fax 978-443-8000, or visit our website, www.jblearning.com.

Substantial discounts on bulk quantities of Jones & Bartlett Learning publications are available to corporations, professional associations, and other qualified organizations. For details and specific discount information, contact the special sales department at Jones & Bartlett Learning via the above contact information or send an email to specialsales@jblearning.com.

26875-1

Production Credits

VP, Product Development: Christine Emerton
Director of Product Management: Laura Pagluica
Product Manager: Sophie Fleck Teague
Content Strategist: Sara Bempkins
Project Manager: Kristen Rogers
Senior Project Specialist: Dan Stone
Senior Marketing Manager: Susanne Walker
VP, Manufacturing and Inventory Control: Therese Connell
Composition: SPi Global

Project Management: SPi Global
Cover Design: Kristin E. Parker
Text Design: Kristin E. Parker
Media Development Editor: Faith Brosnan
Rights Specialist: Maria Leon Maimone
Cover Images/Title Page: (Top) © Sankai/iStock/Getty Images Plus/Getty Images; (Bottom) © PM Images/DigitalVision/Getty Images
Printing and Binding: McNaughton & Gunn

Library of Congress Cataloging-in-Publication Data

Names: Hayden, Joanna, author. Title: Introduction to public health program planning / Joanna Hayden. Description: First edition. | Burlington: Jones & Bartlett Learning, 2021. | Includes bibliographical references and index. | Summary: Identifiers: LCCN 2020050336 | ISBN 9781284175189 (paperback) Subjects: LCSH: Health planning. | Health promotion. | Community health services. Classification: LCC RA394.9 .H39 2021 | DDC 362.1--dc23 | LC record available at https://lccn.loc.gov/2020050336

6048

Printed in the United States of America
25 24 23 22 21   10 9 8 7 6 5 4 3 2 1

Contents

Preface

Program planning is integral to the practice of public health. As such, the intent of this text is to familiarize students preparing for careers in public health with the basics of this essential skill. It is an introduction to, not a compendium of, all that there is on the topic. With its three sections, Planning Foundations, Planning Basics, and Planning Frameworks, the depth and breadth of the content covered in *Introduction to Public Health Program Planning* is meant to provide students with a base from which to build their planning skills.

The first section, Planning Foundations, is comprised of Chapters 1–3. Chapter 1 is an introduction to program planning, its role in public health, and factors that contribute to health that become the focus of programs. Chapter 2 presents a summary of the more commonly used intrapersonal, interpersonal, and community-level behavior theories that serve as the foundation for program development. In Chapter 3, the generic stages of program planning—assessing, planning, implementing, and evaluating—are introduced in preparation of their detailed discussions in the next section. Also covered in this chapter are the preparatory activities inherent in constituting a planning committee and convening a meeting, from developing an agenda to taking minutes.

The second section of the text, Planning Basics, includes Chapters 4–7, with each chapter covering one of the generic stages of planning process. Chapter 4, Assessing Needs, introduces the process of conducting a needs assessment, including data sources and collection methods, and prioritizing results. Chapter 5 presents the activities associated with developing a program plan to address the priority issue identified in the needs assessment, from developing goals, objectives, and program activities to writing a program rationale. Chapter 6, Implementing, explains how programs are implemented, how implementation contributes to outcomes of the program, and the challenges inherent in the process. Chapter 7, Evaluating, addresses program evaluation from the types of evaluation and evaluation designs to developing an evaluation plan and writing an evaluation report.

The third and final section of the text, Planning Frameworks, consists of Chapters 8–13. These chapters cover a mix and array of commonly used planning frameworks, each in its own chapter, which includes a short historical perspective of the framework followed by a detailed discussion of its phases, steps, or tasks. In Chapter 8, the PRECEDE-PROCEED framework is introduced. Each phase of the framework is discussed and, wherever possible, supplemented with examples from the literature. Chapter 9, Mobilizing for Action Through Planning and Partnerships (MAPP), provides a summary of the six phases of the MAPP process with examples of its use in practice. Chapter 10 presents the five steps of the MAP-IT framework—Mobilize, Assess, Plan, Implement, and Track, with questions intended as a guide for using the framework. In Chapter 11, the six core process and six planning steps of Intervention Mapping are summarized and supplemented with figures and tables to enable students to better understand the matrices characteristic of this framework. Chapter 12 presents three planning frameworks used to address specific health issues and methodology to give the student exposure to more focused frameworks. These include the Strategic Planning Framework for programs addressing substance abuse and misuse issues, Protocol for Assessing Community Excellence in Environmental Health (PACE-EH) for programs addressing environmental health issues, and Making Health Communication Programs Work for developing communication campaigns. The stages, steps, and activities comprising each of these frameworks are described and their use in practice demonstrated by examples from the professional literature. The final chapter of the text, Chapter 13, provides direction on how to choose a framework. To this end, a set of guidelines is presented and a chart that compares the generic stages of program planning to the different stages, phases, and steps of the frameworks presented in Chapters 8–12.

Most chapters begin with an analogy to prompt student understanding of the content to be discussed. Each chapter ends with a *Chapter Summary Sentence,* a statement that encapsulates the essence of the chapter contents to substantiate student understanding of what was presented.

Also at the end of every chapter is a *Planning in Practice Chapter Activity.* These activities are based on peer-reviewed journal articles that demonstrate the application of the chapter content in a practice setting to enable students to "see" how the information is used in the real world. The activities in Chapters 1–12 are based on articles in open access journals for which the links are provided. The activity article in Chapter 13 is not open access, but is easily accessed through the university/college library with the information provided.

It is my hope that this text will provide students with a solid foundation in program planning to start their careers in public health. It is also my hope that it will serve as a reference throughout their careers.

Acknowledgments

This book would not have happened had it not been for Mike Brown, my longtime (recently retired) editor at Jones & Bartlett Learning. It was his confidence in my ability to write the text and his guidance during the preliminary stages of the project that enabled it to come to fruition. I cannot thank him enough for this and for his wise counsel over the years.

A special thanks to Sophie Teague, my "new" editor, who took over from Mike without missing a beat, and Sara Bempkins, my content strategist, whose support from start to finish was invaluable. To the Jones & Bartlett Learning editorial and production staff goes a huge thank-you for all their help—Maria Leon Maimone, Praveen Babu, Dan Stone, and Faith Brosnan.

I also want to thank Hollie Gibbons, John Hudson, Christine Malone, Jamie Newman, and Tonya Roberson for making time in their busy schedules to serve as reviewers. Their suggestions were spot-on. I hope they see how much I valued their comments on the pages of this text.

Last but not least, I'd like to thank my husband Roger for his never ending support of my writing and never ending supply of tea, and finally our pup Alfie for making sure I took breaks from sitting at my computer to take him for his walks.

Reviewers

Hollie Gibbons, MPH, RD
Assistant Professor
Cedar Crest College
Allentown, PA

John S. Hudson, PhD, RN, FACHE
University of North Carolina, Chapel Hill
Chapel Hill, NC

Christine Malone, EdD, MBA, MHA, CPHRM, CMPE, FACHE
City University of Seattle
Seattle, WA

Jamie Newman MPH, RT(R)(M)(BD)
Lecturer
California State University, Long Beach
Long Beach, CA

Tonya S. Roberson, PhD, MPH
Director of Community Engagement,
    Program Development and Academic
    Support
Governors State University
University Park, IL

SECTION I

Planning Foundations

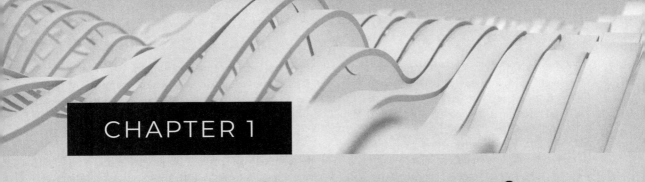

CHAPTER 1

Introduction to Planning

Introduction

Welcome to planning!

Regardless of your professional aspirations, planning skills will serve you well in your public health career. If at first glance the planning process appears overwhelming, relax a little because you've already used it to some degree when you planned your last vacation, party, or camping trip.

So, what exactly is planning? Planning is a process, a series of actions or steps, a systematic approach used to reach a goal or predetermined endpoint. Look at the planning process as a GPS. It gives directions, estimates how long each phase of the trip should take and when you'll arrive at your destination.

Think back to your last party. Why did you have it? The reason for it determined who was invited, where it was held, the time, day,

food, drink, and possibly music or entertainment. The "to-do" list you made kept you on track to get everything done. The decisions you made and the actions you took were all part of planning your party.

While the ability to plan is a handy life skill, for a public health professional it's a necessity. It underlies each of the 10 essential public health services, which include

- Monitoring health status to identify and solve community health problems
- Diagnosing and investigate health problems and hazards in the community
- Informing, educating, and empowering people about health issues
- Mobilizing community partnerships to identify and solve health problems
- Developing policies that support individual and community health efforts

- Enforcing laws and regulations that protect health and ensure safety
- Linking people to health services
- Ensuring a competent public and personal healthcare workforce
- Evaluating the effectiveness, accessibility, and quality of health services
- Conducting research for innovative solutions to health problems (Centers for Disease Control and Prevention [CDC], 2017a)

Why Plan?

We plan because it helps us develop the most logical, organized, effective, and efficient means to accomplish our goal. We plan because success doesn't happen by magic, and in the words of Benjamin Franklin, "failing to plan, is planning to fail."

Planning helps us focus on priorities, formalize efforts, set expectations and timelines, define roles and responsibilities, measure the effectiveness of our actions (CDC, n.d.), use resources wisely, and adjust along the way to improve future programs. It's a process that flows through the entirety of a program, giving it direction, making it more purposeful, being amenable to change, and offering clear understanding of its effectiveness (Steuart, 1993).

So, planning is the process used to create or develop programs or interventions. By definition, a program is a set of related, organized public health actions and activities undertaken to achieve an intended outcome, including policies, interventions, initiatives, preparedness, research, capacity and infrastructure, and other efforts (CDC, 2019).

An *intervention*, by definition, is any combination of elements or strategies designed to assess, improve, maintain, promote, or modify health or health conditions, or produce behavioral change among individuals or entire populations (Missouri Department of Health and Senior Services [DHSS], n.d.; World Health Organization [WHO], n.d.). An intervention,

then, can refer to an educational program or a health promotion campaign, new or improved laws or policies (Missouri DHSS, n.d.), workshops, curricula, screenings, trainings, demonstrations, initiatives, or projects.

Endeavors referred to as interventions are just as likely to be referred to as programs, and vice versa. Although both terms, intervention and program, are used interchangeably in public health, *program* is used throughout this text in reference to any or all of the previous examples.

Programs come in many "sizes." Some are global, such as the World Health Organization's *Global TB (tuberculosis) Program*, which advances universal access to TB prevention, care, and control; guides the global response to threats; and promotes innovation (World Health Organization [WHO], 2018a) or the WHO Program for International Drug Monitoring, which enhances patient care and safety in the use of medicines (WHO, 2018b).

Other programs are national in scope. For example: the CDC's *Safe Water Program*, which aims to decrease environmental threats to water systems and reduce exposure to waterborne contaminants (CDC, 2015) or the Food and Drug Administration's (FDA's) *Real Cost* program, which is a national public education program to discourage young people from using tobacco (FDA, n.d.). A sampling of the many other national programs are the *Supplemental Nutrition Assistance Program—SNAP*; *FAST*, a campaign for stroke awareness; *Great American Smoke Out*; and *Safe to Sleep Campaign* (formerly Back to Sleep) for sudden infant death prevention.

A host of programs at the state level address a wide mix and array of public health issues. For example, the Massachusetts *Childhood Lead Poisoning Prevention Program* aims to prevent, screen, diagnose, and treat childhood lead poisoning (Massachusetts Department of Public Health, 2018), while *Matter of Balance*, a statewide program in New Jersey, reduces the fear of falling and increases the activity levels of older adults (New Jersey Department of

Human Services, 2013). In 2003, Project ECHO (Extension for Community Health Outcomes) was launched in New Mexico to help alleviate a shortage of specialty physicians in rural and remote areas of the state (University of New Mexico, 2018).

There is no lack of public health programming at the local or community level either. Among the many are car seat distribution and demonstration events, cancer screenings, health fairs, mall walking interventions, and rabies clinics for dogs and cats, to name but a tiny fraction of all that are offered.

While a well-thought-out plan is critical to the success of any program, the plans are only as good as the information used to develop them. Key to planning successful programs is understanding what influences health in the first place.

Determinants of Health

Determinants of health are factors that contribute to the state of a person's health (U.S. Department of Health and Human Services [USDHHS], 2018a). It's important to know about the determinants of health in planning programs because it enables us to identify the things we cannot change, plan to change the things we can, and have the wisdom to know the difference (Alcoholics Anonymous, n.d.).

The determinants of health are grouped into five broad categories: individual behavior, social and physical factors, biology and genetics, health services, and policies. The interrelationships among these factors determines the health of a person and, by extension, a population (USDHHS, 2018a).

Behavioral Determinants of Health

The contribution individual behaviors make to health cannot be overstated. The actions people take, the way they live their lives, the choices they make every day, all day, impact health. Just for a moment, think about the health behavior choices you made today. Did you eat breakfast? If you did, what did you eat? Was it oatmeal with a piece of fresh fruit or a bowl of sugar-sweetened cereal with a soda? Did you brush your teeth today? Did you stay up all night playing video games? Was your seat belt buckled on your drive to campus? These are all lifestyle behaviors that affect health.

Studies conducted over the past 50 years on the relationship between lifestyle and disease identify three behaviors strongly associated with morbidity and mortality—cigarette smoking, physical inactivity, and a predominately animal-based diet (Puddu & Menotti, 2015). Other behaviors known to affect health include inadequate sleep, substance abuse, and medication abuse—in particular, antibiotics (Farhud, 2015).

Lifestyle behaviors are important because up to 40 percent of the premature deaths in the United States each year from the five leading causes of death—heart disease, stroke, cancer, chronic lower respiratory diseases, and unintentional injuries—have preventable lifestyle causes. Tobacco use, physical inactivity, and poor diet coupled with inadequate control of high blood pressure, high cholesterol, type 2 diabetes, and weight, as well as excessive alcohol use, contribute to increased risk of heart disease and stroke (CDC, 2014). Tobacco use, poor dietary choices alone and in combination with poor weight management (overweight or obesity), physical inactivity, sun exposure, excessive alcohol use, and exposure to known carcinogens are among the behaviors contributing to premature cancer deaths. Tobacco smoking, exposure to secondhand smoke, and indoor and outdoor air pollution increase the risk of death from chronic respiratory disease (CDC, 2014).

More than a third of the deaths from unintentional injury could be prevented if people changed their behavior, specifically, if people wore seat belts, used a helmet

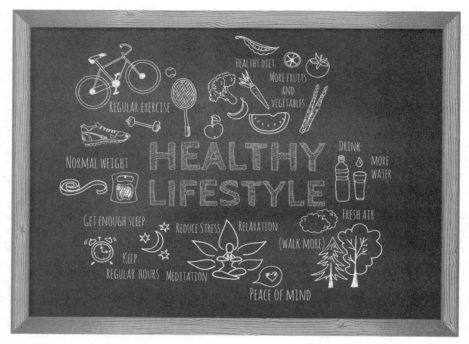

Figure 1-1 Behavioral determinants of health
© Aigel Ber/Shutterstock

when riding a motorcycle, and didn't misuse or abuse drugs and/or alcohol (CDC, 2014). (See **Figure 1-1**.)

Social and Physical Determinants of Health

The behaviors people engage in that affect their health don't happen in a vacuum. They happen within the context of where they live, learn, work, play, and worship, within social and physical environments (USDHHS, 2018a). They are influenced by the social, cultural, and economic realities of their lives (Cockerham, 2000).

The social determinants of health are grouped into five key areas: economic stability, education, social and community context, health and health care, and the neighborhood and built environment (USDHHS, 2018b). They entail the economic and social conditions that influence health (WHO, 2008) and

are contributing factors to health inequities (CDC, 2014). (See **Figure 1-2**.)

Economic Stability

Economic stability encompasses employment status, food availability, stable housing, and poverty. Inconsistent employment or insufficient income from employment can create a situation where people are faced with making choices between subsistence needs and healthcare needs. Sometimes the resulting choice is that healthcare and medication needs are postponed in order to buy food and pay rent (Reid, Vittinghoff, & Kushel, 2008).

Poverty and food insecurity are related to some of the most serious health problems in the United States, including asthma, cancer, depression, hepatitis, high blood pressure, obesity, diabetes, and congestive heart failure, among others. They have significant health consequences across the lifespan, increasing the risk

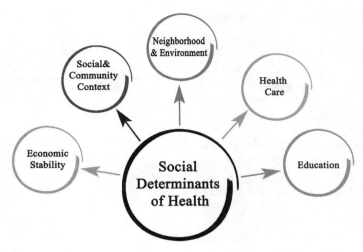

Figure 1-2 Social determinants of health

© Arka38/Shutterstock

of chronic disease and poor mental health (Food Research & Action Center, 2017).

Education

Both formal and informal education impact health and health behavior. Formal education is consistently linked to greater problem-solving skills, information-processing ability, and a personal sense of control over one's actions (Pampel, Krueger, & Denny, 2010). Education teaches people how to obtain, assess, and use information (Mirowsky & Ross, 2003, 2005), thereby increasing health literacy. When people understand their health needs and can read and follow instructions, advocate for themselves, and communicate effectively with their healthcare providers, it leads to healthier behaviors and better health outcomes. In fact, physicians respond differently to patients they see as less educated. They communicate less with them and provide more directive care (Zimmerman et al., 2015), rather than involving the patient in care decisions.

However, more education doesn't always predict healthier behaviors. In some cases, the opposite is true—as education increases—so do some unhealthy behaviors. Two examples of this are binge drinking (Zimmerman et al., 2015) and eating disorders (Goodman, Heshmati, & Koupil, 2014),

Because of the importance of education to individual and public health, it's necessary to emphasize that not all education is attained from formal schooling (Hahn & Truman, 2015). For a moment, think about all the things people learn outside the classroom from family, friends, neighbors, and community. So, when research links knowledge with health, keep in mind that not all consequences might be because of formal education (Feinstein, Sabates, Anderson, Sorhaindo, & Hammond, 2006).

Although education is clearly linked to better health, contrary to what would be expected, programs focused on increasing knowledge alone don't always work well, nor do they necessarily lead to behavior change (Kelly & Barker, 2016; Kollmuss & Agyeman, 2002; Whitehead & Russell, 2004). Just because people know something, doesn't mean they'll change what they do. Knowledge is necessary for behavior change to occur, but it doesn't guarantee it will happen.

Social and Community Context

Civic engagement, discrimination, incarceration, and social cohesion are aspects of the social environment that define our relationships with others. They are reflected in cultural practices and religious beliefs, race relations, and government and power relations (Barnett & Casper, 2001).

Civic engagement enables people to make a difference in their communities, to improve the quality of life in their community through both political and nonpolitical means (Ehrlich, 2000). Civic engagement is both voluntary and autonomously chosen (Goth & Smaland, 2014) and not only has a positive social impact, but also seems to be a significant factor in self-reported health status in many countries across the globe (Kim, Kim, & You, 2015). When people have a voice in the way their communities function, that is, they have a voice in the government and with those in power, they tend to be healthier (National Physicians Alliance, n.d.).

The helping behavior of volunteering boosts both physical and psychological health. Volunteers generally have less depression, lower mortality risks, better psychological well-being, and better physical functioning as compared to those who don't volunteer, even when the health conditions of the two groups are the same (Konrath, Fuhrel-Forbis, Lou, & Brown, 2012).

Religion serves as a social determinant of health in at least three possible ways. It can impact health behaviors through restricting or prohibiting certain foods such as pork, shellfish, or animal products; requiring certain others such as vegetarianism (in Hinduism and Buddhism) and attention to food preparation practices (kosher in Judaism, halal in Islam); and promoting a healthy lifestyle by forbidding alcohol use and smoking (Koenig, 2012; Rumun, 2014).

Second, it might be that religion provides social support for people when they're in crisis through church, synagogue, mosque, or other religious groups (Basu-Zharku, 2011; Koenig, 2012; Oman & Thorensen, 2002). Religion also encourages development of virtues that promote social relationships and social cohesion such as honesty, forgiveness, generosity, altruism, that are associated with marital stability, less crime, and greater social capital (Koenig, 2012).

Religion might also be an individual determinant of health because it supports mental or psychological health by providing its followers with more optimism, encouraging more positive psychological states and less stress (Koenig, 2012; Oman & Thorensen, 2002). It facilitates coping and gives meaning to unfortunate life events, which in turn lessens stress, depression, and anxiety (Koenig, 2012).

Culture represents norms and customs, expected, accepted practices built on common beliefs, values, history, heritage, and language that constitute a way of life. It plays a significant role in health, not only from its impact on behaviors that affect health, but also in how health is defined in the first place. When health is defined without taking culture into consideration, it limits the definition to a body-centered, biomedical viewpoint—that health is biological wellness (Napier et al., 2014), which focuses on disease progression and treatment (Knibb-Lamouche, 2012). But, health through the lens of a culture may be seen as a balance between nature, social relationships, the spirit or supernatural, and the functioning of the human body. Therefore, the concept of health, as it is understood through the lens of a culture, influences health practices (Levesque, 2014).

An excellent example of this is in cultures that believe in a hot/cold theory of disease causation, where health is a state of balance between hot and cold aspects of the body. Illnesses or aliments occur when there is an imbalance between these. When the cause of an illness is "cold," a "hot" treatment is used to bring the body back into balance and vice versa.

Using this definition or concept of health, high blood pressure is a hot disease caused by anger, fear, nervousness, and thick blood. Consequently, it's treated with remedies classified as having cold qualities, including lemon juice and a variety of herbal teas. In contrast, asthma is a cold disease, which calls for treatments with hot qualities to restore balance in the body. Some of the commonly used hot treatments include cod liver oil, honey, olive oil, garlic/onion, and aloe vera juice (Ortiz, Shields, Clauson, & Clay, 2007). Keep in mind that the actual temperature of the treatment is not what determines if it's hot or cold, but rather tradition or belief.

Health and Health Care

Health care as a social determinant of health is about access to care. Access to care means using healthcare services in a timely manner to get the best health outcomes. It entails having health insurance, a usual source of care, and timely care (*Healthy People 2020*, 2020a).

Health insurance enables entry into the healthcare system. Consequently, those without insurance are less likely to receive care and more likely to have poor health (Agency for Health Care Quality [AHCQ], 2018) and more likely to die prematurely (*Healthy People 2020*, 2020a). Compared to those who are insured, the uninsured are also more likely to postpone or not seek health care because of cost and skip preventative screenings, all of which can lead to preventable diseases going undetected and untreated (Garfield, Orgera, & Damico, 2019). (See **Figure 1-3**.)

Having access to a regular or usual healthcare provider leads to better health outcomes (AHCQ, 2018) and a greater likelihood of having preventative screenings (Blewett, Johnson, Lee, & Scal, 2008). It's also associated with an increased likelihood of receiving proper care, lower mortality from all causes, fewer disparities, and lower costs. (*Healthy People 2020*, 2020a).

Access to timely care refers to the healthcare system's ability to provide care quickly when needed. It includes the availability of appointments for an illness or an injury when it's needed and the time spent waiting to see the healthcare provider in both the office and emergency room. A delay in the time it takes to get care increases stress, complications, costs, and the need for hospitalization (*Healthy People 2020*, 2020a).

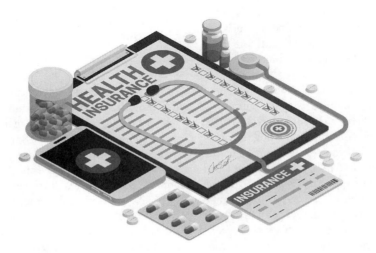

Figure 1-3 Health insurance enables access to care

Neighborhood and Built Environment

The neighborhood and built environment comprise the natural environment or green space, weather, and climate and all things man-made, including buildings, roads, sidewalks, bike lanes, housing and community designs, physical barriers, and exposure to toxic substances (*Healthy People 2020*, 2020b). Where people live and the characteristics of that space significantly affect their health by its influence on physical activity, exposure to toxic substances, and access to healthy food (Perdue, Stone, & Goslin, 2003).

Unfortunately, the built environment in many places is detrimental to health. For example, urban areas often lack safe open spaces for people to walk and children to play. This limits physical activity, which promotes sedentary lifestyles that contribute to diabetes, cardiovascular disease, and obesity (Perdue et al., 2003).

Although open space may be available in suburban areas, these environments have their own set of unhealthy ramifications as they create a dependency on cars. Suburban sprawl not only discourages physical activity because walking or biking from place to place is impractical or even impossible, but it also contributes to air pollution (Perdue et al., 2003).

The built environment isn't always detrimental to health. In fact, it can be conducive to good health. When neighborhoods are built including the natural hills of the terrain (rather than leveling them), it encourages people to walk uphill, which is a physiologically vigorous activity that can contribute to weight control and reduced risk of diabetes (Villanueva et al., 2013).

In addition to the impact the built environment has on our health is the impact of the neighborhood itself. We see this clearly with lead poisoning. Lead poisoning is linked to the unequal distribution of housing in low-income neighborhoods that contain lead paint (Sampson & Winter, 2016). It's a particularly serious problem in urban areas. In fact, exposure to environmental lead is almost four times greater (21 vs. 6 percent) for children living in inner cities than

other children (Lidsky & Schneider, 2003). It's associated with cognitive impairment and lower IQ (Reuben et al., 2017); stunted physical development (Lidsky & Schneider, 2003); increased impulsivity, anxiety, and depression (Winter & Sampson, 2017); and delinquent behavior (Sampson & Winter, 2018). The neurological, physical, and cognitive damage from lead poisoning is irreversible and lifelong.

People living in disadvantaged neighborhoods face daily stressors (Pampel et al., 2010) that trigger drinking, smoking, and overeating (Bjorntorp, 2001; Marmot, 2004), increase the risk of dying prematurely, and contribute to reduced incentive to adopt healthy behaviors (Lawlor, Frankel, Shaw, Ebrahim, & Smith, 2003). It might be that engaging in unhealthy behaviors makes sense when people live in conditions where they expect to die young (Pampel et al., 2010) rather than engaging in healthy ones.

Biological and Genetic Determinants of Health

The biologic and genetic determinants of health include, for example, age, biological sex and/or gender, family history, and inherited or genetic conditions. In theory, along with health behaviors, these factors account for about 25 percent of our health (CDC, 2014). (See **Figure 1-4**.)

Age

Although age is associated with a number of different diseases and conditions—hearing loss, cataracts, osteoarthritis, diabetes, emphysema, dementia (WHO, 2018c), heart disease, and cancers—these are loosely correlated with a person's actual age in years (WHO, 2018c) and are partly the result of lifestyle behaviors, diet, and environment, which are modifiable (Merck Manual, 2016). The point here is that age as a determinant of health shouldn't automatically be associated with "aging" and poor or failing health. Different health issues are associated with different ages across the

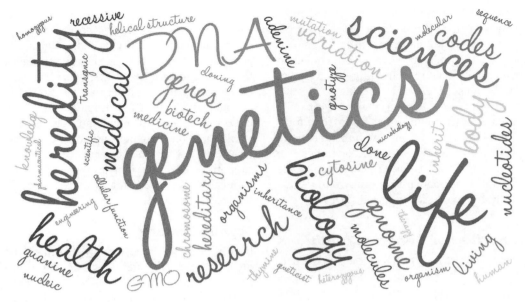

Figure 1-4 Biological and genetic determinants of health

© Arloo/Shutterstock

lifespan. For instance, half of the 20 million sexually transmitted infections that occur each year are in those ages 15–24 (CDC, 2017b). The autoimmune disease lupus is most commonly diagnosed in people 15–44 years old (Lupus Foundation of America, 2017). Asthma is a leading chronic disease of children. Sudden infant death occurs in children under 1 year of age, and chicken pox is one of the most common viral illnesses of childhood (CDC 2017c).

Sex and Gender

Sex and gender are important determinants of health. Sex refers to characteristics that are biologically or genetically created. Gender refers to characteristics that are socially created. Individually and collectively, they result in different health risks, health-seeking behaviors, vulnerabilities to illness, and health outcomes (WHO, 2004).

Sex makes a difference in the incidence of stroke, occurring more frequently in women than in men. It affects the age at which coronary artery disease becomes apparent, with men diagnosed on average 10 years earlier than women. High blood pressure occurs more frequently in young men than in young women, but the incidence of stroke later in life is greater in women than in men. Biologically, women have fewer nephrons in their kidneys than men, which lessens their ability to concentrate urine and increases their risk of end-stage kidney disease. Lung disease such as asthma is seen more often in young boys than young girls but reverses in adulthood, with the incidence and severity of asthma becoming greater in women than men (Regitz-Zagrosek, 2012).

The contribution gender and gender roles make to health occurs in subtle ways. When people don't abide by established gender norms, there is stigma, discrimination, and social exclusion, all of which negatively affect health. Differences in gender norms also affect risk factor exposure, access to and use of health services, and the social impact of illness (WHO, 2015). Women generally take more responsibility for their overall health (Deeks, Lombard, Michelmore, & Teede, 2009), while men focus on health behaviors associated with masculinity (Calasanti, Pietila, Ojala, &

King, 2013). For example, men exercise more than women but also drink more (National Center for Health Statistics, 2018). An emphasis on masculinity or toughness can (and often does) contribute to unhealthy behaviors to avoid signs of physical weakness (Pietila, 2008). This may explain why men generally hesitate to get medical help other than for a health issue that interferes with their ability to perform in the masculine role or to perform sexually (O'Brien, Hunt, & Hart, 2005). Case in point is the popularity of drugs to treat erectile dysfunction (Calasanti et al., 2013).

Inherited or Genetic Conditions

There is no denying the major role genetics play in our health. Genetic disorders or diseases happen when there is a mutation or an abnormality in one or more genes at birth, when there is an interaction between mutated genes and specific environmental factors, when gene mutation occurs from environmental exposure to some agent, or when there is a change in the number (more or less) or the structure of entire chromosomes containing the genes (National Institutes of Health [NIH], 2015).

While some diseases are caused by a single gene mutation present at birth, sickle cell, cystic fibrosis, and Tay-Sachs diseases, for example, most genetic disorders result from an interaction between the genes we are born with and the environment in which we live, work, and play (CDC, 2000; NIH, 2015). Diseases such as diabetes, some cancers, and heart disease fall into this category. They develop over time with exposure to environmental factors such as poor diets, sedentary lifestyles, and stress.

A good example of this is smoking and nicotine addiction. Smoking initiation is very much influenced by the social environment—peers, family members, family dynamics, exposure to tobacco advertising. Once an addiction to nicotine develops, quitting can be very difficult. The difficulty is exacerbated if there is an inherited (genetic) susceptibility to the rewarding effects of the nicotine (Institute of Medicine [IOM], 2006).

After decades of research, we know obesity results from a complex gene–gene and gene–environment interaction. One of the more likely genetic contributions seems to be gene variants that disrupt cellular pathways, which increase energy intake (food) and decrease satiety (Hetherington & Cecil, 2010), leading those with these variations to eat more and not feel full. While this alone may not cause obesity, it may when coupled with a social environment that supports a sedentary lifestyle, consumption of high-calorie fast foods, and supersized portions (Hill & Peters, 1998).

Family History

Even though we don't directly inherit many diseases from our parents, we do share our genetic makeup, lifestyles, habits, and environments with our families, which can positively or negatively affect our health. This is why family medical history might be one of the strongest indicators of disease risk, especially for heart disease, diabetes, asthma, and certain cancers—all of which "run in families" (Genetic Alliance, 2009).

Access to Health Services

Access to comprehensive, quality health services is necessary not only for promoting and maintaining health, but also for early disease detection and treatment, limiting disability, reducing the likelihood of premature death, and increasing life expectancy (*Healthy People 2020* (2020a)). In addition to the need for health insurance coverage and timely care discussed previously under social determinants of health, availability of services and barriers to care also impact access.

Availability of Services

Even with health insurance, if services aren't available, they can't be used. This is a significant issue in rural areas. Seeing a healthcare provider often means traveling long distances for care. Not only does this take time away from a job and may cost lost wages, but it also necessitates having reliable transportation. This is particularly true of mental health providers, as they tend to live and work in urban areas (National Rural Health Association, 2018).

Barriers to Access

Overall, barriers to accessing health services include the high cost of care in terms of insurance premiums, copays or out-of-pocket costs, inadequate or no insurance, and insufficient availability of services. These barriers contribute to unmet health needs and health disparities, delays in receiving care, financial burdens, and preventable illnesses and hospitalizations (USDHHS, 2018c).

Other barriers to access include childcare needs where the parent doesn't have resources for childcare during hours when appointments are available and lack of knowledge about the health care available. Language barriers, customs and religious beliefs, and trust or lack thereof in healthcare providers and the healthcare system contribute to healthcare-seeking behaviors. Other barriers to accessing healthcare are nonfinancial. For example, appointments that are only available during regular work hours or that can only be scheduled online can be problematic, as is a lack of transportation to get to an appointment. Another barrier is not having health professionals available that speak the person's language and understand the cultural or religious beliefs (Kullgren et al., 2012).

Policies, Laws, and Regulations

Policies, laws, and regulations affect health in a variety of ways. For example, the Patient Protection and Affordable Care Act of 2010 made health insurance affordable and available to more people, expanded Medicaid coverage, and supported innovations in healthcare delivery to reduce healthcare costs (Patient Protection and Affordable Care Act, 2010). (See **Figure 1-5**.)

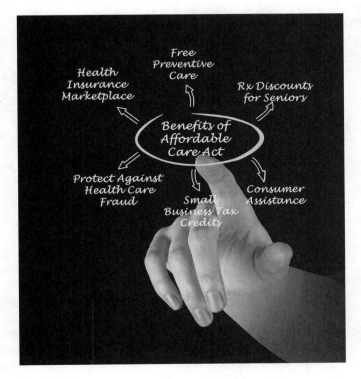

Figure 1-5 Laws affect health

Increased taxes on tobacco products have reduced the number of people who smoke. Regulations at the national level for standard safety features in cars made seat belts mandatory, which in turn reduces the number of injuries and death from accidents (USDHHS, 2018a), as do policies at the state level that prohibit drinking and driving. Policies that address housing inequities by providing vouchers to those in need of financial assistance result in improved mental and physical health of the head of the household (Osypuk, Joshi, Geronimo, & Avecedo-Garcia, 2015).

Regulations also create environments that foster good health. For example, they regulate air and water quality and how roads are planned, which affects the walkability of communities (Pellegrin, 2017).

Less obvious in their effects on health are the policies and regulations that create opportunities for people to attain higher levels of education. For example, scholarships and grant programs that reduce financial barriers to education result in opportunities for better-paying jobs. Higher education levels and greater income are the greatest predictors of better health outcomes (Pellegrin, 2017).

Chapter Summary

Planning is an organized process for developing programs to improve health that recognizes the contribution health determinants make to both the health problem and its solution.

Planning in Practice Chapter Activity

Understanding how the determinants of health contribute to not only a health issue but its solution as well is essential to program planning. To this end, answer the following questions:

1. Think about a health issue you have, for example, lack of sleep, poor diet, or sedentary lifestyle.
2. Which determinants of health are contributing to your health issue?
3. What might you do to change the determinants that are contributing to your health issue?

In the article *The Burden and Social Determinants of Asthma for Adults in the State of Georgia* (Ebell, Marchello, & O'Connor, 2017), the social determinants of health are explored in terms of their contribution to the prevalence of asthma.

Read the article, and then answer the following questions.

Article link: https://www.ncbi.nlm.nih.gov/pmc/articles/PMC5603255/

(Note: Download PDF)

Article Questions

1. What are the demographic and other characteristics of the population in which the prevalence of asthma is the highest?
2. What factors created barriers to appropriate care and ultimately better management of asthma?
3. What solutions did the authors recommended for addressing the issue?

References

Agency for Health Care Quality (AHCQ). (2018). Elements of access to health care. Retrieved June 1, 2020, from https://www.ahrq.gov/research/findings/nhqrdr/chartbooks/access/elements.html

Alcoholics Anonymous. (n.d.). The origin of our serenity prayer. Retrieved August 1, 2018, from http://www.aahistory.com/prayer.html

Barnett, E., & Casper, M. (2001). A definition of "social environment." *American Journal of Public Health*, *91*(3), 465. Retrieved July 23, 2018, from https://www.ncbi.nlm.nih.gov/pmc/articles/PMC1446600/pdf/11249033.pdf

Basu-Zharku, I. (2011). The influence of religion on health. *Inquiries Journal/Student Pulse*, *3*(01), 1–3. Retrieved July 2, 2018, from http://www.inquiriesjournal.com/articles/367/the-influence-of-religion-on-health

Bjorntorp, P. (2001). Do stress reactions cause abdominal obesity and comorbidities? *Obesity Review*, *2*(2), 73–86.

Blewett, L. A., Johnson, P. J., Lee, B., & Scal, P. B. (2008). When a usual source of care and usual provider matter: Adult prevention and screening services. *Journal of General Internal Medicine*, *23*(9), 1354–1360. doi: 10.1007/s11606-008-0659-0 Retrieved June 2, 2020 from https://pubmed.ncbi.nlm.nih.gov/18506542/

Calasanti, T., Peitila, I., Ojala, H., & King, N. (2013). Men, bodily control, and health behaviors: The importance of age. *Health Psychology*, *32*(1), 15–23. doi: http://dx.doi.org/10.1037/a0029300

Centers for Disease Control and Prevention (CDC). (2000). Gene-environment interaction fact sheet. Retrieved July 11, 2018, from https://advancedmedicine.ca/wp-content/uploads/2013/09/The-Gene-Environment-Interaction-Centre-for-Disease-Control.pdf

Centers for Disease Control and Prevention (CDC). (2014). Up to 40 percent of annual deaths from each of five leading causes of death are preventable. Retrieved June 27, 2018, from https://www.cdc.gov/media/releases/2014/p0501-preventable-deaths.html

Centers for Disease Control and Prevention (CDC). (2015). Safe water program. Retrieved August 5, 2018, from https://www.cdc.gov/nceh/ehs/elearn/swpi.html

Centers for Disease Control and Prevention (CDC). (2017a). The public health system and the 10 essential public health services. Retrieved July 18, 2018, from https://www.cdc.gov/stltpublichealth/publichealthservices/essentialhealthservices.html

Centers for Disease Control and Prevention (CDC). (2017b). Sexually transmitted disease: Adolescents and young adults. Retrieved August 1, 2018, from https://www.cdc.gov/std/life-stages-populations/adolescents-youngadults.htm

Centers for Disease Control and Prevention (CDC). (2017c). Healthy schools: Asthma in schools. Retrieved August 1, 2018, from https://www.cdc.gov/healthyschools/asthma/

Centers for Disease Control and Prevention (CDC). (2019). What is program evaluation: Program. Retrieved May 29, 2019, from https://www.cdc.gov/eval/guide/introduction/index.htm

Centers for Disease Control and Prevention (CDC). (n.d.). Worksite health 101: Program planning and implementation. Retrieved June 25, 2018, from https://www.cdc.gov/workplacehealthpromotion/tools-resources/pdfs/Program_Planning_and_Implementation_SLIDES_508.pdf

Cockerham, W. (2000). The sociology of health behavior and health lifestyles. In C. E. Bird, P. Conrad, & A. M. Femont (Eds.), *Handbook of medical sociology* (5th ed., pp. 159–172). Upper Saddle River, NJ: Prentice Hall.

Deeks, A., Lombard, C., Michelmore, J., & Teede, H. (2009). The effects of gender and age on health related behaviors. *BMC Public Health*, *9*(1), 213. doi: 10.1186/1471-2458-9-213 Retrieved July 4, 2018, from https://www.ncbi.nlm.nih.gov/pmc/articles/PMC2713232/pdf/1471-2458-9-213.pdf

Ebell, M., Marchello, C., & O'Connor, J. (2017). The burden and social determinants of asthma for adults in the state of Georgia. *Journal of Georgia Public Health Association*, *6*(4), 426–434.

Ehrlich, T. (Ed.), (2000). *Civic responsibility and higher education*. Westport, CT: American Council on Education/Oryx Press.

Farhud, D. D. (2015). Impact of lifestyle on health. *Iran Journal of Public Health*, *44*(11), 1442–1444. Retrieved on August 3, 2018, from http://ijph.tums.ac.ir

Feinstein, L., Sabates, R., Anderson, T. M., Sorhaindo, A., & Hammond, C. (2006). What are the effects of education on health? Copenhagen, Denmark. Measuring the effects of education on health and civic engagement: Proceedings of the Copenhagen Symposium, OECD. Retrieved July 2, 2018, from http://www.oecd.org/education/innovation-education/37437718.pdf

Food and Drug Administration, Center for Tobacco Products. (n.d.). Public health education campaigns. The Real Cost Campaign. Retrieved August 6, 2018, from https://www.fda.gov/tobacco-products/public-health-education/real-cost-campaign

Food Research & Action Center. (2017). Hunger & health: The impact of poverty, food insecurity and poor nutrition on health and well-being. Retrieved July 23, 2018, from http://www.frac.org/wp-content/uploads/hunger-health-impact-poverty-food-insecurity-health-well-being.pdf

Garfield, R., Orgera, K., & Damico, A. (2019). The uninsured and the ACA: A primer—key facts about health insurance and the uninsured amidst changes to the

Affordable Care Act. *Kaiser Family Foundation.* Retrieved June 1, 2020, from https://www.kff.org/report-section/the-uninsured-and-the-aca-a-primer-key-facts-about-health-insurance-and-the-uninsured-amidst-changes-to-the-affordable-care-act-how-does-lack-of-insurance-affect-access-to-care/

Genetic Alliance. (2009). Understanding genetics: A New York, mid-Atlantic guide for patients and health professionals. Retrieved August 1, 2018, from https://www.ncbi.nlm.nih.gov/books/NBK115560/

Goodman, A., Heshmati, A., & Koupil, I. (2014). Family history of education predicts eating disorders across multiple generations among 2 million Swedish males and females. *PLOS One, 9*(8), e106475. https://doi.org/10.1371/journal.pone.0106475. Retrieved June 28, 2018, from http://journals.plos.org/plosone/article?id=10.1371/journal.pone.0106475

Goth, U. S., & Smaland, E. (2014). The role of civic engagement for men's health and well being in Norway—a contribution to public health. *International Journal of Environmental Research and Public Health, 11,* 6375–6387; doi: 10.3390/ijerph110606375. Retrieved July 18, 2018, from http://www.mdpi.com/1660-4601/11/6/6375

Hahn, R., & Truman, B. I. (2015). Education improves public health and promotes health equity. *International Journal of Health Services, 45*(4), 657–678. doi: 10.177/0020731415585986. Retrieved July 3, 2018, from https://www.ncbi.nlm.nih.gov/pmc/articles/PMC4691207/

Healthy People 2020. (2020a). Access to health services. Washington, DC: U.S. Department of Health and Human Services, Office of Disease Prevention and *Health* Promotion. Retrieved June 2, 2020, from https://www.healthypeople.gov/2020/topics-objectives/topic/access-to-health-services

Healthy People 2020 (2020b). Social determinants of health. Washington, DC: U.S. Department of Health and Human Services, Office of Disease Prevention and Health Promotion. Retrieved October 26, 2020 from https://www.healthypeople.gov/2020/topics-objectives/topic/social-determinants-of-health

Hetherington, M. M., & Cecil, J. E. (2010). Gene-environment interactions in obesity. In W. Langhans & N. Geary (Eds.), *Frontiers in eating and weight regulation* (vol. 63, 195–203). Basel: Karger. doi: http://doi.org/10.1159/000264407

Hill, J. O., & Peters, J. C. (1998). Environmental contributions to the obesity epidemic. *Science 280*(5368), 1371–1374. doi: 10.1126/science.280.5368.1371

Institute of Medicine Committee on Assessing Interactions Among Social, Behavioral, and Genetic Factors in Health, Hernandez, L. M., & Blazer, D. G. (Eds.). (2006). Genetic, environmental, and personality determinants of health risk behaviors. In *Genes, Behavior, and the Social Environment: Moving Beyond the Nature/Nurture Debate.* Washington, DC: National Academies Press. Retrieved July 11, 2018, from https://www.ncbi.nlm.nih.gov/books/NBK19927/

Kelly, P. M., & Barker, M. (2016). Why is changing health related behaviour so difficult? *Public Health, 136*(2016), 109–116. doi: http://dx.doi.org/10.1016/j.puhe.2016.03.030 Retrieved July 23, 2018, from https://www.sciencedirect.com/science/article/pii/S0033350616300178#bib12

Kim, A., Kim, C., & You, M. S. (2015). Civic participation and self-rated health: A cross-national multi-level analysis using the world value survey. *Journal of Preventive Medicine & Public Health, 48,* 18–27. http://dx.doi.org/10.3961/jpmph.14.031. Retrieved July 23, 2018, from https://www.ncbi.nlm.nih.gov/pmc/articles/PMC4322515/pdf/jpmph-48-1-18.pdf

Knibb-Lamouche, J. (2012). Culture as a determinant of health. Roundtable on the promotion of health equity and the elimination of health disparities. Board on Population Health and Public Health Practice; Institute of Medicine. *Leveraging culture to address health inequalities: Examples from native communities: Workshop summary.* Washington, DC: National Academies Press. Retrieved July 23, 2018, from https://www.ncbi.nlm.nih.gov/books/NBK201298/

Koenig, H. (2012). Religion, spirituality, and health: The research and clinical implications. *International Scholarly Research Network Psychiatry, 2012.* doi: 10.5402/2012/278730. Retrieved August 6, 2018, from https://www.hindawi.com/journals/isrn/2012/278730/

Kollmuss, A., & Agyeman, J. (2002). Mind the gap: Why do people act environmentally and what are the barriers to pro-environmental behavior? *Environmental Education Research, 8*(3), 239–260. doi: 10.1080/13504620220145401. Retrieved August 6, 2018, from https://www.tandfonline.com/doi/abs/10.1080/13504620220145401

Konrath, S., Fuhrel-Forbis, A., Lou, A., & Brown, S. (2012). Motives for volunteering are associated with mortality risk in older adults. *Health Psychology, 31*(1), 87–96. doi: 10.1037/a0025226

Kullgren, J.T., McLaughlin, C.G., Mitra, N., & Armstrong, K. (2012). Nonfinancial barriers and access to care for U.S. adults. *Health Services Research, 47*(1 pt 2), 462–485. https://dx.doi.org/10.1111%2Fj.1475-6773.2011.01308.x

Lawlor, D. A., Frankel, S., Shaw, M., Ebrahim, S., & Smith, G. D. (2003). Smoking and ill health: Does lay epidemiology explain the failure of smoking cessation programs among deprived populations? *American Journal of Public Health, 93*(2), 266–270. Retrieved June 28, 2018, from https://www.ncbi.nlm.nih.gov/pmc/articles/PMC1447728/pdf/0930266.pdf

Levesque, A. (2014). The relationship between culture, health conceptions and health practices: A qualitative-quantitative approach. *Journal of Cross-Cultural Psychology*, *45*(4), 628–645. doi: 10.1177/002202211 3519855

Lidsky, T. I., & Schneider, J. S. (2003). Lead neurotoxicity in children: Basic mechanisms and clinical correlates. *Brain*, *126*(1), 5–19. https://doi.org/10.1093/brain/awg014. Retrieved July 4, 2018, from https://academic.oup.com/brain/article/126/1/5/299373

Lupus Foundation of America. (2017). Risk factors for developing lupus. Retrieved August 1, 2018, from https://resources.lupus.org/entry/risk-factors

Marmot, M. (2004). *The status syndrome*. New York, NY: Holt.

Massachusetts Department of Public Health. (2018). Childhood lead prevention program. Retrieved August 4, 2018, from https://www.mass.gov/orgs/childhood-lead-poisoning-prevention-program

Merck Manual. (2016). Physical changes with aging. Retrieved July 9, 2018, from https://www.merckmanuals.com/professional/geriatrics/approach-to-the-geriatric-patient/physical-changes-with-aging

Mirowsky, J., & Ross, C. E. (2003). *Education, social status, and health*. Hawthorne, NY: Aldine DeGuryter.

Mirowsky J., & Ross, C. E. (2005). Education, learned effectiveness and health. *London Review of Education*, *3*(3), 205–220. doi:10.1080/14748460500372366. Retrieved June 28, 2018, from http://www.ingentaconnect.com/content/ioep/clre/2005/00000003/00000003/art00003

Missouri Department of Health and Senior Services (DHSS). (n.d.). What is an intervention? Retrieved May 6, 2019, from https://searchapp.mo.gov/search-missouri/dhss?q=what%20is%20an%20intervention

Napier, A. D., Anacamo, C., Butler, B., Calabrese, J., Chater, A., Chatterjee, H., Guesnet, F., Home, R., ... Woolf, K. (2014). Culture and health. *The Lancet*, *384*, 1607–1639. http://dx.doi.org/10.1016/ S0140-6736 (14)61603-2

National Center for Health Statistics (NCHS). (2018). *Health, United States, 2016*. Retrieved July 9, 2018, from https://www.cdc.gov/nchs/index.htm

National Institutes of Health, National Human Genome Institute. (2015). Frequently asked questions about genetic disorders. Retrieved August 1, 2018, from https://www.genome.gov/19016930/faq-about-genetic-disorders/

National Physicians Alliance. (n.d.). Civic engagement. Retrieved July 12, 2018, from http://npalliance.org/civic-engagement

National Rural Health Association. (2018). About rural health care. Retrieved July 16, 2018, from http://ruralhealthweb.org/about-nrha/about-rural-health-care

New Jersey Department of Human Services. (2013). A matter of balance. Retrieved August 5, 2018, from https://www.nj.gov/humanservices/doas/services/balance

O'Brien, R., Hunt, K., & Hart, G. (2005). It's caveman stuff, but that is to a certain extent how guys still operate: Men's accounts of masculinity and help seeking. *Social Science & Medicine*, *61*(3), 503–516. https://doi.org/10.1016/j.socscimed.2004.12.008

Oman, D., & Thoresen, C. E. (2002). Does religion cause health? Differing interpretations and diverse meanings. *Journal of Health Psychology*, *7*(4), 365–380. doi: 10.1177/1359105302007004326.

Ortiz, B. I., Shields, K. M., Clauson, K. A., & Clay, P. G. (2007). Complementary and alternative medicine use among Hispanics in the United States. *The Annals of Pharmacotherapy*, *41*(6), 994–1004. https://doi.org/10.1345%2Faph.1H600

Osypuk, T. L., Joshi, P., Geronimo, K., & Avecedo-Garcia, D. (2015). Do social and economic policies influence health? A review. *Current Epidemiology Report*, *1*(3), 149–164. https://dx.doi.org/10.1007%2Fs40471-014-0013-5

Pampel, F. C., Krueger, P. M., & Denney, J. T. (2010). Socioeconomic disparities in health behaviors. *Annual Review of Sociology*, *36*, 349–370. https://doi.org/10.1146/annurev.soc.012809.102529

Patient Protection and Affordable Care Act. (2010). Pub. L. No. 111–148, 124 Stat. 119. Retrieved March 24, 2020, from https://www.healthcare.gov/glossary/affordable-care-act/

Pellegrin, M. (2017). 5 ways public policy impacts health. *The Sycamore Institute*. Retrieved March 23, 2020, from https://www.sycamoreinstitutetn.org/5-ways-public-policy-impacts-health/

Perdue, W. C., Stone, L. A., & Gostin, L. O. (2003). The built environment and its relationship to the public's health: A legal framework. *American Journal of Public Health*, *93*(9), 1390–1395. https://doi.org/10.2105/ajph.93.9.1390

Pietila, I. (2008). *Between rocks and hard places: Ideological dilemmas in men's talk about health and gender*. PhD, Tampere University, Tampere, Finland. Retrieved July 9, 2018, from https://trepo.tuni.fi/handle/10024/67877

Puddu, P. E., & Menotti, A. (2015). The impact of basic lifestyle behaviour on health: How to lower the risk of coronary heart disease, other cardiovascular diseases, cancer and all-cause mortality. Lifestyle adaptation: A global approach. *E-Journal of Cardiology Practice*, *13*(32). Retrieved June 27, 2018, from https://www.escardio.org/Journals/E-Journal-of-Cardiology-Practice/Volume-13/the-impact-of-basic-lifestyle-behaviour-on-health-how-to-lower-risk-of-coronary

Regitz-Zagrosek, V. (2012). Sex and gender differences in health. *EMBO Reports, 13*(7), 596–603. Retrieved June 2, 2020, from https://www.ncbi.nlm.nih.gov/pmc/articles/PMC3388783/

Reid, K. W., Vittinghoff, E., & Kushel, M. B. (2008). Association between level of housing instability, economic standing and health care access. *Journal of Health Care for the Poor and Underserved, 19*(4), 1212–1228. https://doi.org/10.1353/hpu.0.0068

Reuben, A., Caspi, A., Belsky, D., Broadbent, J., Harrington, H., Sugden, K., Houts, R., … Moffitt, T. (2017). Association of childhood blood-lead levels with cognitive function and socioeconomic status at age 38 years with IQ change and socioeconomic mobility between childhood and adulthood. *Journal of the American Medical Association, 317*(12), 1244–1251. doi: 10.1001/jama.2017.1712

Rumun, A. J. (2014). Influence of religious beliefs on healthcare practice. *International Journal of Education and Research, 2*(4), 37–48. Retrieved July 2, 2018, from http://www.ijern.com/journal/April-2014/05.pdf

Sampson, R. J., & Winter, A. S. (2016). The racial ecology of lead poisoning. *DuBois Review: Social Science Research on Race, 13*(2), 261–283. https://doi.org/10.1017/S1742058X16000151

Sampson, R. J., & Winter, A. S. (2018). Poisoned development: Assessing childhood lead exposure as a cause of crime in a birth cohort followed through adolescence. *Criminology, 56*(2), 269–301. https://doi.org/10.1111/1745-9125.12171

Steuart, G. (1993). The importance of program planning. *Health Education Quarterly, 20*(1 supp), s21–s27.

U.S. Department of Health and Human Services (USD-HHS), Office of Disease Prevention and Health Promotion (ODPHP). (2018a). Determinants of health. *Healthy people 2020*. Retrieved June 27, 2018, from https://www.healthypeople.gov/2020/about/foundation-health-measures/Determinants-of-Health

U.S. Department of Health and Human Services (USD-HHS), Office of Disease Prevention and Health Promotion (ODPHP). (2018b). Social determinants of health. *Healthy people 2020*. Retrieved June 27, 2018, from https://www.healthypeople.gov/2020/topics-objectives/topic/social-determinants-of-health

U.S. Department of Health and Human Services (USD-HHS), Office of Disease Prevention and Health Promotion (ODPHP). (2018c). Access to health services. *Healthy people 2020*. Retrieved July 16, 2018, from https://www.healthypeople.gov/2020/topics-objectives/topic/Access-to-Health-Services

University of New Mexico. (2018). Project ECHO: A revolution in medical education and care delivery. Retrieved August 5, 2018, from https://echo.unm.edu

Villanueva, K., Knuiman, M., Koohsari, M. J., Hickey, S., Foster, S., Badland, H., … Giles-Corti, B. (2013). People living in hilly residential areas in metropolitan Perth have less diabetes: Spurious association of important environmental determinant? *International Journal of Health Geographics, 12*(1), 59. doi: https://doi.org/10.1186/1476-072X-12-59 Retrieved July 30, 2018, from https://ij-healthgeographics.biomedcentral.com/articles/10.1186/1476-072X-12-59

Whitehead, D., & Russell, G. (2004). How effective are health education programmes—resistance, reactance, rationality and risk? Recommendations for effective practice. *International Journal of Nursing Studies, 41*, 163–172. doi: 10.1016.S0020-7489(03)00117-2

Winter, A. S., & Sampson, R. J. (2017). From lead exposure in early childhood to adolescent health: A Chicago birth cohort. *American Journal of Public Health, 107*(9), 1496–1501. doi:10.2105/AJPH.2017.303903

World Health Organization (WHO). (2004). Gender in mental health research. Retrieved June 2, 2020, from https://www.who.int/gender-equity-rights/knowledge/9241592532/en/

World Health Organization (WHO). (2015). Gender. Retrieved July 9, 2018, from https://www.who.int/gender-equity-rights/news/factsheet-403/en/

World Health Organization (WHO). (2018a). Global TB programme. Retrieved August 5, 2018, from http://www.who.int/tb/about/en/

World Health Organization (WHO). (2018b). The WHO programme for international drug monitoring. Retrieved August 5, 2018, from http://www.who.int/medicines/areas/quality_safety/safety_efficacy/National_PV_Centres_Map/en/

World Health Organization (WHO). (2018c). Ageing and health. Retrieved July 4, 2018, from http://www.who.int/news-room/fact-sheets/detail/ageing-and-health

World Health Organization (WHO). (n.d.). International classification of health interventions. Retrieved May 6, 2019. from https://www.who.int/classifications/ichi/en/

World Health Organization (WHO). Commission on Social Determinants of Health. (2008). *Closing the gap in a generation: Health equity through action on the social determinants of health. Final report of the Commission on Social Determinants of Health.* Retrieved July 3, 2018, from http://www.who.int/social_determinants/thecommission/finalreport/en/

Zimmerman, E. B., Woolf, S. H., & Haley, A. (2015). Understanding the relationship between education and health: A review of the evidence and an examination of community perspectives. *Agency for Healthcare Research and Quality*. Retrieved June 28, 2018, from https://www.ahrq.gov/professionals/education/curriculum-tools/population-health/zimmerman.html

CHAPTER 2

Health Behavior Theories

STUDENT LEARNING OUTCOMES

After reading this chapter, the student will be able to:

- Explain the purpose of using theory in program planning.
- Discuss concepts, constructs, and variables.
- Differentiate between intrapersonal, interpersonal, and community-level theories and models.
- Explain a personal health behavior using a theory from each level.

What Is a Theory?

The aim of program planning is to improve health in some way. Improving health usually involves changing health behavior. To change health behavior, we need to understand why people do what they do in the first place. Rather than rely on guesswork to explain this, we use theories.

So, what is a theory? A theory is "a set of interrelated concepts, definitions, and propositions that present a systematic view of events or situations by specifying relations among variables in order to *explain* and *predict* events or situations" (Glanz, Rimer, & Viswanath, 2008, p. 26). Simply, theories help *explain* behavior and suggest ways to change it, too (Glanz et al., 2008). They do this by giving direction for studying the health problem, identifying the intended program audience, developing methods to resolve the health problem, and suggesting ways to evaluate the success of these endeavors (National Cancer Institute [NCI], 2005).

Certainly, there are programs out there that were planned without a theoretical basis. But, research shows that programs developed with a theoretical base tend to be more successful in achieving their goals (Bluethmann, Bartholomew, Murphy, & Vernon, 2016; Glanz & Bishop, 2010; Tebb et al., 2016).

In addition to theories there are *models*. Models are composites, or a mixture of ideas taken from different theories and used together. They function the same way theories do, (Glanz et al., 2008) and in some cases can be more useful than any one specific theory.

Theory Components

While each theory or model explains health behavior and informs behavior change from a unique perspective, all theories and models are the sum of their parts. These parts or components include a concept, constructs, and variables.

Theory Concept

At the heart of each theory is a *concept*. A concept is the idea from which the theory is developed that explains why people do or don't engage in a particular health behavior. Think about why you brushed your teeth this morning. Was it because you believe brushing prevents dental decay? Or was it because you're afraid of the dentist and want to avoid having to see her. Or maybe you brushed your teeth because it's what our society expects adults to do. Each of these could explain why you brushed your teeth. Each is a theory concept.

Theory Constructs

Constructs emerge from the concept. Constructs are the ways the concept is used in each specific theory (Kerlinger, 1986) to explain or change behavior. For instance, if beliefs are the concept and the health behavior we want to explain or change is dental hygiene, then identifying the specific beliefs related to dental hygiene are the constructs, the ways we use the concept in the theory. An example is the extent to which someone believes dental disease is serious, or how at risk the person believes he/she is for dental caries and gum disease. Another belief might be how beneficial a person believes daily brushing and flossing is. It could also be that the person's beliefs are barriers stopping him/her from practicing good dental care. Fear is a common barrier to good dental care which stems from the belief that going to the dentist is painful.

Variables

Variables are the operationalized concept, or how the concept is measured (Glanz et al., 2008). Using beliefs as the concept and mammogram practices as the health behavior they

influence, a variable or way to measure the concept would be to have women complete a questionnaire that measures their breast cancer beliefs and their mammogram practices. When researchers in Iran asked women to do exactly this, the following beliefs were identified as barriers for having an annual mammogram—not having time, not knowing where to go for screening, and fear that the test was painful and embarrassing (Aflakseir & Abbas, 2012). Their beliefs (the theory concept) were measured (by using a questionnaire), and the results offered an explanation of why they did not have regular breast cancer screening.

Each theory has at least one concept (health influencing factor), a series of constructs that indicate how the concept is used in the theory, and variables to enable measurement of the concept. To use an analogy here, imagine the theory is a house. The concept is brick—brick influences what a house will look like and is used to develop or build the house. The constructs are the ways bricks are used in the house—for the front steps, the walkway, or maybe the fireplace. The brick can be measured (operationalized) by square footage, number, size, or weight. (See **Figure 2-1**.)

Types of Theories

Theories and models are often separated into three types based on their level of influence: intrapersonal, interpersonal, and community. Theories and models at each level explain and suggest ways to change behavior by examining how different factors at each tier influence what people do and why they do it. While it's beyond the scope and purpose of this text to cover the plethora of theories at each level, the more commonly used ones are summarized here.

Intrapersonal Theories

Theories at the intrapersonal or individual level explain behavior by focusing on factors within people that influence what they do, such as knowledge, attitudes, beliefs, motivation, self-concept, developmental history, past

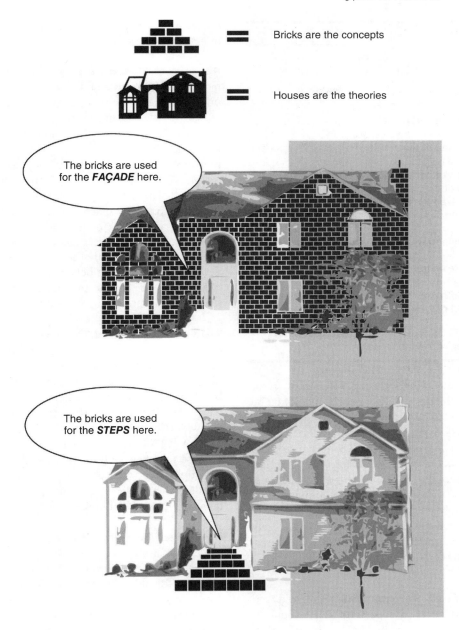

Figure 2-1 Theories, concepts, and constructs

Hayden, J. (2019). *Introduction to Health Behavior Theory* (3rd ed). Burlington, MA: Jones & Bartlett Learning.

experience, and skills (NCI, 2005). The Health Belief Model, Self-Efficacy Theory, Theory of Reasoned Action, Transtheoretical Model, and Protection Motivation Theory are common intrapersonal theories.

Health Belief Model

The underlying concept of the Health Belief Model (HBM) is that personal beliefs or perceptions about an illness and its prevention strategies influence behavior (Hochbaum, 1958).

Table 2-1 Health Belief Model

Concept
Behavior is influenced by personal beliefs or perceptions.

Constructs
Perceived seriousness: Personal opinion as to the severity of the disease.

Perceived susceptibility: Personal assessment disease risk.

Perceived benefits: Personal appraisal of behavior change advantages.

Perceived barriers: Personal judgment of obstacles blocking adoption of new behavior.

Modifying variables: Personal factors that affect whether the new behavior is adopted.

Cues to action: Factors that start a person on the way to changing behavior.

Self-efficacy: Personal belief in one's own ability to successfully do something.

Hayden, J. (2019). *Introduction to Health Behavior Theory* (3rd ed.). Burlington, MA: Jones & Bartlett Learning, p. 57.

According to this theory, a range of factors within the person affect beliefs, including, but not limited to: knowledge, attitudes, experiences, skills, culture, and religion.

The four main original belief constructs of the HBM are perceived seriousness, perceived susceptibility, perceived benefits, and perceived barriers. Each of these, individually or in combination, explain health behavior. Additional constructs of the HBM include cues to action, motivating factors, and self-efficacy. (See **Table 2-1**.)

Perceived Seriousness. Perceived seriousness refers to a person's belief about the seriousness or severity of a disease. While perception of seriousness is often based on medical information or knowledge, it may also be colored by personal experience with an illness. For example, although high blood pressure is a serious condition that increases risk of stroke, heart attack, and kidney failure, people with high blood pressure don't have symptoms or feel "sick," which can skew their perception of its seriousness.

Perceived Susceptibility. One of the more powerful motivators for changing an unhealthy behavior is a person's perception of disease risk. The greater the perceived risk, the greater the likelihood of adopting behaviors to decrease the risk. When people believe they are at risk of skin cancer, they use sunscreen. When people believe they are at increased risk of Lyme disease, they use tick repellant, avoid tall grasses, and check themselves for ticks after being outdoors. When people believe they are at risk of the flu, they get vaccinated. During the Covid-19 pandemic, when everyone believed they were at risk, they wore masks, practiced social distancing, and frequent handwashing.

Perceived Benefits. The construct of perceived benefits is a person's appraisal of how useful a new behavior is in decreasing the risk of developing a disease. For a new behavior to be adopted, the perceived benefits have to outweigh the consequences of continuing the old behavior (Centers for Disease Control and Prevention [CDC], 2004). People use sunscreen because they believe it decreases their risk of developing skin cancer. They quit smoking because they believe continuing to smoke increases their risk of lung cancer.

Perceived Barriers. Perceived barriers are those obstacles a person believes stand in the way of adopting the new healthier behavior or changing the old unhealthy behavior. They are the strongest predictors of behavior of any of the HBM constructs (Janz & Becker, 1984). Barriers can be any number of things from lack of transportation, not having a specialty healthcare provider in rural areas, limited access to fresh fruits and vegetables in urban "food deserts," clinic hours that conflict with working hours, inadequate support from family members, or lack of skill to make the desired change.

Additional Constructs

- *Modifying variables* are the factors that influence a person's perception of the benefits of a health behavior and its adoption or rejection. These include demographic factors such as age, gender, and marital status; sociopsychological factors, which include peers, social class, and personality; and last, the structural factors of knowledge and past experience (Rosenstock, 1974).

- *Cues to action* are those things that trigger people to begin changing their unhealthy behaviors. A cue to action might be an overheard conversation in the grocery store about the benefits of eating less processed foods, a family member's diagnosis of an illness, a Facebook posting about a friend's health scare, a reminder text that it's time for an annual checkup, or a product warning label.

- *Self-efficacy,* or personal belief in one's own ability to carry out an action, is a significant factor in changing behavior. In general, people will try something new if they believe they can do it and won't try it if they believe they can't.

Think about it. Would you try to run a 20-mile marathon if you didn't think you could? Probably not.

Self-Efficacy Theory

Self-efficacy is not only a construct in the Health Belief Model, but it's also a theory unto itself. It's based on the concept that people generally do things they think they can and avoid things they think they can't. The constructs of Self-Efficacy Theory are factors that influence an individual's perception of ability, including mastery experience, vicarious experience, verbal persuasion, and somatic and emotional state (Bandura, 1994, 1997; Pajares, 2002). (See **Figure 2-2**.)

Mastery Experience. Mastery experiences result when a person is successful at or accomplishes an attempted task. These experiences are important because people are more likely to believe they can do something new if it's similar to something they have already done well (Bandura, 1994). For example, if someone can roller skate, he's more likely to believe he can ice skate, than if he can't skate at all.

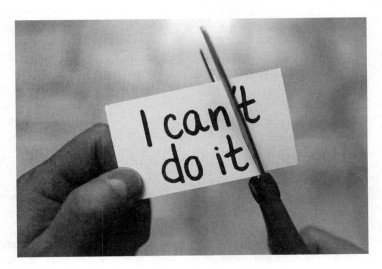

Figure 2-2 Self-Efficacy Theory
© Brian A Jackson/Shutterstock

Vicarious Experiences. When people watch others who are like themselves succeed at or accomplish something they'd like to do, this is a vicarious experience. The extent to which these experiences affect self-efficacy is related to how much a person identifies with or thinks the model (the person being watched) is like him- or herself (Bandura, 1994). The more a person identifies with the model, the greater the influence the vicarious experience has on self-efficacy. While vicarious experiences can strengthen self-efficacy if the model is successful, they can also weaken it if the model fails at the task the person is trying to accomplish.

Verbal Persuasion. Verbal persuasion is what the cheerleaders in people's lives do—coaches, teachers, and parents—with their words of encouragement. Positive comments by others increase self-efficacy and the likelihood of a person attempting a new task or challenging situation. Similarly, negative comments deter from self-efficacy, which can be an obstacle to taking on a new endeavor.

Somatic and Emotional States. Self-efficacy is affected by the physical and/or emotional reaction people have when they think about doing something—that gut reaction. If the thoughts produce an uncomfortable response such as anxiety, fear, embarrassment, nausea, headache, stress, and so on, it diminishes self-efficacy and the likelihood of performing the task (Bandura & Adams, 1977; Pajares, 2002). The responses affect self-efficacy, which in turn affects the decision-making process. But, if the undesirable response is reduced, self-efficacy can improve (Bandura & Adams, 1977).

Not all somatic and emotional states are unpleasant with a negative impact on self-efficacy. For example, the anticipated calm a meditator has when she thinks about her practice or the enjoyment hikers have as they plan their trails through the woods are physically and emotionally positive states of being. When

thoughts of a task elicit pleasant rather than unpleasant results, self-efficacy is enhanced, and the behavior is likely to continue (Bandura & Adams, 1977).

Theory of Reasoned Action and Theory of Planned Behavior

The concept underlying both the Theory of Reasoned Action (TRA) and the Theory of Planned Behavior (TPB) is intention, or a person's inclination to engage in a particular behavior (Ajzen & Fishbein, 1980; Fishbein, 1967). Intention is influenced by a person's attitudes, subjective norms, and volitional control in the TRA, and behavioral control in the TPB. (See **Figure 2-3**.)

Attitudes. Attitudes are formed from a series of beliefs and the value placed on the related behavioral outcome of those beliefs (Ajzen, 2002). If the behavioral outcome is seen as positive—valuable, beneficial, desirable, advantageous, or a good thing—then a person's attitude will be favorable, and there's a greater likelihood of engaging in the behavior. For example, people who believe it's acceptable to be seen with soda, believe in entertaining their friends with soda, and believe soda is a good treat, have a positive attitude toward drinking soda and therefore, drink soda (Madiba, Bhayat, & Nkambule, 2017). Conversely, if people believe it's unacceptable to be seen drinking soda, don't believe in entertaining their friends with soda, and don't believe soda is a good treat, their attitude would be negative, and they're not likely not drink soda.

Another example is sunscreen use. If people believe they are at risk of skin cancer, believe sunscreen use prevents skin cancer, and believe they can incorporate its use into their daily routine, these result in a positive attitude toward sunscreen use and greater likelihood of its use.

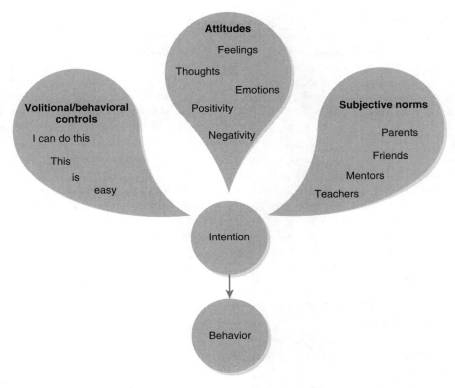

Figure 2-3 Theory of Reasoned Action and Theory of Planned Behavior

Subjective Norms. Intention is also influenced by subjective norms. Subjective norms are the perceived social pressures that people feel push them to engage or not engage in a certain behavior. Subjective norms come from normative beliefs or what people believe important others in their lives expect them to do (Ajzen, 2002). Important others are family members, friends or peers, religious leaders, healthcare providers, teachers, coaches, or others held in high esteem—others that people want to please. Subjective norms are what encourage people to start or quit smoking, drink alcohol or abstain, join a gym, learn yoga, take vitamins, and the list goes on.

Volitional Control. Although intention underlies the TRA and TPB, in order for some-

one to act on their intention, the behavior has to be under volitional control. A behavior under volitional control is one in which a person can decide, at will, to do or not do (Ajzen, 1991). For example, a person can, at will, decide to give up soda, meditate, binge drink, or use seat belts.

For behaviors not under willful control such as eating organic fruits and vegetables—if they are not available or affordable, having protected sex—if the male partner chooses not to use a condom, avoiding secondhand smoke—if someone in the house smokes, the TRA is not useful. Consequently, the TRA was expanded to include the construct of behavioral control, which created the *Theory of Planned Behavior* (Ajzen, 1991, 2002). Behavioral control is the differentiating construct between the TRA and TPB.

Behavioral Control. Behavioral control is an individual's *perception* of the control (power or influence) he or she has over performing a behavior. It's affected by a set of control beliefs, which help or hinder the person to perform the behavior (Ajzen, 2002); that is, they affect the perception of how easy or difficult it is to carry out the behavior (Ajzen, 1991). For example, the designated driver intends not to drink at an off-campus party, has a positive attitude toward not drinking, and wants to abide by the law. But, she may not be able to willfully avoid consuming alcohol, as the bartender's actions are not in her control. In this case, she has behavioral control, not volitional control, over staying sober, believing it's easy to do so if she brings her own beverage.

Transtheoretical Model— Stages of Change

Rather than explaining why people behave in a certain way relative to their health, the Transtheoretical Model (TTM) offers insight into how people change their behavior. It proposes that behavior change occurs in steps or stages. Hence, this model is aptly referred to as Stages of Change.

The three constructs of the TTM are stages of change, processes of change, and self-efficacy. Each stage of change has its own distinct characteristics and time frame and its own processes of change enabled by self-efficacy that facilitate movement to the next stage and eventually behavior change (Prochaska, DiClemente, & Norcross, 1992).

Stages of Change. There are five stages of change: precontemplation, contemplation, preparation, action, and maintenance.

- *Precontemplation* is the stage people are in before they start thinking about changing a behavior. People in this "prethinking" or "not thinking" stage haven't started thinking about making a change yet because they either don't recognize they have an unhealthy behavior that needs to be changed, they are uninformed or underinformed about the health consequences of their behavior, or they just aren't ready to change a behavior they know they should. The stage ends as soon as the person starts thinking about changing the unhealthy behavior (Prochaska et al., 1992).

- *Contemplation* begins as soon as a person starts thinking about changing a behavior. The list of things that prompt a person to begin thinking about changing a behavior is endless (Prochaska et al., 1992). To name but a few, an article in the newspaper, a magazine or online; a TV commercial, documentary, or episode topic of a favorite series; Twitter, Facebook, Instagram, a website, or an app; family, friends, or healthcare professionals; and so on can influence us. These are the same things as the cues to action in the Health Belief Model.

  Thinking about making a change is necessary for change to occur, but thinking alone doesn't change behavior. Behavior changes when a decision is made to adopt a new behavior. The decision to take action or not to take action is called *decisional balance*. Decisional balance entails weighing the perceived pros and cons, or costs and benefits, of the new behavior against the old behavior (Prochaska, 1994). When people can't make a decision and get stuck in "thinking mode" for more than 6 months, this is behavioral procrastination or chronic contemplation (DiClemente, Schlundt, & Gemmell, 2004). You may know people in this stage. They say they want to lose weight, begin an exercise program, get more sleep, or manage their stress better, but after months of thinking and talking about doing something, they can't make the decision to start.

- *Preparation* begins once the decision to change is made. This stage is short, usually lasting only about 1 month because people are generally anxious to get started.

It's during this stage that they make a plan for changing their behavior and gather whatever is needed to put the plan into action (Velicer, Prochaska, Fava, Norman, & Redding, 1998). For example, if the plan is to increase their activity level, to implement the plan they may need new sneakers, a gym membership, and a pedometer.

- *Action* begins when the plan is implemented. Action lasts about 6 months and is the time when people are in the active process of modifying their behavior to address their problem. The goal of this stage is a changed behavior (DiClemente et al., 2004; Prochaska et al., 1992)
- *Maintenance* is the final stage when people work to avoid relapsing to their old behavior Maintenance lasts at least 6 months for some behaviors, and years for others (Prochaska et al., 1992). Maintaining the change and permanently incorporating the new behavior into one's lifestyle can be the most difficult part. Talk to any smoker who has ever tried to quit smoking and he will tell you quitting is the easy part; staying "quit" is the hard part. That's what the maintenance stage is all about.

Processes of Change. The 10 processes of change are stage specific and explain how change occurs as people move from one stage to the next (Prochaska & DiClemente, 1982). They include consciousness raising, dramatic relief or emotional arousal, environmental reevaluation, social liberation, self-reevaluation, stimulus control, helping relationships, counterconditioning, reinforcement management, and self-liberation (Prochaska & DiClemente, 1983).

- *Consciousness raising* is how people become aware of their health problem and its cause, the actions they can take to address it, and the consequences if they don't (Prochaska et al., 1992; Velicer et al., 1998).

- *Dramatic relief,* also called emotional arousal, is how a person reacts emotionally to the behavior in need of changing (Prochaska et al., 1992; Velicer et al., 1998).
- *Environmental reevaluation* is when people consider how their unhealthy behavior impacts or affects the physical and or social environment (Prochaska et al., 1992; Velicer et al., 1998). For example, how does my smoking affect the air my child breathes in the house?
- *Social liberation* is the process people use when they look for opportunities or situations to support their new behavior (Prochaska et al., 1992; Velicer et al., 1998). For example, a person whose new behavior is walking 30 minutes a day might look for a mall nearby to enable her to walk in inclement weather.
- *Self-reevaluation* is the process people use when they assess differences in their self-esteem before and after they changed the unhealthy behavior (Prochaska et al., 1992; Velicer et al., 1998).
- *Stimulus control* is how people remove or avoid triggers or cues for the old behavior from their environment (Prochaska et al., 1992; Velicer et al., 1998). A common trigger for smoking is coffee. By switching to tea instead, the "smoking" stimulus is controlled.
- *Helping relationships* are connections with others who form a support network for the person undergoing a behavior change (Prochaska et al., 1992; Velicer et al., 1998).
- *Counterconditioning* is the process that helps people replace an unhealthy behavioral response to a stimulus with a healthier one (Prochaska et al., 1992; Velicer et al., 1998). For instance, if thirst is the stimulus that triggers the unhealthy behavior of drinking soda, in counterconditioning, the person replaces the unhealthy soda with unsweetened iced tea.
- *Reinforcement management* is the process that supports continuation of the new

behavior, either through rewards for doing it, or punishments for not (Prochaska et al., 1992; Velicer et al., 1998). An example of a reward for an ex-smoker might be a massage for every week she remains "quit."

- *Self-liberation* is how people free themselves from or let go of a behavior they no longer want. They choose to change their behavior, believe they can, and commit to making the change (Prochaska et al., 1992). Choosing to stop texting while driving, believing it can be done, and committing to pulling over before using the phone is an example of self-liberation from an unsafe behavior.

Because the processes of change facilitate movement through the stages of change, different processes are used in different stages. Consciousness raising, dramatic relief, and environmental reevaluation move people from precontemplation to contemplation. Self-reevaluation, social liberation, helping relationships, and dramatic relief move people from contemplation to preparation. Self-liberation helps people move to action and maintenance. Counterconditioning helping relations, reinforcement management, and stimulus control all help people implement their change plans and maintain the changed behavior. (See **Figure 2-4**.)

Self-Efficacy. Self-efficacy is the extent to which a person is confident in his or her ability to do something. In the TTM, that "something" is working through the stages to change a behavior. Once the change occurs, self-efficacy helps people maintain their new behavior in situations that could cause them to relapse to the old behavior.

Protection Motivation Theory

In Protection Motivation Theory, the concept underlying behavior is fear, the threatening thoughts it triggers, and the desire to protect

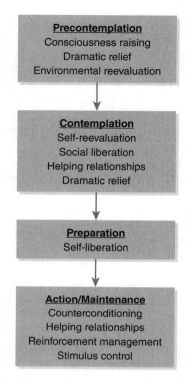

Figure 2-4 Transtheoretical model stages and processes of change

Hayden, J. (2019). *Introduction to Health Behavior Theory* (3rd ed). Burlington, MA: Jones & Bartlett Learning

oneself from the threatening outcome (Floyd, Prentice-Dunn, & Rogers, 2000). The extent of motivation to protect oneself from the threat comes from threat appraisal and coping appraisal (Maddux & Rogers, 1983). (See **Figure 2-5**.)

Threat Appraisal. Threat appraisal entails two perceptions—the perception of how serious or severe a threat is and the perception of vulnerability or probability the threatened outcome will happen. The more serious a threat is perceived to be, and the greater the perception of personal vulnerability to it, the greater the likelihood of the person adopting behaviors to prevent the feared outcome (Floyd et al., 2000). Simply put, when people believe something serious is likely to happen to them, they are more apt to change their behavior.

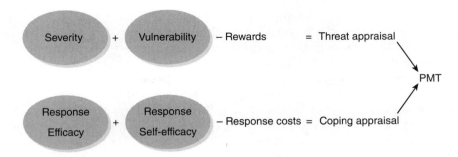

Figure 2-5 Protection Motivation Theory

Modified from Floyd, D.L., Prentice-Dunn, S. & Rogers. R. (2000). A meta-analysis of research on protection motivation theory. *Journal of Applied Social Psychology*, 30(2), 407–429.

Coping Appraisal. Coping appraisal is an assessment of the protective or new behavior in terms of its coping response efficacy, which is its effectiveness in preventing or reducing the threat, and response self-efficacy, which is a personal belief in the ability to carry it out the protective behavior (Rogers, 1975) and the cost of doing so, whether it's monetary, personal time, or personnel (Floyd et al., 2000).

When people believe a recommended behavior works and that they can carry it out, the chances of them adopting the new behavior increases. However, if the cost of the new behavior is too high, adoption is less likely (Floyd et al., 2000). For example, if people believe exercise can help control their type 2 diabetes, and they believe they have the ability to exercise, chances are they will, unless it means joining a gym, which may be too expensive financially or cost too much time getting there.

Interpersonal Theories

Theories at the interpersonal level explain behavior by focusing on factors that occur within relationships that influence what people do. They explain that behavior results from the influence of other people, such as family, friends, peers, healthcare providers, coworkers, teachers, coaches, and religious or spiritual leaders, among others. These "others"

influence behavior by sharing their thoughts and feelings, giving advice, and providing emotional support or assistance. A commonly used interpersonal theory in public health is Social Cognitive Theory.

Social Cognitive Theory

Reciprocal determinism is the underlying concept in social cognitive theory. It explains that behavior results from a dynamic back-and-forth relationship among three elements—personal factors, the environment, and the behavior, and that a change in any one of them changes them all. These three elements are influenced by self-efficacy, expectations, expectancies, self-regulation, observational learning, and reinforcement, all of which serve as the most often used theory constructs (Bandura, 1977). (See **Figure 2-6**.)

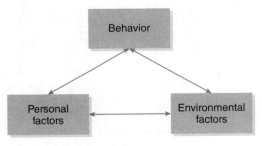

Figure 2-6 Social Cognitive Theory

Reproduced from Pajares, F. (2002). Overview of social cognitive theory and of self-efficacy. Retrieved from http://www.emory.edu/EDUCATION/mfp/eff.html.

- *Self-efficacy*, as discussed previously, is the extent to which a person is confident in his or her ability to do something. Given this, it's understandable that behavior changes when self-efficacy changes.
- *Expectations* are the outcomes people anticipate or expect will result from a particular behavior that causes them to engage in or avoid the behavior (Bandura, 1977). For instance, people use condoms because the expectation of this behavior is disease prevention. People avoid texting while driving because the expectation is that it will prevent an accident.
- *Expectancies* reflect the value people assign to or associate with the anticipated outcome (expectations) of a behavior. Generally, people engage in a behavior if they value the outcome as positive or rewarding and avoid the behavior if they associate it with being negative, unrewarding, or undesirable (Bandura, 2001). For example, if a person expects that quitting smoking will cause weight gain (negative or undesirable expectancy), then it's less likely she will try. On the other hand, if a person expects that quitting smoking will decrease the risk of lung cancer and heart disease (positive expectancy or desirable), then it's more likely she'll try to quit.
- *Self-regulation* or self-control in regard to a behavior is based on a person's own personal (internal) standards. This internal or self-control comes from beliefs people form about what they can do, the likely outcome of their behavior, the goals they set, and the plan of action they take that results in the expected outcomes (Bandura, 1991). For example, a person with type 2 diabetes believes he can control his blood sugar, which will reduce his risk of heart disease. He sets a goal of getting his blood sugar to the level recommended by his healthcare provider. He develops a plan to modify his carbohydrate intake within the guidelines of the American Diabetes Association, which will result in better blood sugar control and reduced risk of complications.
- *Observational learning* is learning by watching others. How much people learn this way depends on how much attention they give to the person being watched (the model). The degree of attention given depends on the power and attractiveness of the model, the circumstances under which the model is being observed, the person's motivation for learning the new behavior, how important it is for the behavior to be learned, and the complexity of the behavior (Bandura, 1977; Grusec, 1992). Observational learning works best when the model is considered a powerful person, is well respected, or is someone to whom the observer can relate (NCI, 2005).
- *Reinforcement* explains that people engage in certain behaviors because they are either seeking a reward (positive reinforcement) or want to avoid a punishment (negative reinforcement) (Bandura, 1977). Positive reinforcement is a desirable incentive that encourages the continuation or repetition of a behavior—praise, recognition, a shopping trip, flowers, a new hockey stick, a vacation. Negative reinforcement is a punishment that discourages the continuation or repetition of a behavior—no dessert, scolding, embarrassment, extra chores, restricted screen time, loss of car keys.

We tend to think of rewards being for desirable behaviors and punishments for undesirable, but this isn't necessarily true all of the time. An undesirable behavior can be rewarded, and when it is, it continues. For instance, binge drinking is an undesirable behavior rewarded by the cheering-on of friends. Overspending on credit cards is rewarded by having credit extended.

Community-Level Theories

Community-level theories explain behavior by focusing on factors within social systems that influence our behavior, such as the communities in which we live, the organizations and institutions we are part of, regulations, legislation, norms, and policies (Cottrell, Girvam, & McKenzie, 2009; NCI, 2005). The theories at this level include Diffusion of Innovation, Social Capital Theory, and the Social Ecological Model.

Diffusion of Innovation

Diffusion of Innovation is the process by which new ideas spread. Why some become part of the social fabric and others do not is explained by four constructs—the innovation, the ways in which the innovation is communicated, the time it takes different groups to adopt it, and the social system in which those groups live (Rogers, 2003).

Innovation. An *innovation* is something new or novel. It can be a practice, a program, a method, an idea, a device—anything that is different than what existed before. The success or failure of an innovation (the likelihood of its adoption or rejection) is affected by its advantage over what is already available, the extent to which it is compatible with social norms and values, its trialability or suitability for use on a limited basis, its complexity or ease of use, and observability of the results of its use. Innovations that are advantageous, compatible, triable, and easy and have observable results are adopted more rapidly than those that are not (Rogers, 2003; Rogers & Scott, 1997).

Communication Channel. The *communication channel* is the format people use to share the information, to spread the word of about an innovation. Diffusion is the social process people engage in when they share information about something new (Rogers, 2003).

An effective and rapid communication channel for diffusing information about something new is mass media, namely social media/online, newspaper, radio, magazines, and television. This communication channel can reach a very large audience very quickly, making a considerable portion of a society rapidly aware of a new product or idea. Depending on the innovation, sometimes a conversation between two people, word of mouth, is equally as effective. One friend telling another about a new product would have an impact on the latter trying something new that the former has already tried (Hayden, 2019).

Time. *Time* refers to how long it takes different groups or segments of a society to adopt an innovation and the steps they go through in the process. The rate of adoption by the different population segments follows a bell-shaped adoption curve that sorts people into five categories or segments: innovators, early adopters, early majority, late majority, and laggards. (See **Figure 2-7**.) Where people fall on the curve depends on a number of factors, for example, comfort with risk taking, socioeconomic status, extent of social networks, and leadership and the innovation.

- *Innovators* are in the first segment of the adoption curve. These are the risk takers. They are the small percentage of a population who like to take chances and can cope with the unpredictability of an innovation (Rogers, 2003).
- *Early adopters* are next on the curve. These are the opinion leaders in a community—well respected individuals with intricate communication networks who know a lot of different people (Rogers, 2003).
- The *majority* follows next on the curve. It's divided into two segments, the *early majority* on the upward side of the curve

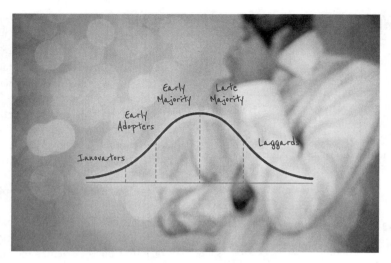

Figure 2-7 Adoption curve

© Jirsak/Shutterstock

and the *late majority* on the downward side. The early majority are influenced by opinion leaders and mass media, and when they begin to adopt an innovation, it's on its way to becoming mainstream.

- The *late majority*, although strongly influenced by their peers, wait until an innovation is an established norm or necessity before they adopt (Rogers, 2003).
- *Laggards* are at the end of the end of the downward side of the curve. People in this group tend to be conservative, traditional, suspicious of innovation, and risk adverse. They wait a long time before adopting an innovation (Rogers, 2003).

The length of time it takes the different segments of a population to make a decision about adopting an innovation is the outcome of the innovation-decision process. This process follows a sequence of steps that includes knowledge, persuasion, decision, implementation, and confirmation (Rogers, 2003).

Because people can't make a decision about adopting something new if they don't know about it, *knowledge* of an innovation's existence is the necessary first step in the innovation-decision process. Knowledge is gained through a communication channel (Rogers, 2003).

Once people know about an innovation, they can begin developing an attitude (either positive or negative) toward it. Their eventual attitude comes from thinking about and mentally applying the innovation to a present or future situation, which helps persuade them one way or another as they formulate their attitude toward the innovation (Rogers, 2003).

Armed with knowledge of the innovation and after having developed an attitude toward it, people make a *decision* to engage in activities that will either lead them to adopt or reject the innovation (Rogers, 2003). After engaging in the activities, the decision to either adopt or reject the innovation is made. For example, if the innovation is a soap that changes color after 20 seconds of handwashing, and after learning about how it works, the attitude toward it is positive, the activity would be to buy it and try it. After trying it, the decision would be made to either continue using it (adoption) or never buying it again (rejection). Sometimes this completes the innovation-decision process, but on occasion people need confirmation from others that the decision they made was a good one (Rogers, 2003).

Social System. The fourth and final construct in Diffusion of Innovation is the *social system*. The social system is any group of people, informal or formal, working together to accomplish a goal. Social systems embody the norms, values, beliefs, attitudes, and other common characteristics of the people in the system and is the conduit through which diffusion takes place (Rogers, 2003).

Social Capital

The concept underlying *social capital* explains it's the trusting and reciprocal interactions people have with each other that influences behavior. Networks and relationships are the constructs of this theory (Putnam, 2000; Putnam, Leonardi, & Nanetti, 1993).

Networks. Networks are the connections people have with other people through which they gain access to all the resources of the others in the network. These networks come in all sizes from those as large as whole societies or communities to as small as a nuclear family. But, before network resources can be accessed, there must be trust and reciprocity between the members of the network (Carpiano, 2006).

Once trust and reciprocity are established, they give rise to the expectations and obligations of membership in the network (Hawe & Shiell, 2000). It's this sense of connectedness and obligation to others in the network that leads to the behaviors and attitudes beneficial to the person and the greater group (Putnam, 2000).

Relationships. Relationships are the scaffolding upon which networks are built. In social capital theory there are three types of relationships—bonding, bridging, and linking, differentiated by the nature of the association between the people who make up the social network.

- *Bonding* social capital relationships are those between people who have similar demographic characteristics, social identity, origin, status, resources, and so on (Claridge, 2018; Szreter & Woolcock, 2004). These are the relationships that exist between family members, friends, and neighbors and in companies where employees share a sense of identify and belonging (Claridge, 2018).
- *Bridging* social capital relationships are those formed between people who differ sociodemographically (age, education, ethnicity), but have shared goals and interests (Wakefield & Poland, 2005). These relationships allow people to participate in activities with mutually beneficial outcomes that are not possible within their bonding relationships (Szreter, 2002). For instance, bridging relationships are those between people in a church choir, volunteer fire department, or community theater group.
- *Linking* social capital relationships are those between people who interact across power or authority gradients (Szreter & Woolcock, 2004), where one person has dominance, control, or influence over the other. The relationships between teacher and student, clergy and parishioner, judge and criminal are examples of linking social capital relationships. (See **Figure 2-8**.)

Social Ecological Model

The underlying concept of the Social Ecological Model (SEM) explains behavior as the result of a dynamic interplay among various factors at differing levels of influence. These levels were originally identified as intrapersonal, interpersonal, institutional, community, and societal (Stokols, 1992), visualized as a target with concentric circles—the smallest in the center (intrapersonal) expanding to the widest (societal). (See **Figure 2-9**.)

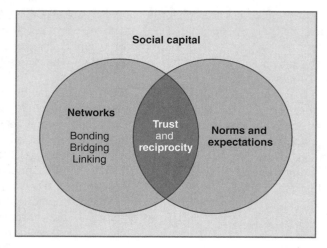

Figure 2-8 Social capital

Hayden, J. (2019). *Introduction to Health Behavior Theory*, (3rd ed). Burlington, MA: Jones & Bartlett Learning.

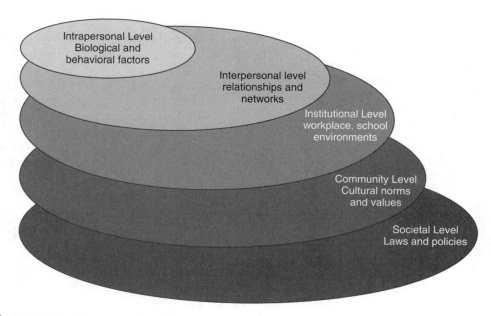

Figure 2-9 Social-ecological model

Data from Baral, S., Logie, C. H., Grosso, A., Wirtz, A. L., & Beyrer, C. (2013). Modified social ecological model: A tool to guide the assessment of the risks and risk contexts of HIV epidemics. *BMC Public Health*, 13(1), 1–8.

Intrapersonal or Individual Level. The intrapersonal or individual level identifies personal factors that affect behavior. These include personal history, knowledge, attitudes, beliefs, personality, self-efficacy, skills, perceptions, age, gender, and education level, among others.

Interpersonal or Relationship Level. The behavioral influences at the interpersonal level are the relationships we have with others. These relationships provide our social identity, and support systems and define roles within the social structure (WHO, 2006). They are the relationships we have with family friends, peers, coworkers, healthcare providers, and so on.

Institutional or Organizational Level. This set of behavioral influences are at the institutional or organization level. These are the rules, regulations, and policies usually associated with the workplace environment (Eddy, Donahue, Webster, & Bjornstad,

2002) but can include religious organizations (Haughton et al., 2015) and other informal or formal organizations or institutions that have behavioral expectations for members of the group.

Community Level. Community level influences are the formal or informal norms, standards, and expectations of individuals, groups, or organizations comprising the community (WHO, 2006). It includes the built environment as community structures often determine how people behave (Poux, 2017). Some examples, are the availability of parks, safe playgrounds, and walking paths.

Societal or Public Policy Level. At the societal or public policy level, health is influenced by law, regulations and policies, social or cultural norms, and attitudes (CDC, 2015; WHO, 2006). These are broad societal factors at the local, state, and federal levels that affect not only health, but economics and education as well (CDC, 2015).

Chapter Summary

Health behavior theories explain why people do what they do relative to their health and form the basis of programs to change behavior and improve health.

Planning in Practice Chapter Activity

Understanding why people engage in unhealthy behaviors is critical to developing programs that help them change their behaviors and improve their health. To this end, in small groups, complete the following:

1. Use the Theory of Reasoned Action to explain what might account for the higher rates of drinking among women in sororities compared to those not in sororities. Record your group's responses.

2. Read the article below, and answer the questions that follow.

Article: *An Application of the Theory of Planned Behavior to Sorority Alcohol Consumption* (Hutching, Lac, & LaBrie, 2008). (Note: Read the "Discussion" section at the end of the article.) Article link: https://www.ncbi.nlm.nih.gov/pmc/articles/PMC2387076/

   (Note: Download PDF.)

Article Questions

1. What did the authors find predicted alcohol use?
2. How did the authors' findings compare with your group's explanation of drinking among sorority women?
3. What suggestions did the authors make for developing programs based on the predictors of alcohol use they found?

References

Aflakseir, A., & Abbas, P. (2012). Health beliefs as predictors of breast cancer screening behavior in a group of female employees in Shiraz. *Iranian Journal of Cancer Prevention, 5*(3), 124–129. Retrieved August 17, 2018, from https://www.ncbi.nlm.nih.gov/pmc/articles/PMC4294534/

Ajzen, I. (1991). The theory of planned behavior. *Organizational Behavior and Human Decision Process, 50,* 179–211. https://doi.org/10.1016/0749-5978(91)90020-T

Ajzen, I. (2002). *Theory of planned behavior.* Retrieved October 24, 2004, from https://people.umass.edu/aizen/tpb.html

Ajzen, I., & Fishbein, M. (1980). *Understanding attitudes and predicting social behavior.* Englewood Cliffs, NJ: Prentice-Hall.

Bandura, A. (1977). *Social learning theory.* Englewood Cliffs, NJ: Prentice-Hall.

Bandura, A. (1991). Social cognitive theory of self-regulation. *Organizational Behavior and Human Decision Processes, 50*(2), 248-287. https://doi.org/10.1016/0749-5978(91)90022-L

Bandura, A. (1994). Self-efficacy. In V. S. Ramachandran (Ed.), *Encyclopedia of human behavior* (Vol. 4, pp. 71–81). New York, NY: Academic Press. (Reprinted from *Encyclopedia of mental health,* by H. Friedman, Ed., 1998, San Diego, CA: Academic Press)

Bandura, A. (1997). *Self-efficacy: The exercise of control.* New York, NY: Freeman.

Bandura, A. (2001). Social cognitive theory: An agentic perspective. *Annual Review of Psychology, 52,* 1–26. doi: https://doi.org/10.1146/annurev.psych.52.1.1

Bandura, A., & Adams, N. (1977). Analysis of self-efficacy theory of behavior change. *Cognitive Therapy and Research, 1*(4), 287–310.

Bluethmann, S. M., Bartholomew, L. K., Murphy, C. C., & Vernon, S. W. (2016). Use of theory in behavior change interventions: An analysis of programs to increase physical activity in posttreatment breast cancer survivors. *Health Education and Behavior.* Advanced online publication. https://doi.org/10.1177%2F1090198116647712

Carpiano, R. M. (2006). Toward a neighborhood resource-based theory of social capital for health: Can Bourdieu and sociology help? *Social Science and Medicine, 62,* 165–175. https://doi.org/10.1016/j.socscimed.2005.05.020

Centers for Disease Control and Prevention (CDC). (2004). Program operations guidelines for STD prevention: Community and individual behavior change interventions. Retrieved September 15, 2018, from https://www.cdc.gov/std/program/community.pdf

Centers for Disease Control and Prevention (CDC). (2015). The social ecological model: A framework for prevention. Retrieved June 3, 2020, from https://www.cdc.gov/violenceprevention/publichealthissue/social-ecologicalmodel.html

Claridge, C. (2018). What is bonding social capital? Retrieved September 15, 2018, from https://www.socialcapitalresearch.com/what-is-bonding-social-capital/

Cottrell, R. R., Girvan, J. T., & McKenzie, J. F. (2009). *Principles & foundations of health promotion and education* (4th ed.). San Francisco, CA: Pearson/Benjamin Cummings.

DiClemente, C.C., Schlundt, D. & Gemmell, L. (2004). Readiness and stages of change in addition treatment. *American Journal of Addiction, 13*(2), 103-119. https://doi.org/10.1080/10550490490435777

Eddy, J. M., Donahue, R. E., Webster, R. D., & Bjornstad, E. (2002). Application of an ecological perspective in worksite health promotion: A review. *American Journal of Health Studies, 17*(4), 197–202. Retrieved from: https://libres.uncg.edu/ir/uncg/listing.aspx?id=2960

Fishbein, M. (1967). *Readings in attitude theory and measurement.* New York, NY: Wiley.

Floyd, D. L., Prentice-Dunn, S., & Rogers, R. W. (2000). A meta-analysis of research on protection motivation theory. *Journal of Applied Social Psychology, 30*(2), 407–429. https://doi.org/10.1111/j.1559-1816.2000.tb02323.x

Glanz, K., & Bishop D. B. (2010). The role of behavioral science theory in development and implementation of public health interventions. *Annual Review of Public Health, 31,* 399–418. https://doi.org/10.1146/annurev.publhealth.012809.103604. Retrieved August 13, 2018, from https://www.annualreviews.org/doi/pdf/10.1146/annurev.publhealth.012809.103604

Glanz, K., Rimer, B. K., & Viswanath, K. (Eds.). (2008). *Health behavior and health education* (4th ed.). San Francisco, CA: Jossey-Bass.

Grusec, J. E. (1992). Social learning theory and developmental psychology: The legacies of Robert Sears and Albert Bandura. *Developmental Psychology*, *28*(5), 776–786. https://psycnet.apa.org/doi/10.1037/0012-1649.28.5.776

Haughton, J., Ayala, G. X., Burke, K. H., Elder, J. P., Montanez, J., & Arredondo, E. (2015). Community health workers promoting physical activity. *Journal of Ambulatory Care Management*, *38*(4), 309–320. https://doi.org/10.1097/JAC.0000000000000108. Retrieved May 8, 2019 from https://www.ncbi.nlm.nih.gov/pmc/articles/PMC4565764/

Hawe, P., & Shiell, A. (2000). Social capital and health promotion. A review. *Social Science & Medicine*, *51*, 871–885. https://doi.org/10.1016/S0277-9536(00)00067-8

Hayden, J. (2019). *Introduction to health behavior theory* (3rd ed.). Burlington, MA: Jones & Bartlett Learning.

Hochbaum, G. M. (1958). *Public participation in medical screening programs: A socio-psychological study* (Public Health Service Publication No. 572). Washington, DC: Government Printing Office.

Janz, N. K., & Becker, M. H. (1984). The health belief model: A decade later. *Health Education Quarterly*, *11*(1), 1–47. https://doi.org/10.1177/109019818401100101

Kerlinger, F. N. (1986). *Foundations of behavioral research* (3rd ed.). New York, NY: Holt, Rinehart & Winston.

Madiba, T. K., Bhayat, A., & Nkambule, N. R. (2017). Self-reported knowledge, attitude and consumption of sugar-sweetened beverages among undergraduate oral health students at a university in South Africa. *Journal of International Society of Preventive & Community Dentistry*, *7*(suppl 3), 137–142. doi: 10.4103/jispcd.JISPCD_306_17. Retrieved August 29, 2018, from https://www.ncbi.nlm.nih.gov/pmc/articles/PMC5730975/?report=printable

Maddux, J. E., & Rogers, R. W. (1983). Protection motivation and self-efficacy: A revised theory of fear appeals and attitude change. *Journal of Experimental Social Psychology*, *19*, 469–479. https://doi.org/10.1016/0022-1031(83)90023-9

National Cancer Institute [NCI]. (2005). *Theory at a glance: A guide for health promotion practice*. Bethesda, MD: U.S. Department of Health and Human Services, Public Health Services, National Institutes of Health, National Cancer Institute. Retrieved August 13, 2018, from https://cancercontrol.cancer.gov/brp/research/theories_project/theory.pdf

Pajares, F. (2002). Overview of social cognitive theory and of self-efficacy. Retrieved May 8, 2019, from http://www.uky.edu/~eushe2/Pajares/eff.html

Poux, S. (2017). Social ecological model offers new approach to public health. Retrieved June 3, 2020, from https://borgenproject.org/social-ecological-model/

Prochaska, J. O. (1994). Strong and weak principles for progressing from precontemplation to action on the basis of twelve problem behaviors. *Health Psychology*, *13*, 47–51. https://psycnet.apa.org/doi/10.1037/0278-6133.13.1.47

Prochaska, J. O., & DiClemente, C. C. (1982). Transtheoretical therapy: Toward a more integrative model of change. *Psychotherapy: Theory, Research and Practice*, *20*, 161–173. https://psycnet.apa.org/doi/10.1037/h0088437

Prochaska, J. O., & DiClemente, C. C. (1983). Stages and processes of self-change of smoking: Toward an integrative model of change. *Journal of Consulting and Clinical Psychology*, *51*, 390–395.

Prochaska, J. O., DiClemente, C. C., & Norcross, J. C. (1992). In search of how people change: Applications to addictive behaviors. *American Psychologist*, *47*(9), 1102–1114. https://psycnet.apa.org/doi/10.1037/0003-066X.47.9.1102

Putnam, R. D. (2000). *Bowling alone: The collapse and revival of American community*. New York, NY: Simon and Schuster.

Putnam, R. D., Leonardi, R., & Nanetti, R. Y. (1993). *Making democracy work: Civic traditions in modern Italy*. Princeton, NJ: Princeton University Press.

Rogers, E. M., & Scott, K. L. (1997). The diffusion of innovations model and outreach from the National Network of Libraries of Medicine to Native American communities. Retrieved October 30, 2004, from http://communitas.co.za/wp-content/uploads/2008/09/DiffusionofInnovationModelofChange.doc

Rogers, E. M. (2003). *Diffusion of innovation*. New York, NY: Free Press.

Rogers, R. W. (1975). A protection motivation theory of fear appeals and attitude change. *The Journal of Psychology*, *91*, 93–114. https://doi.org/10.1080/00223980.1975.9915803

Rosenstock, I. (1974). Historical origins of the health belief model. *Health Education Monographs*, *2*(4), 328–335. https://doi.org/10.1177%2F109019817400200403

Stokols, D. (1992). Establishing and maintaining healthy environments: Toward a social ecology of health promotion. *American Psychologist*, *47*(1), 6–22. https://psycnet.apa.org/doi/10.1037/0003-066X.47.1.6

Szreter, S. (2002). The state of social capital: Bringing back in power, politics, and history. *Theory and Society*, *31*(2), 573–621.

Szreter, S., & Woolcock, M. (2004). Health by association? Social capital, social theory and the political economy of public health. *International Journal of Epidemiology*, *33*(4), 650–667. https://doi.org/10.1093/ije/dyh013

Tebb, K. P., Erenrich, R. K., Jasik, C. B., Berna, M. S., Lester, J. C., & Ozer, E. M. (2016). Use of theory in computer-based interventions to reduce alcohol use among adolescents and young adults: a systemic review. *BMC Public Health, 16*(1), 517. https://doi.org/10.1186/s12889-016-3183-x Retrieved May 8, 2019 from https://www.ncbi.nlm.nih.gov/pmc/articles/PMC4912758/

Velicer, W. F., Prochaska, J. O., Fava, J. L., Norman, G. J., & Redding, C. A. (1998). Smoking cessation and stress management: Applications of the transtheoretical model of behavior change. *Homeostasis, 38,* 216–233.

Wakefield, S. E. L., & Poland, B. (2005). Family, friend or foe? Critical reflections on the relevance and role of social capital in health promotion and community development. *Social Science & Medicine, 60,* 2819–2832. https://doi.org/10.1016/j.socscimed.2004.11.012

World Health Organization (WHO). (2006). Ecological framework. Retrieved January 2, 2017, from http://www.who.int/violenceprevention/approach/ecology/en

CHAPTER 3

Preparing to Plan

STUDENT LEARNING OUTCOMES

After reading this chapter, the student will be able to:

- Explain the benefits of working with a planning committee.
- Write an invitation letter to potential planning committee members.
- Form a planning committee.
- Develop a meeting agenda.
- Explain the generic stages of program planning.

Introduction

Imagine you want to have a Super Bowl party, or a wedding reception, or maybe you want to surprise your significant other with a vacation on an exotic island in the South Pacific. All of these "events" take planning, and planning takes preparation. Before you can begin planning, you'll likely ask a few other people to help because these types of events are group efforts. There are so many tasks to get done, it's almost impossible for one person to handle everything and have a successful outcome.

The same is true when planning a health program. It's a group effort, and the earlier in the process the group is formed, the more committed the members are likely to be since they're involved in decision making from the very beginning.

Planning Groups

Planning groups go by any number of titles, including planning committee, advisory board, steering committee, commission, working group, task force, ad hoc committee, and coalition. Each of these can differ somewhat in their role, structure, and composition, but all such groups have a common focus—the members work together to find a solution for an identified problem.

For example, a steering committee, as the name implies, guides or steers a program at its inception. It develops action plans, considers political and other implications of the program, and may develop vision and mission statements and an organizational structure. Typically, a steering committee has a finite lifespan of not more than 6 months (Center for Community Health and Development [CCHD], 2020).

An advisory committee, on the other hand, provides advice. Advisory committee members are knowledgeable about the community and the issue of concern. They are usually well respected in their field and well known in the community, and because of this, they lend prestige to an initiative. Advisory committees are often established when an initiative is the "baby" of one person who wants and needs support but is not looking for guidance (CCHD 2020).

A commission is a group of people who are brought together and officially charged with a task (commission, 2018). A working group, task force, coalition, or ad hoc committee are all similar in that they are formed to address a specific issue or for a limited purpose.

For consistency and clarity, planning committee is the term used throughout this text. It's defined as: a group of people with knowledge, expertise, and interest in a specific health issue and or population that can contribute in a meaningful way to assessing, planning, implementing, and evaluating programs to address needs and improve health.

Benefits of a Planning Committee

In addition to sharing the considerable amount of work that goes into planning a program, having a planning committee has other benefits. For example, generating ideas, community support and networking opportunities, and sharing expertise (CCHD, 2020).

- *Generating ideas:* The more people invested in finding a solution to a problem, the more interesting and effective those solutions can be (CCHD, 2020).
- *Generating community support:* When a variety of representatives from the community are involved in the program, there is greater likelihood of community ownership or buy in, which often means a greater chance of success. The more

engagement from different facets of the community—agencies, organizations, individuals—the greater the opportunity to educate those they represent about the issues (CCHD, 2020).

- *Generating networking opportunities:* Each member of the planning committee brings to the group access to the all people in their networks—or their connections, which can number in the hundreds. These are far more connections than would be possible from any one person on the committee contacting others on their own. When people are contacted by those they know, they are often more willing to help when asked. The networking possibilities are endless (CCHD, 2020).
- *Sharing expertise:* People who work for other organizations and agencies in the community have knowledge and experience to offer a newly formed committee. Business owners in the community or people who serve on other boards and similar committees also bring valuable insight and expertise (CCHD, 2020).

Forming a Planning Committee

Because members of a planning committee are involved in all aspects of planning the program, the composition of the committee is critical to its success. Following are tips for whom to include on the committee:

> **TIP 1** Include people with an interest in the health problem.

It's most important for the planning committee to be composed of people from a variety of community organizations and individual community members with an interest in the health issue. When people have something to gain either personally or professionally from a successful program, it increases the likelihood of program "ownership," which in turn contributes to its success. For example, the Estancia Water Planning Committee in New Mexico, whose goal is to protect the quality and preserve the quantity of water resources of the Estancia Basin for future generations, includes the following people: three county government representatives; three representatives from municipal, developer, and county interest groups; three representatives for agriculture enterprises; three representative appointees from the Soil and Water Conservation Districts; one citizen-at-large; and one representative from the New Mexico State Engineer Office and Land Office (Bernalillo County, n.d.).

> **TIP 2** Include people outside the intended audience who may be affected by the program.

These are people the program would affect indirectly because of their status and/or connections in the community (CCHD, 2020) or to the intended audience. For example, depending on the issue being addressed, representatives from law enforcement or the small business community might be appropriate because of their connections with the community. Parents would be appropriate if children were the intended audience.

> **TIP 3** Include "doers" and "influencers."

Doers do the work. They are the worker bees. Just as a beehive has thousands of worker bees to keep the colony alive, the same is true of a planning committee. The committee and the program will never get off the ground if no one does the work. (See **Figure 3-1**.)

The hive also needs a queen. So, too the planning committee needs at least one influencer. Influencers are people whose names alone will garner support for the program (CCHD, 2020). Think about who these "influencers" might be in your community, perhaps the mayor, superintendent of schools, police chief, hospital president, executive director of a nonprofit agency, or a business leader.

While there should be enough doers and influencers on the committee to get the work done, the actual number of people should be small enough to reach decisions and come to a consensus. Although there is no magic number as to how many people this is, in business five to seven seems to be the number that maximizes productivity (Threlfall, 2016), with every member over seven reducing decision-making effectiveness by 10 percent (Blenko, Mankins, & Rogers, 2010).

To constitute the planning committee, potential members are invited either by letter (on agency letterhead paper) or email that contains the following information:

– A brief explanation of the issue or problem the planning committee will address.
– A request for a representative from their agency/organization to participate on the planning committee.
– The day, time, and location of the first meeting (scheduled for at least 2–3 weeks from the date of this initial letter or email) or a request for available dates/times.
– An approximate duration of the committee commitment (weeks, months, years?).
– An approximation of meeting frequency and length.
– A response by date (7 days after the date of the letter or email is sufficient).
– A request for the name, phone number, and email address of the agency's representative, if the agency will participate.

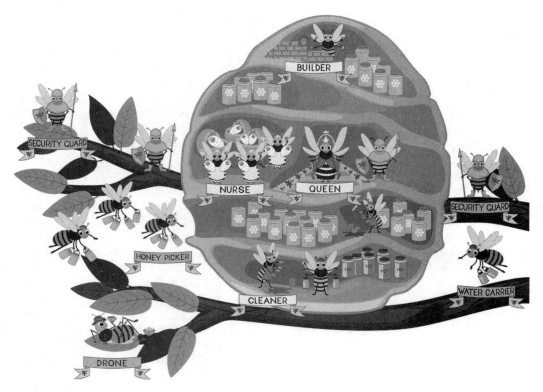

Figure 3-1 Structure of a beehive
© Kazakova Maryia/Shutterstock

- Email and phone number of person the invitee can contact for more information.
- Signature and official title of person sending the letter (email).

(See **Figure 3-2**.)

Following are some possible entities from which planning committee members might be recruited:

- Schools (preschools, elementary, high school).
- Local colleges or universities (students, faculty, and or administrators).
- Local, county, or state government officials.
- Local agencies and organizations.
- Civic organizations or service clubs.
- Social clubs, sports clubs, and community centers.
- Local or county Chamber of Commerce and other business organizations.
- Social service agencies.
- Youth groups and organizations.
- Faith communities (churches, mosques, synagogues, etc.) (CCHD, 2020).

Within a week of sending the invitation letter, most, if not all, the people contacted should have replied. People who didn't reply should be contacted by phone. Once responses are obtained from everyone invited, a preliminary committee membership list is compiled.

Anywhere Health Department
1234 Main Street
Anywhere, U.S.A

May 17, 2020

Michael Miller, Vice President Community Services
Anywhere Medical Center
567 Avenue A
Anywhere, U.S.A. 11111

Dear Mr. Miller:

As Director of the City of Anywhere Health Department, I am pleased to invite you to serve as a member of our community health assessment planning committee. The goal of the community health assessment is to identify the priority health needs and issues of the residents of Anywhere through a collaborative and systematic data collection and analysis process. The role of the Planning Committee is to serve as a representative for our community and the local public health system and to work with Anywhere Health Department staff to guide and oversee the community health assessment process. We know that no single entity or agency can make a community healthy, so we are delighted to work with you towards a shared goal of assessing and improving health for all those who live and work in Anywhere.

Our community health assessment process is expected to begin with our first Planning Committee meeting in June 2020 and be completed in September 2021. During this time, as a Planning Committee member, we ask that you commit to participating in all monthly in-person meetings as determined by the Committee and planned around schedules. If you are unable to serve on the Committee but are still interested in having your organization be represented, we would appreciate it if you could send us the name, title, and email address of your designee. We ask that your designee be someone in a senior leadership position within your organization or who is otherwise authorized to represent the organization.

We would be honored to have you serve on the Committee. Please consider our invitation, and email Jane Smith, Program Associate, at jsmith@anywhere.gov with your decision no later than Monday, May 29th 2020. If you decide to participate, please fill out the survey at this link (linkto survey.com) by May 29th indicating your availability for our first meeting, which will be held in mid to late June.

If you have questions or concerns, please contact John Brown, Director of Planning, at jbrown@anywhere.gov

Thank you for your time and we look forward to hearing back from you.

Sincerely,

Dr. Mary Davis
Executive Director and Health Officer
Anywhere Health Department

Figure 3-2 Planning committee invitation letter

Reproduced from National Association of County and City Health Officials (NACCHO). (2017). Steering committee invitation letter. Retrieved from https://www.naccho.org/uploads/downloadable-resources/Steering-Committee-Invitation-Letter-Draft-5.18.17.docx.

One week before the initial meeting is scheduled and again the day before, send an email reminder with the date, start and end time, location (or if using an online platform, the meeting link), and preliminary agenda. Use the blind copy email option for two reasons: (1) some people may not want their email addresses shared, and (2) if the list is long, it takes up too much space on the page before the message.

The convener of the initial planning meeting prepares the agenda. An agenda is an outline of the topics to be addressed during the meeting. It helps keep the discussion on track and move the planning process along. It also acts as a guideline for minutes or notes of the meeting and a historical record of what was addressed and when.

While there is no one correct template for an agenda, it should be written on agency letterhead (even if it's sent out electronically) and contain the following information:

– Name of the committee.
– Meeting date, time, location.
– List of topics to be discussed along with the person responsible for leading the discussion.

Figure 3-3 is one example of an agenda template.

Although there are many formats for holding a meeting—conference call, video call, Skype, Zoom, etc.—face-to-face is most advantageous when the people work in close geographic proximity to each other. Given that more than 90 percent of human communication occurs through body language, and only 7 percent through words (Borg, 2010), spending the extra time and effort it takes to arrange an in-person meeting, at least for the first meeting, is time well spent.

Face-to-face meetings also allow for more effective discussions, sharing of opinions, and relationship building. The downside of these, however, is that the conversation can veer off topic more easily, and side conversations between members can be distracting.

A committee chairperson is usually selected at the first meeting of the planning committee. This person is not always the planner who convened the meeting but can be. However, if the chairperson is chosen by the members from the membership, it encourages committee ownership of the project.

The planning committee chairperson is critical to the success of the program. The chairperson is responsible for presiding over the committee meetings and holding people accountable for the timely completion of tasks they agreed to complete. Consequently, not everyone can be a chairperson. Just because someone volunteers for the position, doesn't mean he or she should be selected.

As a guide, a good chairperson should be:

– knowledgeable about and interested in the health issue or affected population.
– enthusiastic about seeing the program come to fruition.
– creative and open to thinking out of the box.
– a people person who works well with others.
– assertive enough to keep the meeting agenda moving along and the members on task.
– open to discussions of ideas he/she does not agree with.
– a good communicator, both verbally and in writing.
– respected by the committee members.
– able to mitigate disagreements when/if they arise (Volunteer Now, n.d.).

In addition to the committee chairperson, it's important to have someone responsible for meeting minutes. Meeting minutes are a summary of what happens at each committee meeting. They serve as a reference for why decisions were made, actions taken, and tasks delegated. The committee members can decide to select one person to take minutes or rotate the responsibility among them all with a different person taking the minutes at each meeting. It's the responsibility of the chairperson to provide guidance on how detailed the minutes should be, specifically the degree of discussion

Anywhere County Health Department
Office of Public Health Initiatives
Elder Health Improvement Planning Committee
January 2, 2020

Time: 1 – 2 p.m.
Location: Meeting Room A
Anywhere County Health Department Complex
1234 Main Street
Anywhere, USA

Agenda

1. Welcome and introductions – John Smith, BS (convener)

2. Accept agenda

3. Overview of elder health issues – Sally Jones, MPH, County Health Officer

4. Overview of committee charge – Sally Jones

5. Chairperson selection – John Smith

6. Adjournment

Figure 3-3 Sample meeting agenda

to be recorded. Some minutes are limited to only actions taken; others have detailed accounts of who-said-what. However, all minutes follow the order of the agenda.

Although there is no one best way to record minutes, the following items are usually recorded:

- Committee title
- Meeting date
- Names of those in attendance and absent
- Meeting start time
- Name of person who called the meeting to order (usually the chairperson)
- Outcome of the vote to accept the agenda or changes made to the agenda, if any
- Outcome of vote to accept the minutes from previous meeting and corrections to the previous meeting minutes, if any
- A narrative that follows the format of the agenda
- Old business—topics or issues from previous meetings needing further discussions and the person's name who raised the issue

- New business—topics or issues not addressed at the meeting that a member wants addressed, and the person's name who raised the issue
- Adjournment time
- Signature of person taking minutes

(See **Figure 3-4** for an example of meeting minutes.)

Planning Process

With the planning committee formed, work on planning the program can begin. Planning includes:

- engaging the community.
- developing a vision and goals.
- conducting community assessments.
- prioritizing health issues and needs.
- developing a program plan.
- implementing the plan.
- evaluating the plan's outcomes and impact (Centers for Disease Control and Prevention [CDC], 2015).

Anywhere County Health Department
Office of Public Health Initiatives
Improving Senior Health Planning Committee

January 12, 2020
Meeting Minutes

Present: K. Connors, L. Doe, S. Jones, W. Monroe, J. Peters, J. Smith, S. Stevens
Absent: J. Oliver

Meeting called to order at 1:00 p.m. by J. Smith, Chairperson

1. Welcome and introductions – J. Smith
   J. Smith welcomed and introduced members of the group.

2. Acceptance of agenda – moved by S. Jones, seconded by S. Agenda unanimously accepted
   without changes.

3. Overview of senior health issues – S. Jones
   S. Jones presented information about health issues facing older adults in the community, particularly
   the increasing rates of health issues related to dementia. Discussion followed about how these issues
   were being addressed by attendees' agencies.

   K. Connors – Helping Hands Home Care Agency provides on-going training
   for their care aides specifically on how to address the nutritional and personal
   hygiene needs of aggressive or combative patients.

   L. Doe – Senior Housing Center provides monitor bracelets for all residents as a
   stipulation of housing.

   W. Monroe – Anywhere Community Hospital and Medical Center offers a seniors
   only clinic once a week staffed by geriatricians that provide assessments.

   J. Peters – Physical Therapy Center of Anywhere holds free monthly workshops for
   seniors and their family members/care givers on fall prevention.

   S. Stevens – State University at Anywhere, Department of Public Health partners
   with community agencies to collect and analyze data for needs assessments and
   program evaluations.

4. Overview of committee charge and responsibilities– S. Jones

   S. Jones explained that the committee is charged with:
   a. completing a needs assessment of older adults to identify gaps in services or
      missing services.
   b. using the information from the needs assessment to develop interventions to
      address the identified needs.

Figure 3-4 Sample meeting minutes

(continues)

5. Chairperson selection – J. Smith
   J. Smith distributed materials outlining the role and responsibilities of the committee chairperson. After a short discussion, nominations from the group were solicited. Two attendees were nominated with both accepting the nomination, S. Stevens, and W. Monroe. Each nominee was given 3 minutes to present his/her qualifications for being selected chairperson, which was followed by a secret ballot vote counted by S. Jones. The results were 5 votes for S.Stevens, and 2 votes for W. Monroe.

   S. Stevens is the newly elected committee chairperson.

6. Adjournment – meeting adjourned at 2:06 p.m.

Minutes respectfully submitted by:
J. Smith

Figure 3-4 (Continued)

These planning tasks are subsumed within four broad generic stages of planning: assessing, planning, implementing, and evaluating.

Assessing *need* is the first stage of planning. It's through a needs assessment that the problems and unmet needs of a specific population are identified. It entails collecting data from and about the people who comprise the population of concern, analyzing it, and using the results to determine the priority problem or greatest need that will be the focus of the program.

Planning is the stage in which decisions are made about how to address the priority problem identified in the needs assessment. It entails using the needs assessment results to establish the intended audience of the program (also called target audience, target population, or priority population), develop the program goals and objectives, and the strategies and actions to accomplish them.

Implementing is the action stage. It entails putting the program into practice, delivering it to the intended audience, and maintaining it.

Evaluating is the stage in which the results and effectiveness of the program are established. It entails collecting data from or about the intended audience, analyzing it, and interpreting it. The results are used as the basis for verifying efficacy, making revisions, or discontinuing the program.

The generic stages of planning encompass the following seven principles of program planning:

– *Plan with people* by establishing a planning committee.
– *Plan with data* generated from a needs assessment.
– *Plan for priorities* based on the results of the needs assessment and available assets/resources.
– *Plan with a process* by following a planning model or framework.
– *Plan for measurable outcomes* to enable effectiveness to be determined.
– *Plan for evaluation* to establish efficacy.
– *Plan for permanence* to ensure the program continues (Minelli & Breckon, 2009).

Chapter Summary

Program planning is a group effort undertaken by a diverse representation of community members, agencies, and organizations, collaborating throughout the four generic stages of the planning process.

Planning in Practice Chapter Activity

Forming a planning committee with the right mix and array of people is the first step in the program planning process. Its composition is critically important to the success of the program. Read the article below, and answer the questions that follow.

Article: *Adapting the WHO package of essential noncommunicable disease interventions, Samoa* (Bollars, Naseri, Thomsen, Varghese, Sorensen, DeVries, & Meerten. 2018)

Article link: https://www.who.int/bulletin/volumes/96/8/17-203695/en/

Article Questions

In small groups, answer the following questions:

1. What health issues were the Samoan people at increased risk of that prompted the adaptation of the WHO programs?
2. What determinants of health contributed to the health issues of the Samoan people?
3. Who was on the National Steering Committee, and what were their responsibilities?
4. What community asset was used to facilitate the program in the villages, and how?
5. How was information about the program shared with village members?
6. What indicates there was a commitment to a long-term process?

References

Bernalillo County. (n.d.). Boards and commissions: Estancia Basin Water Planning Committee. Retrieved May 10, 2019, from https://www.bernco.gov/boards-commissions/estancia-basin-water-planning-committee.aspx

Blenko, M. W., Mankins, M. C., & Rogers, P. (2010). *Decide & deliver*. Watertown, MA: Harvard Business Review Press.

Borg, J. (2010). *Body language: 7 easy lessons to master the silent language*. Upper Saddle River, NJ: Pearson Education, Inc.

Center for Community Health and Development (CCHD). (2020). Chapter 9, Section 2: Creating and gathering a group to guide your initiative. University of Kansas. Retrieved October 27, 2020 from the Community Toolbox https://ctb.ku.edu/en/table-of-contents/structure/organizational-structure/group-to-run-initiative/main

Centers for Disease Control and Prevention (CDC). (2015). Assessment & planning models, frameworks & tools. Retrieved April 1, 2020, from https://www.cdc.gov/publichealthgateway/cha/assessment.html

commission. (2018). In Merriam-Webster.com. Retrieved December 5, 2018, from https://www.merriam-webster.com/dictionary/commission

Minelli, M. J., & Breckon, D. (2009). *Community health education: Settings, roles and skills*. Sudbury, MA: Jones and Bartlett Learning.

Threlfall, D. (2016). What is the ideal team size to maximize productivity? Retrieved November 28, 2018, from https://www.teamgantt.com/blog/what-is-the-ideal-team-size-to-maximize-productivity

Volunteer Now. (n.d.), Characteristics of a good chairperson. Retrieved March 27, 2020, from https://www.diycommitteeguide.org/resource/characteristics-of-a-good-chairperson

SECTION II

Planning Basics

CHAPTER 4

Assessing Needs

STUDENT LEARNING OUTCOMES

As a result of reading this chapter the student will be able to:

- Collect primary and secondary data
- Develop qualitative and quantitative data collection instruments
- Conduct a survey
- Prioritize health issues
- Conduct a needs assessment
- Explain community-based participatory research

Introduction

The overall purpose of planning is to improve the public's health by developing programs to solve problems or address unmet needs that either directly or indirectly impact health. For example, climate change, community design, housing, and transportation (American Public Health Association [APHA], 2018) are problems or needs that impact health in some way.

Logically then, the first step in the planning process is to identify the problems or the unmet needs. In some situations, this is easy—the "problem" is the organization's raison d'être. For example, the American Heart Association addresses the problems of heart disease and stroke (American Heart Association, n.d.),

and the March of Dimes focuses on meeting the needs of pregnant women, mothers, and babies (March of Dimes, n.d.).

In situations where health problems and unmet needs are not as obvious or focused, as in a school or community or at a worksite, they are identified through a needs assessment. A *needs assessment* is a systematic way of finding out if there are gaps between "what is" and "what should be" (Kaufman, 1988). It's a method for collecting the information necessary to make decisions (Watkins, West Meiers, & Visser, 2012) about what the most pressing problems or needs are, guide decision making in the course of developing a program, and then serve as baseline data for evaluating how effective the program was in solving the problem or filling the need.

Following are general reasons for doing a needs assessment:

- To learn more about the needs of a specific group or community.
- To learn detailed information from a larger and more representative group of people than you could get from observation alone.
- To get more honest and objective description of needs than people might tell you publicly.
- To become aware of needs that are not obvious.
- To document needs as is required in many funding applications and as is almost always helpful in advocating or lobbying for your cause.
- To ensure any actions eventually taken are in line with needs expressed by the intended audience (Center for Community Health and Development [CCHD], 2018a).

Conducting a Needs Assessment

While the setting, reason for, and intended audience of needs assessments will vary and influence aspects of how they're done, the following five steps are generic to conducting all needs assessments (CCHD, 2018a; McCawley, 2009; Watkins et al., 2012).

Step 1—Clarify the Reason for Doing the Needs Assessment

If the reason for doing the needs assessment isn't clear, don't go any further. You can't collect information unless you know what you're collecting information about.

In this first step, answer the following questions:

- What issue, problem, or population is of concern (CCHD, 2018a)?
- What information is the needs assessment intended to produce (CCHD, 2018a)?

- What decisions will the needs assessment information inform (Watkins et al., 2012)?
- What questions will the needs assessment answer (Watkins et al., 2012)?

Step 2—Compile the Known Data, and Determine What Data Are Missing

In this step, information is gathered to establish what is already known about the issue, problem, or population of concern identified in Step 1 and programs that successfully addressed them. By collecting the available information, what's missing becomes evident. You don't know what's missing until you see what you have.

In this step, answer the following questions:

- What information is known?

"What is known" is answered by secondary data—data previously generated by someone else for another purpose, but applicable to the needs assessment being conducted (CCHD, 2018b). Secondary data are available from a plethora of sources, including government reports; local, county, and state health department statistics; registries; disease-specific associations and organization; and in studies and the professional literature (see **Table 4-1**).

- What information is missing?

"What is missing" is the information that is needed but not available in any of the secondary data sources. The contribution secondary data makes to identifying missing information was evident when health professionals at a women's shelter wanted to develop a shelter-based medical program to improve maternal and child health outcomes of pregnant homeless women (Ake et al., 2018). The review of secondary data sources from the local health department on infant mortality showed a rate of 9.1 deaths per 1,000 births,

Table 4-1 Secondary data sources

Source	Information	Access
Behavioral Risk Factor Surveillance System	Information on health conditions and risk behaviors in the United States	https://www.cdc.gov/brfss/
CDC Wonder	Databases for the analysis of public health data	https://wonder.cdc.gov/
Disability and Health Data System	State-level, disability-specific data	https://www.cdc.gov/ncbddd/disabilityandhealth/dhds
U.S. Census	Population, housing, economic, and geographic information	https://factfinder.census.gov/
Centers for Medicare & Medicaid Services Research and Data Clearinghouse	Statistics, trends, and reports on all aspects of Medicare and Medicaid services	https://www.cms.gov/Research-Statistics-Data-and-Systems/Research-Statistics-Data-and-Systems
Environmental Public Health Tracking Network	Data on health, exposure, and hazard information and from a variety of national, state, and city sources	https://ephtracking.cdc.gov/
Health Research and Services Administration Data Warehouse	Information on primary care and health centers, programs, health workforce, rural health	https://data.hrsa.gov/
National Center for Health Statistics	Statistical information to guide actions and policies	https://www.cdc.gov/nchs/
Pregnancy Risk Assessment and Monitoring System	State-specific, population-based data on maternal attitudes and experiences before, during, and shortly after pregnancy	https://www.cdc.gov/prams/
Web-based Injury Statistics Query and Reporting System (WISQARS)	Injury-related data	https://www.cdc.gov/injury/wisqars/index.html
Youth Risk Behavior Surveillance System	Data on behaviors contributing to the leading causes of death and disability among youth and adults	https://www.cdc.gov/healthyyouth/data/yrbs/index.htm
National Institutes of Health	Disease-specific health information and data	https://www.nih.gov/
Centers for Disease Control and Prevention (CDC)	Disease-specific health information and data	https://www.cdc.gov/

(continues)

Table 4-1 Secondary data sources   *(continued)*

Source	Information	Access
National health associations and organization, ex: American Heart Association American Cancer Society American Lung Association	Disease-specific health information	https://www.heart.org/; https://www.cancer.org/; https://www.lung.org/
Professional journals	Data from original research and evaluation studies	

Data compiled from: Centers for Disease Control and Prevention (CDC). (2017). Public Health Professionals Gateway, Data and Benchmarks. Retrieved May 13, 2019, from https://www.cdc.gov/publichealthgateway/cha/data.html

which was substantially higher than the national average of 5.8 deaths per 1,000 births gleaned from CDC data. Secondary data from studies in professional journals showed higher rates of cigarette, alcohol, and drug use among pregnant homeless women associated with birth complications (Cutts et al., 2015; Little et al., 2005), while other studies reported data showing homeless women experienced higher rates of physical injury, mental illness, and pregnancy complications that range from common mild ones to those associated with prematurity and low birth-weight that may have long-term effects (Clark et al., 2019).

Although information from the secondary data sources pointed to a need for programs addressing substance abuse, pregnancy prevention, and stress management, the information the health professionals didn't have was about the needs of the pregnant homeless women at *their* shelter. As it turned out, their needs assessment identified pregnancy education, access/transportation, baby care, advocacy, and material necessities as the unmet needs of the women in their shelter (Ake et al., 2018).

In another example, although national statistics (secondary data) documented ethnic/minority-related health disparities, public health professionals in southwest Kansas did not find information about minority health in rural areas they could use for chronic disease prevention programming (Bopp et al., 2012).

However, the secondary data did enabled them to pinpoint what they needed to find out—the specific unmet needs related to chronic disease prevention of the Hispanic community in *their* part of their state.

Step 3—Identify from Whom Data are Missing

The focus of this step is to determine from whom information is missing and who can provide it. For example, if the missing information is in compliance with CDC childhood vaccination recommendations, this information is missing from children, but it's their parents or guardians who can provide it.

To complete this step, answer the following questions:

- Whose input is needed?
- Whose behaviors affect the problem (Watkins et al., 2012)?

The people whose input is needed are those who can provide the missing information. These are primary data sources. Primary data sources are people from whom original information is directly collected. You ask, they answer, no middleperson involved.

In a needs assessment, primary data sources usually include the people with the health problem or whose needs you're trying to determine, "others" whose behavior impacts them, and those who are knowledgeable about the problem or the people with the problem. Sometimes these are one and the same but not always. For example, if the problem is childhood obesity, the people whose needs you're trying to determine are the obese children, the others whose behavior impacts them are their parents, those who are knowledgeable about them are school personnel, and those knowledgeable about childhood obesity are healthcare professionals.

The specific sources of primary data vary depending on the population in which the problem exists. For example, if the problem is low influenza vaccination rates in the preschool population, the primary data sources are different than if low vaccination rates are in the older adult population. In the case of children, the primary data sources are their parents or guardians, pediatric healthcare practitioners, and perhaps day care or preschool personnel, depending on their age. In the case of older adults, primary data sources are the older adults themselves, perhaps senior center personnel, and healthcare professionals.

A real-world example of this occurred in Amsterdam when public health professionals concluded from secondary data that in order to address unhealthy behaviors and poor health outcomes of children from lower-income families, they needed to find out the specific lifestyle-related issues of the children in their city. To fill in this information gap, they identified three primary data sources—children living in the low-income areas, their parents, and the healthcare professionals who interacted with them (Anselma, Chinapaw, & Altenburg, 2018).

Step 4—Decide How to Collect the Missing Data

There are a number of methods or ways to collect data. Determining which method will produce the missing data depends on the type of data that're missing.

To complete this step, answer the following questions:

- What type of data are missing (Watkins et al., 2012)?

There are two types of data, quantitative and qualitative. Quantitative data are numerical and answer questions of "how many" or "how much." They are analyzed statistically to produce means/averages, ratios, percentages, and correlations, among other outcomes (New South Wales [NSW] Department of Education, 2019).

Qualitative data are narrative, words, sentences and answer questions of "what," "how," and "why." They provide more in-depth details of a person's thoughts, feelings, and opinions (Kabir, 2016; NSW, 2019) and are analyzed by identifying themes or patterns in the responses.

- What methods will be used to collect and analyze the missing data (Watkins et al., 2012)?

Methods for collecting needs assessment data include: survey (questionnaire or interview), focus groups, and observation. The method used is driven by the type of data that is missing. Questionnaire surveys are used to collect quantitative data, focus groups to collect qualitative data, and interviews and observation to collect either or both. (See **Table 4-2.**)

Surveys. The term *survey* is frequently used for both the method of data collection and the form used to record the data, which can get confusing. For clarity purposes, the term *survey* in this text refers to the data collection method. The terms *questionnaire* or *instrument* refer to the forms used to record the data.

Surveys collect data from a group of people through their responses to questions (Check & Schutt, 2012). They are conducted using self-administered paper or electronic (online) questionnaires that ask questions and provide a set of answers or response options for the person to choose from, as in a

Table 4-2 Comparison of qualitative and quantitative methods

Qualitative methods	Quantitative methods
Answers "What?" and "Why?" questions to explore or explain an occurrence.	Answers the questions Who? What? When? Where? "How many?" to confirm an occurrence.
Produces narrative data.	Produces numerical (statistical) data
Uses interviews, observations, focus groups to collect data.	Uses questionnaires, tools, equipment to collect data.
Uses open-ended questions to explore an issue.	Uses closed-ended questions to get quantifiable results.

Data from Canyon University, Center for Innovative Research and Teaching, (n.d.). When to use quantitative methods
Original source: Grand Canyon University, Center for Innovative Research and Teaching, (n.d.). When to use quantitative methods. Retrieved February 16, 2020 from https://cirt.gcu.edu/research/developmentresources/research_ready/quantresearch/whentouse

multiple-choice test. Surveys can also be conducted by in-person or phone interviews in which the person is read the questions and answers and responds verbally.

The following are common tasks associated with conducting a needs assessment survey (CCHD, 2018d):

Task 1—Identify the population.

The first task is to identify the population that can best provide the needed data. For example, if the needs assessment is being done to identify gaps in adult health service needs in the community, then the intended audience is any adult living in the community. But, if the needs assessment is being done to identify gaps in the health service needs of children in the community, then the intended audience is parents or guardians, pediatric healthcare providers (pediatricians, pediatric nurse practitioners, child psychologists, school nurses), and school personnel.

Deciding who will participate in the survey is one task; determining how many people will participate is another. If the needs assessment is focusing on adult health service needs of the community, there may be a population of tens of thousands of adults in the community. While surveying all of them may be possible, it's not practical or probable given the time and money it would take. Instead, a sample or part of the adult population is surveyed. The challenges with this are to make sure that every adult in the population has a chance to be in the sample, and then having enough people in the sample to be confident that the results accurately reflect what the results would have been if the entire population had been surveyed. The number of people needed for this confidence is the sample size.

The easiest way to calculate the size of the sample needed is to use an online calculator. Two free resources for calculating sample size are:

Survey System's Sample Size Calculator (https://www.surveysystem.com/sscalc.htm)

UCLA's Sample Size Calculator (http://statistics.ucla.edu/)

(For a more in-depth explanation of sample size, see Chapter 7, Evaluating.)

Task 2—Develop data collection instrument.

With the population of the needs assessment decided and the sample size determined, the next task is developing a data collection instrument. This begins with the planning committee creating a set of questions and response options to generate the missing data.

Following are guidelines for developing a simple needs assessment instrument:

Guideline 1—Know what information is needed.

Be careful to distinguish between "need to know" information and "nice to know" information (Losby & Wetmore, 2012). Questions that generate "nice to know" information are irrelevant (Edwards et al., 2009) and should not be included in the questionnaire. To determine which questions to include and which to leave out, ask if the question will generate missing information. If the answer is "no," don't include the question.

Guideline 2—Decide on question (item) format.

Questions, also called items, are written in two formats, closed-ended and open-ended. The format used is determined by the type of data to be collected.

◆ Closed-ended questions

Closed-ended questions are those in a multiple-choice test. They are answered by choosing from a set of response options. For example: Did you get a flu vaccine this year?— is a closed-ended question with two response options to choose from—"yes" or "no." Which of the following vaccinations have you received? Choose all that apply—Hepatitis A, Hepatitis B, MMR (Measles, Mumps, Rubella), Shingles, DTaP (Diphtheria, Tetanus, Pertussis), influenza, is a closed-ended question with many response options.

Because closed-ended questions are used to collect quantitative (numerical) data, the response options are assigned a number. For example, Yes = 1, No = 2. These numbers don't reflect a value. "No" could just as well be assigned 1, and "Yes," 2. The responses correspond to a number for analysis purposes.

Two benefits of using closed-ended questions are that it's easy to assign a number to the response options for statistical analysis, and the questions are standardized so all respondents are asked the same questions in the same order. On the downside, closed-ended questions

force respondents to choose from a set of responses that may or may not accurately reflect their answer (McLeod, 2018).

Closed-ended questions can also use scaled responses. For example, on a scale of 1 to 5, with 1 = strongly disagree, 2 = disagree, 3 = not sure or neutral, 4 = agree, 5 = strongly agree, to what extent do you agree with the following statement—"I don't use the park because I am concerned about my safety." These types of questions, referred to as **Likert scale**, are used to collect quantitative data about attitudes, beliefs, or feelings.

The most common scale is the five-point agree/disagree scale, but scales can range anywhere from two to seven (Losby & Wetmore, 2012) and measure a variety of concerns such as likelihood, satisfaction, frequency, quality, and importance. (See **Table 4-3**.)

◆ Open-ended questions

Open-ended questions don't provide response options but rather ask respondents to provide their own answers in their own words, as in an essay exam. These questions require the respondents to have writing skills good enough to construct coherent sentences (McLeod, 2018), making them difficult for those with limited English language abilities to answer. They also tend to take longer to complete and analyze and are more likely to be left unanswered.

Analyzing open-ended questions is not quick or easy. If qualitative software is not used, it entails reading each written response, identifying themes, and categorizing or coding the data so a meaningful interpretation can be made. If using open-ended questions is the best way to collect the missing data, the extra time needed for analysis should be taken into consideration (Boynton & Greenhalgh, 2004).

Neither type of data, qualitative or quantitative, is necessarily better than the other, overall. In most cases, both types of data are collected to ensure the missing information is uncovered.

Table 4-3 Likert rating scales

2 point scale	3 point scale	4 point scale	5 point scale	7 point scale
Agreement				
Disagree Agree	Disagree Neutral Agree	Strongly disagree Disagree Agree Strongly agree	Strongly disagree Disagree Neutral Agree Strongly agree	Strongly disagree Disagree Slightly disagree Neutral Slightly agree Agree Strongly agree
Frequency				
Never Always	Never Sometimes Always	Never Infrequently Sometimes Always	Never Infrequently Sometimes Frequently Always	Never Very infrequently Infrequently Sometimes Frequently Very frequently Always
Importance				
Unimportant Important	Unimportant Not sure Important	Unimportant Fairly important Important Very important	Unimportant Slightly important Not sure Important Very important	Unimportant Minimally important Slightly important Not sure Somewhat important Important Very important
Quality				
Poor Excellent	Poor Acceptable Excellent	Poor Fair Good Excellent	Poor Fair Good Very good Excellent	Very poor Poor Fair Acceptable Good Very good Excellent
Likelihood				
Very unlikely Very likely	Very unlikely Unsure Very likely	Very unlikely Unlikely Likely Very likely	Very unlikely Unlikely Not sure Likely Very likely	Very unlikely Unlikely Not sure Probably Likely Very likely

Data from Brown, S. (2010). Scale examples for surveys. Iowa State University Extension Center. Retrieved May 20, 2019 from https://www.extension.iastate.edu/Documents/ANR/LikertScaleExamplesforSurveys.pdf;
Vagias, W. M. (2006). Likert-type scale response anchors. Clemson International Institute for Tourism & Research Development, Department of Parks, Recreation and Tourism Management. Clemson University. Retrieved February 26, 2020 from http://media.clemson.edu/cbshs/prtm/research/resources-for-research-page-2/Vagias-Likert-Type-Scale-Response-Anchors.pdf

<u>Guideline 3</u>—Follow the BRUSO model to create questions.

The BRUSO model is a guide for creating questions that are **B**rief, **R**elevant, **U**nambiguous, **S**pecific, and **O**bjective (Price, Jhangiani, & Chiang, 2015). Each of these characteristics makes it easier and faster for respondents to complete a questionnaire.

Questions are

Brief, to the point and written in plain language without technical terms (Price et al., 2015) or jargon. For example, instead of using "hypertension," use "high blood pressure"; instead of "influenza vaccination," use "flu shot"; and instead of "myocardial infarction," use "heart attack."

Relevant, focused on the topic, and provide missing needs assessment information. Relevance avoids bothering respondents with what they may perceive as unrelated or even "nosy" questions (Price et al., 2015).

Unambiguous with only one possible interpretation (Price et al., 2015). To avoid ambiguity, define or explain what you mean. When asking about drinking habits, for example, state that an alcoholic drink is 1 and ½ ounces of hard liquid (approximately a shot), a 5-ounce glass of wine, or a 12-ounce bottle of beer. When asking about flossing behaviors, define regular flossing as at least once a day. Don't assume everyone reading the question will interpret it the same way, or the way you meant.

Specific, address one issue and make it clear to respondents what they are responding to and about. A common problem with specificity happens with double-barreled closed-ended items—items asking about two separate issues but allowing only one response (Price et al., 2015). For example, "How likely are you to attend classes about diet and exercise?" If someone is very likely to attend classes about diet, but not likely to attend classes about exercise, they wouldn't be able to answer the question. This should be split into two separate questions, one about diet the other about exercise.

Objective, present the issue in a nonbiased way that doesn't reflect the opinion of those on the planning committee or lead respondents to a particular answer (Price et al., 2015). For example, "As a parent of a middle school student, do you support 30 minutes of daily mandatory physical activity during school hours to address the childhood obesity problem?" Yes or no? What parent would say no?

Following are specific tips for creating Likert scale questions.

> **TIP** Write explicitly worded questions and statements (Survey Monkey, 2020).

If questions and statements are not worded clearly and can be interpreted in different ways, the response data are not useful. For example, if the purpose of a needs assessment is to identify gaps in student health services on campus, and students are asked to indicate the extent of their agreement with the following statement—"Student Health Center services meet the needs of students on campus," what does this mean? Does it mean that students need the services available, or does it mean the Student Health Center provides all the services students need or does it mean the mission of the Student Health Center is to meet the health needs of students on campus? A more explicit statement to tease out gaps in services would be "The Student Health Center provides the range of mental health services students need."

> **TIP** Use scales that make sense with the statement or question.

Although the traditional Likert scale, strongly disagree–strongly agree continuum, is commonly used (Losby & Wetmore, 2012), it may be illogical depending on the statement or question asked. Continuing with the campus health services example, asking for agreement/ disagreement with the following question is illogical—"How likely are you to use the mental health services at the student health center if weekend hours were available?" This calls for the likelihood response scale.

> **TIP** Label all response options, and assign each a numeric value.

All response options are labeled and given a number value. For commonly used response option labels, see **Table 4-3**.

Assigning a numeric value to the responses enables the data to be analyzed statistically. For example, if a mean of 4.3 was computed on a five-point agree/disagree scale (1 = strongly disagree—5 = strongly agree), for all the students' responses to the statement "The Student Health Center provides the range of mental health services students need," this would indicate that most students agreed with the statement. On the other hand, a mean of 1.3 would indicate most students disagreed. (See **Figure 4-1**.)

> **TIP** Use odd scales with no more than seven options

An even-numbered scale is referred to as a forced choice scale because it doesn't have a midpoint or neutral response. For example, a four-point agreement scale would be: strongly agree, agree, disagree, strongly disagree. The neutral or "I don't know" option is missing, which forces the respondent to either agree or disagree to some extent.

Sometimes forcing people to think about their response to a question prevents them from taking the easy way out and choosing the middle, resulting in more accurate data. On the other hand, people who genuinely "don't know" end up randomly choosing any response (Holbrook, 2008), resulting in less-accurate data.

People also tend to randomly choose an answer when a scale has more than seven response options. The plethora of responses is confusing and leads to haphazard answers, which again reduces the accuracy of the data (Survey Monkey, 2020).

Guideline 4—Consider other issues.

Other issues to consider when developing an instrument include the following:

◆ *Instrument completion time*

The more questions on an instrument, the more time it takes to complete, but the less time people spend answering each question. An instrument with 26–30 questions takes about 10 minutes to complete. An instrument with 10 questions takes about 5 minutes to complete. The longer the instrument, the greater the risk of it not being completed. When instruments take more than about 8 minutes to complete, up to 20 percent of people stop filling it out (Chudoba, 2020). Bottom line, if possible, keep the instrument to less than 20 questions and taking no more than about 8 minutes to complete.

Please circle the number that corresponds to your level of agreement with the following statement:

I feel safe walking around my neighborhood.

1 – Strongly disagree
2 – Disagree
3 – Not sure
4 – Agree
5 – Strongly agree

Figure 4-1 Example of rating scale question

◆ Order of the questions

It's best to start with the easiest to answer questions and move to those that are more difficult and to group questions addressing the same issue together. Questions addressing sensitive issues such as sexual behavior, drug use, and abuse are best placed at the end of the instrument to allow respondents to become comfortable answering the questions.

◆ Anonymity versus confidentiality

It's important to inform respondents of how the data are being collected, that is, anonymously or confidentially. When data are collected anonymously, responses *cannot* be linked to the person providing them. In contrast, when information is collected confidentially, responses *can* be linked to the person providing them. Unless there is a specific reason for collecting data confidentially, it should be collected anonymously. However, anonymous data collection is not possible with focus groups and interviews. This data is always confidential because the person collecting it knows who provided it.

◆ Demographic data

Demographic data are characteristics of the intended audience, typically age, gender, marital status, income, educational level, race, and employment status (). However, as with all questions on a questionnaire, if the answer is "nice to know," but not needed or is irrelevant, don't ask it. For example, if you want to know the perceived health risks of men in your community and you're only contacting men to participate in the needs assessment, there is no need to ask for sex, it's irrelevant. Demographic information should only be collected if it has a bearing on the outcome of the needs assessment.

◆ Instructions

Instructions for completing the questionnaire are a key factor for getting back usable questionnaires, filled out correctly. The instructions should be written in clear, concise language explaining exactly how to complete the form.

For example:

- Please circle the number next to your response.
- Please click the box next to your answer.
- Please put a check mark in the box next to all that apply.
- Please print your responses in the blank spaces provided.

Sometimes individual questions need specific instructions, such as those that ask respondents to rank a list of concerns, or Likert scale items. To make it easier and faster for people to complete the questionnaire, group questions together that have the same instructions. For example, put all scale questions together, or all open-ended questions together.

◆ Introduction

Every questionnaire needs a short introductory paragraph that explains its purpose and acknowledges the importance of the respondent's participation. It should also include the sponsoring organization, keeping in mind that university-sponsored surveys tend to yield higher questionnaire response rates (Price et al., 2015).

The introduction also establishes informed consent. At the very least, the introduction should describe the topics covered in the questionnaire, the option to withdraw or stop completing the questionnaire at any time without consequences, confidentiality versus anonymity, and an estimated amount of time it's likely to take to complete.

Because written consent forms are not typically used for surveys, it's important for the introduction to be clearly written so every respondent can read and understand it (Price et al., 2015). This is particularly important when the intended audience has limited English language skills. See **Figure 4-2** for an example of an introductory paragraph.

Task 3—Determine how the survey will be conducted.

Surveys are conducted in a number of ways, including in-person or phone interview,

Any City University Medical Center and the Any City Health Department are working on a project to improve the health knowledge of people living or working in our community. The aim of the project is to set up a Health Information Center at the medical center where people can get health information, go to classes to learn about different health problems or learn how to make changes so they can live healthier lives. This survey is the first step in the project.

While your participation is very important to us, it is up to you to answer the questions or not. If you choose not to answer the questionnaire, just tear it up and add it to your paper recycling bin. There is no way for us to know if you choose not to participate.

If you choose to answer the questions, fill out the questionnaire and return it to us in the enclosed envelope. Please **do not** write your name on the form. All your answers are anonymous.

We do not foresee any risks to you if you choose to participate in this survey. The benefits of your participation will be in the long term when the project is completed and the Health Information Center is up and running.

Your input in this survey is voluntary. No compensation is offered for your participation.

Figure 4-2 Sample introductory paragraph for a questionnaire

Data from Centre for Health Literacy (n.d.) (2019). Health literacy project. Appendix 3. Informed consent form. Retrieved May 21, 2019 from http://www.centreforliteracy.qc.ca/health/finalsum/rr/rra3.html

direct mail paper-and-pencil questionnaires, emailed questionnaires, or links to online questionnaires (CCHD, 2018e). Each survey method has its own set of pros and cons. There is no perfect method. (See **Table 4-4**.)

In deciding how to conduct the survey, consider the following:

The type of data needed

If qualitative data are needed, then interviews using open-ended questions will likely provide the missing information. If quantitative data are needed, then a written questionnaire (paper and pencil or electronic) or an interview using closed-ended questions will provide the missing information.

The intended audience

With which method is the intended audience more likely to answer questions, an interview or in a written questionnaire (CCHD, 2018d)? Input from members of the intended audience or those on the planning committee with in-depth knowledge of the intended audience is key in making this determination.

The method response rate

Response rate is a percent that reflects the number of people who complete the questionnaire divided by the total who received it, multiplied by 100 (to give the percent). For

example, if 1,500 people receive the questionnaire, and 654 complete and return it, the response rate is 43.6 percent (654/1,500 = .436 × 100 = 43.6%). The response rate is important because if it's too low, the results won't accurately represent the population, and the data may not be useful, which would defeat the whole purpose of doing the needs assessment.

In general, the response rate for all survey methods is 33 percent, with the average rate ranging from 57 percent for in-person interviews to 13 percent for in-app surveys (Lindermann, 2018). These rates are not specific to health needs assessment surveys, but rather for surveys in general. According to the Gallup Poll and Pew Research Center (2020), in 2017, landline telephone survey response rates were as low as 9 percent, with cell phone rates a bit lower at 7 percent (Keeter, Hatley, Kennedy, & Lau, 2017; Marken, 2018). Online questionnaire response rates are between 20 and 30 percent (Porter, 2019).

Overall, interviews produce the highest response rates. For example, the CDC's National Health Interview Survey (2019) has an annual response rate of 70 percent (CDC, 2019). (See **Figure 4-3**.)

Table 4-4 Pros and cons of survey methods

Method	Pros	Cons
Surveys	<ul><li>Can complete anonymously.</li><li>Can administer to large groups at the same time.</li><li>Can provide data on behaviors, opinions, attitudes, and beliefs.</li><li>Can standardize.</li><li>Can provide data for statistical analysis.</li></ul>	<ul><li>Closed-ended (forced) responses can prevent true participant response.</li><li>Wording of questions can bias responses.</li><li>Impersonal.</li><li>Low response rate.</li></ul>
Interviews (individual/ in-depth)	<ul><li>Can build rapport with participant.</li><li>Can clarify questions.</li><li>Can personalize the discussion.</li></ul>	<ul><li>Time consuming.</li><li>Expensive.</li><li>Interviewer skills and comments can affect responses.</li><li>Cannot complete anonymously.</li><li>Cannot use with large groups.</li></ul>
Focus Groups	<ul><li>Can get common impressions. quickly.</li><li>Can clarify questions.</li><li>Can get breadth and depth of information in a short time frame.</li><li>Can personalize</li></ul>	<ul><li>Need experienced facilitator.</li><li>Difficult to schedule a group of 6–8 people.</li><li>Time consuming to analyze responses.</li><li>Anonymous or confidential participation not possible.</li><li>Group members can influence responses.</li></ul>
Observation	<ul><li>Can view participants in natural setting as behaviors occur.</li><li>Can maintain observer anonymity.</li><li>Can generate quantifiable data.</li></ul>	<ul><li>Difficult to interpret observed behaviors.</li><li>Observation can influence behaviors (Hawthorne effect).</li><li>Time consuming to recording and analyze each individual event observed.</li><li>Cannot use with large groups.</li></ul>

Data from: Salabarría-Peña, Y, Apt, B.S., Walsh, C.M. (2007). Practical Use of Program Evaluation among Sexually Transmitted Disease (STD) Programs, Atlanta (GA): Centers for Disease Control and Prevention; Retrieved from https://www.cdc.gov/std/program/pupestd.htm February 16, 2020.
State of Michigan, (n.d.). Pros and cons of data collection methods. Retrieved February 17, 2020 from https://www.michigan.gov/documents/mentormichigan/Data_Collection_Methods--pros_and_cons_2_403346_7.pdf.

Response rates for mailed questionnaires improve when the mailing address is handwritten, the mailing includes a stamped, self-addressed envelope to return the questionnaire, a prenotification letter is sent, a reminder letter is sent with an additional questionnaire in case the original one was misplaced, there is university sponsorship, and there are no sensitive questions (Harrison, Henderson, Alderdice, & Quigley, 2019; Jones, Baxter, & Kanduja, 2013).

To improve the response rate of online surveys, avoid using the word *survey* in the subject line, offer to share results, use a white background for the questionnaire, and keep it short (Harrison et al., 2019; Jones et al., 2013).

The available resources

The availability of resources, or lack thereof, can make the best survey method unrealistic. Resources include not only funding, but also staff, infrastructure to support data

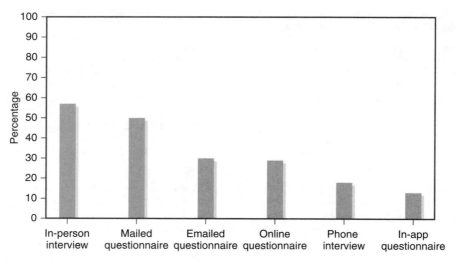

Figure 4-3 Survey method response rates

analysis, access to contact information for the intended audience, and space for in-person interviews, among others.

Contracting with an external agency or firm to conduct the survey can remove most of the resource needs other than funding. For example, a 2018 community assessment survey of older adults conducted by an external firm that entailed a sample of 1,400 people, license to use a proprietary survey template, data collection and analysis using a paper-and-pencil questionnaire, and benchmark comparisons with over 30,000 adults in nearly 200 communities across the country was estimated to cost more than $14,000 (National Research Center, 2019).

The time available to complete the survey

How long the survey takes to complete (CCHD, 2018d) and how much time is available to complete it depend on how much information is needed, the sample size, and the available resources (funding and personnel), and if the survey is being conducted by interview or self-reported questionnaire.

If an interview is used with a large sample and limited resources, it could take months to complete. On the other hand, if the sample is small and there are sufficient resources

(CCHD, 2018d)), or if the questionnaire is self-administered, the survey could be completed in a few weeks.

Special considerations for interviews

If using interviews to collect data, how will they be conducted, in-person or by phone? If in-person, where will the interviews take place? If by phone, does the committee have access to phone numbers? Who will conduct the interviews? How will interviewers be located? Who will train the interviewers? Which type of interview will be conducted: structured, semistructured, or unstructured?

Structured interviews use a verbally administered questionnaire to collect (quantitative) data (Gill, Stewart, Treasure, & Chadwick, 2008). Instead of a respondent filling out the questionnaire form him/herself, an interviewer reads each question and response option to the respondent, the respondent tells the interviewer which response option he/she chooses, and the interviewer records it on the questionnaire. There is no discussion or explanation of the questions or responses.

Semistructured interviews use a set of key questions to collect (qualitative) data (Gill et al., 2008) in the same way questions are used in a focus group script. Similarly, semi-structured interview questions are open-ended, neutral, and understandable and should begin with those that are easy to answer and progress to more difficult or sensitive ones (Gill et al., 2008). The interviews are recorded using a recording device or by written notes, which are transcribed verbatim in preparation for analysis (Parcell & Rafferty, 2017).

Unstructured interviews are not guided by predetermined questions. Rather, they start with a simple opening question and go wherever the conversation leads from there. For example, if the aim of a needs assessment is to determine mental health needs of students on campus, an opening question might be "Please tell me about your past experiences when you met with a counselor." Responses are again recorded and transcribed in preparation for analysis.

By the very nature of their unstructured format, these interviews can last for hours and be difficult to manage. Their use for data collection is usually limited to situations when a substantial depth of information about an issue is necessary or as a starting point when nothing is known about an issue (Gill et al., 2008).

Special considerations for questionnaires:

◆ **Validity and reliability**

Validity and reliability are ways to determine the accuracy of a measurement instrument, such as a questionnaire. Validity is the extent to which an instrument measures what it's supposed to measure. Reliability is the extent to which an instrument consistently measures what it's supposed to measure.

For example, if a bathroom scale is supposed to accurately measure weight, it's a valid instrument if in fact, it does accurately measure weight. It's reliable if it consistently measures accurate weight.

Assessing the extent to which an instrument measures what it purports to measure, that is its validity, is a judgment made based on evidence (Price et al., 2015). Two ways of accomplishing this are to assess the instrument for face validity and content validity.

Face validity is the extent to which an instrument *looks* like it measures what it's intended to measure (face validity, 2020). It's established by having people—experts, the intended audience, and others, make a determination about the relevance of the instrument as it appears to them relative to its purported purpose (Bannigan & Watson, 2009; McLeod, 2013). Because face validity is based on judgment it's not usually assessed through quantitative or statistical analysis (Price et al., 2015).

Content validity is the extent to which an instrument covers the information or subject matter (content) relevant to what it's intended to measure (Bannigan & Watson, 2009; Price et al., 2015). It's established by having an expert panel review the instrument and or by comparing the instrument to those in the literature (Bannigan & Watson, 2009). Content validity, like face validity, is usually not assessed through quantitative means (Price et al., 2015).

As an example, face validity and content validity were used to validate a needs assessment instrument for an African-American college student suicide prevention program. The instrument was assessed by a panel of six experts, which included two subject experts and two college student experts (Bridges et al., 2018).

While there are a number of ways to assess reliability, a commonly used method is test-retest. This entails administering the instrument two separate times to the same group of people who are representative of the intended audience and analyzing the results. Because no test will produce the exact same results even when given repeatedly to the same group of people, the difference between the results from the two tests are analyzed using a statistical procedure to determine the extent of correlation between the two scores (Price et al., 2015). The closer the results are to 1.00 (a perfect correlation, meaning the results are identical) the less of a difference there is, and the greater the reliability. Therefore, an instrument with a reliability coefficient of 0.75 is more reliability than an instrument with a coefficient of 0.47. In general, a test-retest correlation of 0.80 or greater indicates good reliability (Price et al., 2015).

Test-retest reliability was used by the developers of a needs assessment instrument to measure predisposing, enabling and reinforcing factors for a suicide prevention program. The instrument was administered two separate times to the same group of students at a university not involved in the program. The reliability coefficient for the scales measuring the different factors, ranged from 0.73 to 0.97 (Bridges et al., 2018).

◆ *Distribution and collection*

- How will paper questionnaires be distributed?

  If by direct mail, does the committee have access to an updated accurate address list and enough funding for copying and postage?

  If hand delivered, by whom and to where?

  If at community events, which ones draw a large enough crowd from the intended audience?

  If at the health department, how will the intended audience be contacted and asked to pick them up?

- How will paper questionnaires be returned?

  If by mail, is there enough funding for return postage?

  If in person, where and how?

- How will electronic questionnaires be distributed?

  If by email attachment or an emailed link, does the committee have access to accurate email addresses?

  If by social media or posted on the community website, does the intended audience usually access these communication networks?

- Does the intended audience have sufficient computer skills to enable completion of an electronic/online questionnaire?

Task 4—Pilot test.

The importance of pilot testing the questionnaire cannot be overstated. A pilot test is a dry run, a dress rehearsal. It's like a final draft of a term paper your professor reads and hands back with comments and corrections that need to be addressed before the final paper is submitted for a grade. Pilot testing the questionnaire entails having representatives from the intended audience complete the questionnaire and point out any problems they had.

The pilot test identifies the ambiguous, unclear, confusing, irrelevant, and poorly worded questions. It provides information on how long the questionnaire takes to complete and if the instructions are clear.

A pilot test also provides data that can be used to find any potential problems or glitches with data entry or analysis. For example, if responses to open-ended questions are not legible, the instructions for those questions may need to be changed to "please print clearly."

Task 5—Decide how results will be analyzed, distributed, and used.

Data collected from a survey are meaningless unless they are analyzed (tabulated and summarized). For quantitative data this is satisfied by computing descriptive (summary) statistics (at the least means and frequency). Qualitative data are coded or categorized and summarized. (For information on data analysis, consult a statistics or research text.)

Results of the data analysis are interpreted to tease out what they mean, and the actions they suggest. Typically, this is done by a subgroup of planning committee members. The results and interpretations are shared with the entire planning committee to get their input, decide how they'll be used, and plan the next steps (CCHD, 2018d).

Focus Groups. A **focus group** is a guided small-group discussion used to collect qualitative data that cannot be obtained through a survey. For example, opinions about or attitudes toward a health problem, suggestions about how to overcome barriers to a solution,

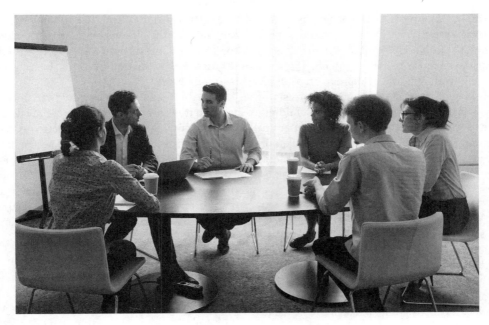

Figure 4-4 Focus group

© Fizkes/Shutterstock

or insight into the cause of a problem. (See **Figure 4-4**.)

A focus group is indicated when action on a problem should be guided by public opinion (CCHD, 2018b). For example, if information is needed about the types of services to provide at school-based health clinics, a focus group is appropriate. However, its use is not restricted to only issues warranting public opinion. It's used to collect qualitative data whenever opinions, feelings, or beliefs are needed.

Conducting a focus group takes planning, people, and resources. Planning begins with clarifying the information needed and developing questions to elicit the information. The people needed to conduct a focus group include:

- A facilitator—This is someone with experience facilitating groups who will lead the group discussion.
- A recorder—This is either someone taking notes during the session or recording the session for later transcription and interpretation.

- A group—These are the people specifically chosen and invited to be part of the group because their input is needed. Ideally, they are from the intended audience or are knowledgeable about the intended audience, are knowledgeable about the problem, or have some other stake in the outcome. A typical focus group is usually 6 to 12 people. To ensure this number attends, it helps to invite a few more people anticipating some will not be able to participate.

The resources needed include a venue and funding. The venue itself should be a known, safe, nonthreatening environment in a location that's convenient to get to, accessible in terms of mass transportation (if applicable), with sufficient parking, and large enough to accommodate the group comfortably.

Deciding on the date, day, and time of the meeting is also important, as these can hamper the participation of the people whose input you want. For example, if you're trying to assemble a group of small-business owners, a meeting early in the morning before regular business hours on Tuesday, Wednesday, or Thursday would be better attended than a meeting in the middle of the day on Monday or Friday. However, if the group consists of stay-at-home parents of school-age children, then a midday meeting would be better. To minimize the chances of poor participation because of logistics, solicit input from members of the intended audience when making these decisions.

Funding is needed because food and beverages are provided during the typical 60- to 90-minute focus group session (CDC, 2018a). In addition, incentives are usually given to the participants at the end of the session in the form of cash or a thank-you gift. Funding may also be needed if an outside consultant is hired to conduct the focus group and analyze the data.

To elicit the information wanted from the focus group, the facilitator follows a script, which helps to control the discussion, keep it on track and focused on the topic. The focus group script has three parts, introduction, questions, and closing.

◆ *Introduction*

The introduction is the first part of the script. It welcomes the participants, introduces everyone, and explains the purpose of the focus group and how the information they share will be collected (by voice recording or written notes) (Boston College, n.d.).

◆ *Key questions*

The second part of the script contains the key questions along with probing and follow-up questions to encourage further comments. These questions are specifically written to prompt discussion. They are open-ended, neutral (don't imply they should be answered one way or another), worded in terms the group will understand, and asked in order from the general to the specific (Boston College, n.d.).

◆ *Closing*

The closing is the last part of the script. It's used at the end of the allotted session time frame to wrap up the meeting, thank participants for their participation and contributions, and explain how the information they provided will be analyzed and shared (Boston College, n.d.). **Figure 4-5** is an example of a focus group script.

If the focus group is audio-recorded, a written transcript is made. If notes are taken, a written summary is made. It helps to have more than one person taking notes or transcribing the audio-recording to avoid bias. The summaries are interpreted to identify response patterns, themes, and new questions and culminate in conclusions (CCHD, 2018b) that are used to inform the planning committee's decisions.

Observation. Observation is a systematic way of collecting data using the senses, usually vision and hearing, about behavior or events where they naturally happen, or to examine the physical condition of a setting (CDC, 2018b; Cohen & Crabtree, 2006). Watching and/or listening allows for documentation of what people are doing while they're doing it rather than relying on people to recall what they did on a questionnaire or during an interview (Paradis, O'Brien, Nimmon, Bandiera, & Martimianakis, 2016). (See **Figure 4-6**.)

Observation is used to collect data about an ongoing situation or process, or how people interact with each other (CDC, 2018b). For example, the way teachers handle a bullying situation on the playground, or the process for following up with clinic patients.

It's used when information about a physical environment is needed (CDC, 2018b), such as the condition of a park, senior center, or lake. It's also used when collecting data directly from the intended audience is not realistic or possible because of their inability or unwillingness (CDC, 2018b). One example of this is how a change in schedule affects people with Alzheimer's disease at an adult day care center.

To collect data through observation:

<u>Determine the focus of the observation.</u>

Clarify exactly what information is needed (CCHD, 2019) from the observation, what behavior can provide the information,

(Part one – Introduction)

Welcome, and thank you all for agreeing to participate in this discussion about how the Any Town Health Department can better serve families caring for those with disabilities. Specifically, we want to know from you which services work, which don't, and which are missing. Once we better understand were our strengths, weaknesses, and missing pieces are, we'll be able to make modification to improve services. This is why we're asking for your input today.

To get started, let me introduce myself. I'm Jenn Dean. I'll be guiding the discussion today. The format we're using is called a focus group. It's called that because it's a discussion or conversation focused on a particular issue. In our case today, the issue is improving health department services for families caring for those with disabilities. I'll guide the discussion by asking a few specific questions for each of you to respond to. There are no right or wrong answers and it's okay not to answer a question, if you don't want to. Feel free to respond to each other's comments, too, just like you would in an ordinary conversation. It's my job to keep things going and to make sure everyone gets a chance to comment. Speaking of comments, they will be voice recorded by James English sitting at the table over there. No one other than James and I hear the recording.

Before we get started, there are two things I want you to know. First, the information you share with use today will be summarized and made into a report. That's why we record the conversation, so we can make sure your comments are summarized correctly. The report will be shared with the health department staff. Secondly, to protect your privacy, the comments you make today will remain confidential. They will not be connected with your name in the report or anywhere else. I hope when you leave here, you'll also respect each other's privacy in the same way. Since there is no way for me to guarantee this, please don't say anything in the group today that you absolutely need to keep private.

Now, going around the room starting on my right, please tell us your name and how long you've been caring for the person with the disability.

Okay, let's get started.

(Part 2 – Questions and discussion)

Transition question: Think back to the first time you used a health department service. Did it meet your expectations?

Key Question 1 – Which of the health department services have you used since?
Follow-up question – Has anyone not used a service since the first time?

Key Question 2 – Which services have you used that worked well?
Follow-up question – What was it that made them work well?

Key Question 3 – Are there services you used that didn't work very well?
Follow-up question – What would have made them better?
Probing question – Does anyone else feel the same way?

Key Question 4 – Are there any services you "wished" were provided?

Key Question 5 – What's the most important recommendation you can make to improve services?

(Part 3 – Closing)

Our time is up. I want to thank everyone again for coming today and for sharing your comments. The information you gave us will be very useful to the health department staff in planning for next year. On behalf of the health department, I have a small gift thank you gift for everyone.

Figure 4-5 Sample focus group script

Data from University of Arizona. (n.d.). Focus group script example. Retrieved February 21, 2020 from http://saem-aiss.arizona.edu/sites/saem-aiss.arizona.edu/files/Focus%20Group%20Template.pdf

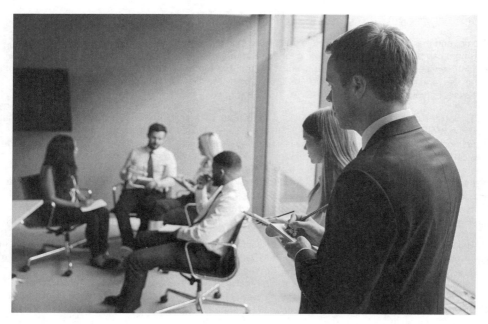

Figure 4-6 Observation
© Monkey Business Images/Shutterstock

and the criteria for determining when the behavior has occurred (Lammers & Badia, 2004). For instance, if the behavioral focus of the observation is texting while driving, the criterion is that it includes texting while stopped at a red light or in bumper-to-bumper traffic, not just when the car is in motion.

Choose the observation type

There are two ways of observing—overtly or covertly. Overt, or participant, observation is when the people being observed know they are being watched and/or the observer interacts with them in some way or is actively involved in what is being observed (Lammers & Badia, 2004). For example, at a farmer's market the participant observer might introduce himself to the vendors, or chat with customers about their purchases and explain what he is doing.

Covert observation, also called nonparticipant observation, is when the observation is made from a distance, without the knowledge of those being watched (CCHD, 2019; Lam-

mers & Badia, 2004). Some examples are standing on a street corner watching how many people drive through an amber light, or sitting in the back of a high school cafeteria watching students interacting with one another. The benefit of covert observation is that people behave naturally when they don't know someone is watching. However, depending on the behavior, covert observation can violate privacy and raise ethical issues (CDC, 2018b).

Design a data recording system

Data collected by observation must be recorded or documented. The three methods used for this are recording sheets, observation guides, and field notes (CDC, 2018b; Taylor-Powell & Steele, 1996).

- *Recording sheets or checklists* are forms (electronic or paper) on which observed behaviors or actions are marked as yes (observed) or no (not observed), or on a rating scale (CDC, 2018b; Taylor-Powell & Steele, 1996). See **Figure 4-7** for an example of a recording sheet.

Dog park observation

1. Day of week: Mon _____, Tues____Wed ____Thur ____Fri____Sat____Sun
2. Time of day: Between 9 a.m.- 12 noon ___, 12 noon – 5 pm,___ 5 pm – 8 p.m. ____
3. Estimated age: <20 _____, 20 – 40 _____, 40 – 60 _____ > 60
4. Gender: male _____ female_____
5. Brought more than one dog: yes _____ (how many _____) no_____
6. Paid attention - watched dog while loose: yes _____ no_____ intermittently _____
7. Corrected dog's inappropriate behavior: yes _____ no _____ n/a _____
8. Picked up dog's feces: yes _____ no _____ n/a_____
9. Properly disposed of dog's feces: yes _____ no_____ n/a

Figure 4-7 Observation recording sheet

Example 1 - Well baby clinic observation guide

Time observation began _____ and ended _____
Date of observation: _____

1. How many adults (parents/guardians) were in the waiting room at the beginning of the observation?____
2. How many children were in the waiting room at the beginning of the observation? _____
3. Were there toys, books or TV to keep children occupied while waiting? Yes _____ No____
4. Were adults generally attentive to their children? Yes _____ No _____ Somewhat____
5. Were adults kept apprised of delays in the appointment schedule? Yes _____ No ___N/A___
6. Were staff accommodating when making follow-up appointments? Yes ___ No ___
7. Did staff treat the adults respectfully? Yes _____ No _____ Sometimes_____
8. Did the adults treat the staff respectfully? Yes _____ No_____ Sometimes_____

Example 2 - Well baby clinic observation guide

Time observation began _____ and ended _____
Date of observation: _____

Record actions observed and comments heard related to the following:

1. Keeping children occupied while waiting.
2. Handling of late appointment arrivals.
3. Process for follow-up appointments.
4. Interactions between staff and adults.

Figure 4-8 Observation guide

- *Observation guides* are forms (electronic or paper) that list the interactions, processes, or behaviors to be observed with space for comments (CDC, 2018b). They can be structured and contain closed-ended questions, or unstructured with open-ended questions. (See **Figure 4-8** for an example of an observation guide.)

- *Field notes are the* least structured way to record observation data. These are descriptions or narratives the observer enters into a notebook or voice records. They don't provide guidance on the behavior to observe but rather contain whatever the observer deems important at the time (CDC, 2018b; Taylor-Powell & Steele, 1996). (See **Figure 4-9** for an example of field notes.)

Date: March 24, 2020

Location: Station Park walking path

Time: 2 – 3:30 p.m.

When I arrived at the park there was only one older couple walking on the path. I began walking and caught up with them, introduced myself and asked them how often they use the park. The woman said they try to walk at least three times a week but that it gets difficult once school is out. The path is overrun with kids on dirt bikes who fool around. The man said the path is a mess during the summer because of geese droppings. He wished there was some way to control the geese, and the kids so older people could use the path all year. I asked if they had ever mentioned any of this to the Recreation Committee. They hadn't.

Figure 4-9 Field notes

Select observation sites

Identify sites or locations where the intended audience engages in the behavior to be observed (CDC, 2018b). Depending on the sites and the focus of the observation, permission may be needed to use them.

Select and train observers

Collecting data through observation is time intensive and takes significant person-power in the form of observers. Observers can be anyone interested in the project who has time and the desire to be trained on how to collect and record the data. For example, volunteers, stakeholders, representatives from the intended audience, and interns from a local university all make good observers.

Schedule the observations

Since there is no way to guarantee when people will do what you want to observe, an observation schedule is developed. In addition to the locale of the observation, it includes the following:

◆ **Duration of each observation session**

How long each observation session lasts depends on the behavior being observed and the site. For example, observing students on the playground during recess can only last as long as they are outside on the playground, but observations of people speeding through amber traffic lights can last for hours.

◆ **Frequency of observations**

How often the observations take place depends on the behavior, who is being observed, and where. For example, observing client–staff interactions at a well-baby clinic can only occur as frequently as the clinic is open, but observing client–staff interaction in an emergency room can happen around the clock, every day.

Step 5—Determine How the Data will Be Analyzed and by Whom

The aim of this step is to make the data, usable. Raw data, the answers on the actual questionnaires or the notes from a semistructured interview, must be analyzed before it can be used.

Answer the following questions to complete this step:

◆ **What type of data analysis will be done?**

Because the type of analysis that can be done depends on the type of data collected, it's wise to seek guidance from the person who will do the analysis *before* the data are collected.

In general, quantitative data from a needs assessment are analyzed statistically for the following:

Frequencies a count of the number of times a response was chosen

Percentages an expression representing a part of the whole

Mean the average of the scores or values for a particular variable

Median the midpoint of the scores or response values that is at the center of the distribution of the scores—with half the response scores above and half below

Mode the most commonly chosen response, score, or value for a particular question

Minimum and maximum values (range) the highest and lowest values or scores for any question response (Grand Canyon University, n.d. a)

Qualitative data analysis is commonly done by completing the following five steps:

Reading and rereading the data, writing down impressions, looking for meaning, and determining which pieces of data are useful.

Focusing the analysis on the answers to a particular question or topic, or examining the data as it relates to a potential target group.

Categorizing or coding the data to identify themes or patterns of ideas, concepts, behaviors, interactions, phrases and so forth.

Identifying patterns or response themes, identifying relationships between themes, and attempting to find explanations from the data.

Interpreting the data and explaining findings after themes, patterns, and relationships are identified. List key ideas gleaned from the data, create diagrams, or use models to explain the findings (Grand Canyon University, n.d.).

◆ *Who will analyze the data?*

Data analysis is a skill unto itself and best done by a statistician or someone with expertise in analyzing, interpreting, and putting the results into a useful format. If no one at the agency or organization leading the needs assessment has this expertise, partnering with a university for this step is a feasible solution. Ideally, the person responsible for data analysis is identified prior to developing or revising the questionnaire. This is done to ensure the data analysis will produce usable results.

Step 6—Prioritize the Needs

With the data analyzed, this last step looks at the needs it revealed. Because there are usually more needs identified than can realistically be addressed, they are prioritized. This enables decisions to be made about which needs can be addressed, and how. The process used to figure this out is prioritization.

The following questions guide the prioritization process:

◆ *Who will prioritize the needs?*

The first question to ask in the prioritization process is who will be involved in the process. Ideally, it should be all stakeholders—those affected by or concerned about the issues, community members, and people with expertise in health fields related to the issues (CCHD, 2018c). It can be all the members of the planning committee or a select group that serves as a prioritization committee. Regardless of the group's title, it should include people affected by the issues revealed in the needs assessment, organizations/agencies/institutions that serve them, those who will be responsible for implementing any programs that are planned to address the priority needs, community members interested or concerned about the issues, and funders (foundations, state agencies, and local funding sources) (CCHD, 2018c).

◆ *What criteria will be used to prioritize the needs?*

With the question about who will prioritize the needs answered, the next question is on what basis or criteria will they prioritize the needs? While the prioritization criteria may vary somewhat depending on the issues being prioritized, the following are common criteria that can serve as a starting point for brainstorming and discussion:

- Seriousness of the need/issue
- Cost and/or return on investment of addressing the need/issue
- Availability of solutions to meet the need/issue
- Impact on the community of the unmet need/issue
- Availability of resources (staff, time, money, equipment) to address the need/issue

Table 4-5 Example of prioritization criteria definition chart

Criterion	Definition
Seriousness of the issue	The extent to which the unmet need is life threatening and/or debilitating.
Size of the problem	The rate of occurrence in the target audience.
Solutions are available	The availability of effective interventions to address the problem that are applicable to the target audience.
Resources are available	The extent to which there are enough resources (personnel, time, equipment, space) available to implement an intervention.
Costliness	The benefits outweigh the costs; addressing the problem costs less than not.
Reasonable time frame for addressing the need	Results of an intervention are possible within 12 months of implementation.

Data from Kuthy, R.A., Siegal, M.D., & Phipps, K. (2003) Assessing oral health needs: ASTDD seven step model. [PDF] Retrieved May 22, 2019 from https://www.astdd.org/docs/step-6.pdf

JM Associates (2017) Prioritization toolkit. Retrieved November 6, 2018 from https://www.jmassociates.com/wp-content/uploads/2017/07/Prioritization-Toolkit-JM-Associates-2017.pdf

- Size of problem or the number of people affected by this unmet need
- Urgency for meeting this need or addressing the issue
- Reasonable time frame for addressing the need
- Amenable

(Association for Community Health Improvement, 2017; National Association of County and City Health Officials [NACCHO], n.d.)

Once a list of possible criteria is identified, it should be defined to avoid variation in how the criteria are interpreted. For example, what does "Reasonable time frame for addressing the need" mean? Is it 3 weeks, 6 months, 5 years? A reasonable amount of time for a stakeholder may be too long for a funder. Making sure everyone agrees on what the criteria mean is critical to the prioritization outcomes. This discussion may reveal that two criterion are essentially the same or that an important criterion people *thought* was

included wasn't. To ensure the finalized criteria are consistently used, it helps to develop a criteria definition chart. (See **Table 4-5** for an example of a prioritization criteria definition chart.)

◆ *How will the needs be prioritized?*

The question of how the needs will be prioritize refers to the method or process the group will use to arrive at the priority needs. There are several that can be used, some more complex than others, but there is no one best method. They all work in a similar way in that each need/issue is viewed through the lens of the predetermined criteria with the goal of identifying the priority issues. (See **Table 4-6**.)

Multivoting and nominal group technique (NGT) are good to use for group decision making because they allow for equal say among all participants regardless of their position in an agency or the community (NACCHO, n.d.). They typically work best with between 6 and 20 participants and a moderator.

Table 4-6 Prioritization methods

Method	Description
Multivoting technique	Decide on priorities by agreeing or disagreeing in group discussions and continuing process/rounds until a final list is developed.
Strategy lists	Determine if the health needs are of "high or low importance" by placing an emphasis on problems whose solutions have maximum impact, with the possibility of limited resources.
Nominal group technique	Rate health problems from 1 to 10 through group discussion.
Hanlon method	List those health needs viewed as priorities based on baseline data, numeric values, and feasibility factors
Prioritization matrix	Weigh and rank multiple criteria for prioritization with numeric values to determine health needs with high importance.

Data from National Association of County and City Health Officials [NACCHO], (n.d.) Guide to prioritization techniques. Retrieved November 5, 2018 from https://www.naccho.org/uploads/downloadable-resources/Gudie-to-Prioritization-Techniques.pdf

The following NACCHO (n.d.) multivoting and NGT processes have been adapted for application to the results of a needs assessment.

- **Distribute and review forms**

  The moderator distributes and reviews the forms or materials specifically developed for prioritizing the needs assessment results, including a priority grid with a list of the issues/needs (see **Table 4-7**) and a prioritization criteria and definition chart.

- **Conduct round one priority assessment.**

  Participants are given time to read the materials and complete their initial assessment of the need/issue against the prioritization criteria. Once they have completed this and determined which issues best meet the criteria, they place a check mark in the box on the priority grid next to the issue under Round 1. Limiting the number of issues each person can vote

Table 4-7 Priority voting grid

Health issue identified in needs assessment	Round 1 Vote	Round 2 Vote	Round 3 Vote
Physical inactivity			
Texting while driving			
Childhood obesity			
Depression			
Access to health care			
Neighborhood safety			

Table 4-8 Round one voting results of six-person committee

Health issue identified in needs assessment	Round 1 Rank	Round 2 Rank	Round 3 Rank
Physical inactivity	5 votes		
Texting while driving	4 votes		
Childhood obesity	2 votes		
Depression	2 votes		
Access to health care	5 votes		
Neighborhood safety	6 votes		

for as a priority prevents someone from voting for all the issues. For example, if there are six issues to be prioritized, each person has four votes, if there are 11 issues, each person has seven votes.

- **Conduct round <u>one</u> vote**
  In round-robin order, each participant tells the group which issues they are voting for. These results are recorded with a check mark on an enlarged ranking grid on a flip chart or projected computer image in the front of the room. (See **Table 4-8**.)

- **Revise priority list**
  Once all the Round 1 votes are recorded, the issues that did not generate any votes or those with votes less than half the number of people voting, are eliminated from the list.

- **Conduct round <u>two</u> vote**
  In round two, the number of votes allotted to each participant is equal to half the number of issues remaining on the list. For example, if six issues remain, then each participant can vote for the three they view as the highest priorities. (See **Table 4-9**.)

Table 4-9 Round two voting results

Health issue identified in needs assessment	Round 1 Vote	Round 2 Vote	Round 3 Vote
Physical inactivity	5 votes	3 votes	
Texting while driving	4 votes	2 votes	
Childhood obesity	2 votes		
Depression	2 votes		
Access to health care	5 votes	3 votes	
Neighborhood safety	6 votes	4 votes	

Table 4-10 Round three voting results

Health issue identified in needs assessment	Round 1 Rank	Round 2 Rank	Round 3 Rank
Physical inactivity	5 votes	3 votes	1 vote
Texting while driving	4 votes	2 votes	
Childhood obesity	2 votes		
Depression	2 votes		
Access to health care	5 votes	3 votes	2 votes
Neighborhood safety	6 votes	4 votes	3 votes

- **Revise priority list**
  The issues that did not generate any votes or those with votes less than half of the number of people voting, are eliminated from the list.
- **Conduct round three vote**
  Once again, participants are allotted the number of votes equal to half the number of remaining issues on the list. For example, if there are two remaining issues, then each participant can vote for one issue.
- **Identify priorities**
  The priority issues are those that receive votes from at least half the participants. For example, if six people are voting, the priority issues are those with at least three votes. (See **Table 4-10**.)

Assessing Need Using Community-Based Participatory Research Principles

Community-based participatory research (CBPR) is a partnership approach to research that includes community members, organizational representatives, and partnering agencies and recognizes them as equals contributing expertise and sharing in all aspects of decision making (Israel et al., 2005). It supports the principle of "planning with people" and engaging the community. Using this approach to assess need ensures that the results are what the community believes it needs rather than what the committee conducting the assessment believes it needs (Horn, McCracken, Dino, & Brayboy, 2008).

CBPR is based on the following nine principles:

PRINCIPLE 1—Recognize community as a unit of identity.

Recognize the community as a unit of identity, and acknowledge the connectedness people have with others through the sharing of common values and norms, interests, and commitments to meeting each other's needs. Communities defined in this way may be geographically bound such as a neighborhood, or geographically dispersed but connected by a common identity or interest (Israel, Eng, Schultz, & Parker, 2012) such as members of a church, synagogue, or mosque or students on a campus. This principle guides the definition of "community," which is central to the needs assessment process.

PRINCIPLE 2—Build on strengths and resources within the community.

Address health concerns by building on the existing strengths, resources, and assets in the community such as individual skills, social networks, and organizations (Israel et al., 2012). This principle addresses the use of a community's assets to guide development of a program to solve its health problems.

PRINCIPLE 3—Facilitate a collaborative, equitable partnership.

Share decision making and control over all aspects of the research (needs assessment) process, such as defining the problem, collecting and interpreting data, disseminating findings, and applying the results to address community issues with all partners (Israel et al., 2012). This principle guides the collaborative relationships between all members of the planning committee, including community members, throughout all stages of the planning process.

PRINCIPLE 4—Foster colearning and capacity building among all partners.

Support the exchange of skills, knowledge, and capacity among all partners involved, and recognize the diverse skills, expertise, and different perspectives and experiences they each bring to the partnership (Israel et al., 2012). This principle addresses the importance of interactions among planning committee members in all stages of the planning process for them to value what each brings to the process.

PRINCIPLE 5—Achieve a balance between generating knowledge and programs (interventions).

Balance the contribution research makes to the knowledge base with the contribution it makes when translated into programs and policies that benefit all partners (Israel et al., 2012). This principle reinforces that while the results from the needs assessment and evaluation stages add to the general body of knowledge of public health, the information is equally as important as the foundation for program and policy development.

PRINCIPLE 6—Focus on health problems, recognizing the multiple determinants of health.

Consider the multiple determinants of health and disease, including biomedical, social, economic, cultural, and physical environmental factors and the need for an interdisciplinary team of community partners to address the local health problems (Israel et al., 2012). This principle addresses the need to acknowledge there are multiple reasons why problems exist in a community and that representatives from many sectors of the community are needed to develop solutions for its problems.

PRINCIPLE 7—Involve systems development.

Address systems development, in which the system such as a partnership draws on the abilities of each partner to engage in a cyclical process that includes all the stages of the planning process, including community assessment, problem definition, data collection and analysis, data interpretation, dissemination, determination of program, and policy strategies (Israel et al., 2012). This principle addresses the development of a means to enable all planning committee partners to share their abilities in all phases of the planning process.

PRINCIPLE 8—Disseminate program results to all partners.

Share all program results with partners and communities involved in ways that are understandable, respectful, and useful (Israel et al., 2012). This principle addresses the distribution of results from the needs assessment and evaluation phases to planning committee partners and the community at large.

PRINCIPLE 9—Commit to long-term process and sustainability.

Establish trust among the partners necessary to successfully carry out CBPR endeavors to achieve the aims of addressing multiple determinants of health by recognizing it requires a long-term process that includes partner commitment to sustainability of the partnership relationship (Israel et al., 2012). This principle addresses the need to develop trusting relationships among the people involved in all stages of the planning process, which is needed for their long-term commitment to the process.

Chapter Summary

A needs assessment is a collaborative endeavor undertaken by stakeholders to identify a community's health problems, which serves as the basis for developing programs to address the problems and improve the community's health.

Planning in Practice Chapter Activity

A needs assessment eliminates guessing, assuming, or supposing what the health needs of a community are by providing data that identify its actual needs.

In small groups—

1. Brainstorm what you assume, guess, or suppose a health needs assessment on a campus would reveal about the issues of importance to the students.
2. Identify who should be on a planning committee to conduct a campus needs assessment.
3. Select a data collection method for conducting the needs assessment, and provide a rationale as to why it was chosen.

Read the article below and answer the questions that follow.

Article: *Ask and ye shall plan: A health needs assessment of a university population* (Katz, Davis, & Findlay, 2002)

Article link: https://www.ncbi.nlm.nih.gov/pmc/articles/PMC6979890/

(Note: Download the PDF to access the full article.)

Article Questions

1. Why was the needs assessment conducted?
2. Who was on the needs assessment planning committee?
3. Was the composition of the planning committee in keeping with the principles of community-based participatory research?
4. What data collection method was used?
5. What health program issues/topics were identified by the majority of students?
6. What health issues did the authors anticipate would be of interest that were not?
7. What issues were of interest to a small percent of students that the authors did not anticipate?
8. How closely did your brainstorming issues match with the health issues of interest revealed in this needs assessment?

9. Who did your group identify for the needs assessment committee that was not on the committee discussed in the article?

10. How did your data collection method differ from the one used by the authors?

References

Ake, T., Diehr, S., Ruffalo, L., Farias, E., Fitzgerald, A., Good, S. D., … Meurer, L. N. (2018). Needs assessment for creating a patient-centered, community-engaged health program for homeless pregnant women. *Journal of Patient Centered Research and Reviews*, 5(1), 36–44. DOI: 10.17294/2330-0698.1591. Retrieved October 3, 2018, from https://digitalrepository.aurorahealthcare .org/cgi/viewcontent.cgi?article=1591&context =jpcrr

American Heart Association. (n.d.). About us. Retrieved May 13, 2019, from https://www.heart.org/en/about-us

American Public Health Association [APHA]. (2018). Topics & issues. Retrieved September 28, 2018, from https:// www.apha.org/topics-and-issues

Anselma, M., Chinapaw, M. J. M., & Altenburg, T. M. (2018). Determinants of child health behaviors in a disadvantaged area from a community perspective: A participatory needs assessment. *International Journal of Environmental Research and Public Health*, 15(4), 644–658. DOI: 10.3390/ijerph15040644. Retrieved October 3, 2018, from https://www.ncbi.nlm.nih.gov/ pmc/articles/PMc5923686/pdf/ijerph-15-00644.pdf

Association for Community Health Improvement. (2017). Step 5: Prioritizing community health issues. Retrieved November 5, 2018, from http://www.healthycommu nities.org/Education/toolkit/files/step5-select-priority .shtml#.W-BzUOJOnIU

Bannigan, K., & Watson, R. (2009). Reliability and validity in a nutshell. *Journal of Clinical Nursing*, 18, 3237–3243. https://doi.org/10.1111/j.1365-2702.2009.029 39.x. Retrieved May 27, 2020, from https://onlinelibrary .wiley.com/doi/pdf/10.1111/j.1365-2702.2009 .02939.x

Bopp, M., Fallon, E. A., Bolton, D. J., Kaczynski, A. T., Lukwago, S., & Brooks, A. (2012). Conducting a Hispanic health needs assessment in rural Kansas: Building the foundation for community action. *Evaluation and Program Planning* 35(4), 453–460. DOI: 10.1016/j.evalprogplan.2012.02.002. Retrieved October 22, 2018, from https://www.ncbi.nlm.nih.gov/ pubmed/22417673

Boston College Office of Vice President of Student Affairs. (n.d.). Focus group protocol. Retrieved February 21, 2020, from https://www.bc.edu/content/dam/files/ offices/vpsa/pdf/assessment/focus.pdf

Boynton, P., & Greenhalgh, T. (2004). Hands on guide to questionnaire research: Selecting designing, and developing your questionnaire. *British Medical Journal*, 328, 1312–1315. DOI: https://doi.org/10.1136/ bmj.328.7451.1312. Retrieved November 12, 2018, from https://www.researchgate.net/publication/8540549 _Hands-on_guide_to_questionnaire_research_ Selecting_designing_and_developing_your_ques tionnaire

Bridges, L. S., Sharma, M., Sung, J. H., Bennett, R., Buxbaum, S. G., & Reese-Smith, J. (2018). Using the PRECEDE-PROCEED model for an online peer-to-peer suicide prevention and awareness for depression intervention among African-American college students: Experimental study. *Health Promotion Perspectives*, 8(1), 15–24. https://doi.org/10.15171/hpp.2018.02

Center for Community Health and Development (CCHD). (2018a). Chapter 3, Section 4: Collecting information about the problem. University of Kansas. Retrieved November 7, 2018 from the Community Tool Box https://ctb.ku.edu/en/table-of-contents/assessment/ assessing-community-needs-and-resources/collect -information/main

Center for Community Health and Development (CCHD). (2018b). Chapter 3, Section 4: Conducting focus groups. University of Kansas. Retrieved November 14, 2018 from the Community Tool Box https://ctb .ku.edu/en/table-of-contents/assessment/assessing -community-needs-and-resources/conduct-focus -groups/main

Center for Community Health and Development (CCHD). (2018c). Chapter 3, Section 23: Developing and using criteria and processes to set priorities. University of Kansas. Retrieved November 7, 2018 from the Community Tool Box: https://ctb.ku.edu/en/table-of-contents /assessment/assessing-community-needs-and -resources/criteria-and-processes-to-set-priorities/ main

Center for Community Health and Development (CCHD). (2018d). Chapter 3, Section 7: Conducting needs assessment surveys. University of Kansas. Retrieved May 14, 2019 from the Community Tool Box https://ctb.ku.edu/ en/table-of-contents/assessment/assessing-communi ty-needs-and-resources/conducting-needs-assess ment-surveys/main

Center for Community Health and Development (CCHD). (2018e). Chapter 3, Section 13: Conducting surveys. University of Kansas retrieved May 15, 2019 from the Community Tool Box https://ctb.ku.edu/en/table-of

-contents/assessment/assessing-community-needs-and
-resources/conduct-surveys/main

Center for Community Health and Development (CCHD), (2019), Chapter 37, Section 3: Data collection: Designing an observational system. University of Kansas retrieved February 22, 2020 from the Community Tool Box https://ctb.ku.edu/en/table-of-contents/evaluate/evaluate-community-interventions/design-observational-system/main

Centers for Disease Control and Prevention, Adolescent and School Health (CDC). (2018a). Data collection methods for program evaluation: Focus groups. Retrieved May 14, 2019, from https://www.cdc.gov/healthyyouth/evaluation/index.htm

Centers for Disease Control and Prevention, Adolescent and School Health (CDC). (2018b). Data collection methods for program evaluation: Observation. Retrieved February 22, 2020, from https://www.cdc.gov/healthyyouth/evaluation/pdf/brief16.pdf

Centers for Disease Control and Prevention, National Center for Health Statistics (CDC). (2019). National health interview survey. Retrieved May 16, 2019, from https://www.cdc.gov/nchs/nhis/about_nhis.htm

Check J., & Schutt, R. K. (2012). Survey research. In J. Check & R. K. Schutt (Eds.), *Research methods in education* (pp. 159–185). Thousand Oaks, CA: Sage Publications.

Chudoba, B. (2020). How much time are respondents willing to spend on your survey? Retrieved April 26, 2020, from https://www.surveymonkey.com

Cohen, D., & Crabtree, B. (2006). Qualitative research guidelines project, Robert Wood Johnson Foundation. Retrieved February 22, 2020, from, http://www.qualres.org/index.html

Clark, R.E., Weinreb, L., Flahive, J.A., & Seifert, R.W. (2019). Homelessness contributes to pregnancy complications. *Health Affairs*, 38(1), 139–146. https://doi.org/10.1377/hlthaff.2018.05156

Cutts, D. B., Coleman, S., Black, M. M., Chilton, M. M., Cook, J. T., Ettinger de Cuba, S., ... Frank, D. A. (2015). Homelessness during pregnancy: A unique, time-dependent risk factor of birth outcomes. *Maternal Child Health Journal*, 19(6), 1276–1283. doi: 10.1007/s10995-014-1633-6. Retrieved October 8, 2018, from https://link.springer.com/article/10.1007%2Fs10995-014-1633-6

Edwards, P. J., Roberts, I., Clarke, M. J., Diguiseppi, C., Wentz, R., Kwan, I., Cooper, R., ... Pratap, S. (2009). Methods to increase response to postal and electronic questionnaires. *Cochrane Database*, 8(3), MR000008.

face validity. (2020). *APA dictionary of psychology*. Retrieved May 27, 2020, from https://dictionary.apa.org/face-validity

Gill, P., Stewart, K., Treasure, E., & Chadwick, B. (2008). Methods of data collection in qualitative research: Interviews and focus groups. *British Dental Journal*, 204, 290–295. DOI: 10.1038/bdj.2008.192. Retrieved

February 21, 2020, from https://www.nature.com/articles/bdj.2008.192

Grand Canyon University, Center for Center for Innovation in Research and Teaching. (n.d. a), Analyzing quantitative data. Retrieved October 31, 2018, from https://cirt.gcu.edu/research/developmentresources/research_ready/quantresearch/analyze_data

Harrison, S., Henderson, J., Alderdice, F., & Quigley, M. A. (2019). Methods to increase response rates to a population-based maternity survey: A comparison of two pilot studies. *BMC Medical Research Methodology*, 19(1), 65. DOI: https://doi.org/10.1186/s12874-019-0702-3. Retrieved May 15, 2019. from https://bmcmedresmethodol.biomedcentral.com/articles/10.1186/s12874-019-0702-3#Sec2

Holbrook, A. (2008). Forced choice. In P. Lavrakas (Ed.), *Encyclopedia of survey research methods Thousand Oaks*, CA: Sage Publications. Retrieved October 27, 2020 from https://methods.sagepub.com/reference/encyclopedia-of-survey-research-methods/n193.xml

Horn, K., McCracken, L., Dino, G., & Brayboy, M. (2008). Applying community based participatory research principles to the development of a smoking cessation program for American Indian teens: "Telling our story." *Health Education and Behavior*, 35(1), 44–69. https://doi.org/10.1177/1090198105285372

Israel, B.A., Parker, E.A., Rowe, A., Salvatore, A., Minkler, M.,Lopez,J.,Butz,A.,...Halstead,S.(2005). Community-based participatory research: Lessons learned from the Centers for Children's Environmental Health and Disease Prevention Research. *Environmental Health Perspectives*, 113(10), 1463–1471. DOI: https://dx.doi.org/10.1289%2Fehp.7675

Israel, B.A, Eng, E., Schulz A.J, & Parker E.A. (2012). *Methods for community-based participatory research for health*. San Francisco, CA:Jossey-Bass,

Jones, T. L., Baxter, M. A. J., & Khanduja, V. (2013). A quick guide to survey research. *Annals of the Royal College of Surgeons of England*, 95, 5–7. doi: 10.1308/003588413x13511609956372. Retrieved May 16, 2019, from https://www.ncbi.nlm.nih.gov/pubmed/23317709

Kabir, S. M. S. (2016). Methods of data collection. In *Basic guidelines for research: An introductory approach for all disciplines* (pp. 201–275). Chittagong: Book Zone Publications. Retrieved February 17, 2020, from https://www.researchgate.net/publication/325846997_METHODS_OF_DATA_COLLECTION

Kaufman, R. (1988) Needs assessment: A menu. *Educational Technology*, 28(7), 21–23. doi https://www.jstor.org/stable/44426572

Keeter, S., Hatley, N., Kennedy, C., & Lau, A. (2017). What low response rates mean for telephone surveys. Retrieved May 16, 2019, from https://www.pewresearch.org/methods/2017/05/15/what-low-response-rates-mean-for-telephone-surveys/

Lammers, W. J., & Badia, P. (2004). *Fundamentals of behavioral research*. Retrieved February 23, 2020, from https://

uca.edu/psychology/fundamentals-of-behavioral-research-textbook/

Lindermann, N. (2018). What's the average survey response rate? Retrieved May 15, 2019, from https://surveyanyplace.com/average-survey-response-rate/

Little, M., Shah, R., Vermeulen, M. J., Gorman, A., Dzendoletas, D., & Ray, J. G. (2005). Adverse perinatal outcomes associated with homelessness and substance use in pregnancy. *Canadian Medical Association Journal, 173*(6), 615–618. doi: 10.1503/ cmaj.050406. Retrieved October 8, 2018, from https://www.ncbi.nlm.nih.gov/pmc/articles/PMC1197161/pdf/20050913s00023p615.pdf

Losby, J., & Wetmore, A. (2012). CDC coffee break: Using Likert scales in evaluation survey work. Retrieved November 12, 2018, from https://www.cdc.gov/dhdsp/pubs/docs/cb_february_14_2012.pdf

March of Dimes. (n.d.). About us. Retrieved May 13, 2019, from https://www.marchofdimes.org/mission/about-us.aspx

Marken, S. (2018). Still listening: The state of telephone surveys. Retrieved May 16, 2019, from https://news.gallup.com/opinion/methodology/225143/listening-state-telephone-surveys.aspx)

McCawley, P. (2009). Methods for conducting an educational needs assessment. University of Idaho Extension. Retrieved October 29, 2018, from https://www.cals.uidaho.edu/edcomm/pdf/bul/bul0870.pdf

McLeod, S. A. (2013). What is the meaning of validity in research? Retrieved May 27, 2020, from https://www.simplypsychology.org/validity.html

McLeod, S. A. (2018). Questionnaire. Retrieved November 12, 2018, from https://www.simplypsychology.org/questionnaires.html

National Association of County and City Health Officials [NACCHO]. (n.d.). Guide to prioritization techniques. Retrieved November 5, 2018, from https://www.naccho.org/uploads/downloadable-resources/Gudie-to-Prioritization-Techniques.pdf

National Research Center. (2019). Community assessment survey for older adults. Retrieved February 19, 2020, from https://www.n-r-c.com/2018-pricing-community-assessment-survey-older-adults/

New South Wales (NSW), Department of Education, Evaluation Hub. (2019). Data types strengths and limitations. Retrieved February 19, 2020, from https://education.nsw.gov.au/teaching-and-learning/professional-learning/evaluation-resource-hub/turning-data-into-evidence/data-types-strengths-and-limitations#Quantitative0

Paradis, E., O'Brian, B., Nimmon, L., Bandiera, G., & Martimianakis, M. A. (2016). Design: Selection of data collection methods. *Journal of Graduate Medical Education, 8*(2), 263–264. https://dx.doi.org/10.4300%2FJGME-D-16-00098.1

Parcell, E. S., & Rafferty, K. A. (2017). Interviews, recording and transcribing. In M. Allen (Ed.), *The SAGE encyclopedia of communication research methods*. Thousand Oaks, CA: Sage Publications. https://dx.doi.org/10.4135/9781483381411.n275

Pew Research Center. (2020). Questionnaire design. Retrieved April 26, 2020, from https://www.pewresearch.org/methods/u-s-survey-research/questionnaire-design/

Porter, B. (2019). Tips and tricks to improve survey response rates. Retrieved May 16, 2019, from https://www.surveymonkey.com/curiosity/improve-survey-response-rate/

Price, P. C., Jhangiani, R. S., & Chiang, I. A. (2015). *Research methods in psychology*. Retrieved May 20, 2019, from https://opentextbc.ca/researchmethods/

Survey Monkey. (2020). What is a Likert scale? Retrieved February 26, 2020, from https://www.surveymonkey.com/mp/likert-scale/

Taylor-Powell, E., & Steele, S. (1996). Collecting evaluation data: Direct observation. Retrieved February 23, 2020, from https://learningstore.extension.wisc.edu/products/collecting-evaluation-data-direct-observation-p1144?_pos=1&_sid=8ee2364c5&_ss=r

Watkins, R., West Meiers, M., & Visser, Y. L. (2012). A guide to assessing needs: Essential tools for collecting information, making decisions, and achieving development results. World Bank. Retrieved October 1, 2018, from https://openknowledge.worldbank.org/handle/10986/2231

CHAPTER 5

Planning

STUDENT LEARNING OUTCOMES

After reading this chapter, the student will be able to:

- Write a mission statement, goals, and objectives.
- Assess readability level.
- Explain different types of objectives.
- Develop strategies and actions.
- Create a logic model.
- Prepare a basic budget.
- Write a rationale.

Introduction

Planning the program is the second stage of the program planning process. It's in this stage that the program plan is created—the detailed written proposal for solving the problems and addressing the unmet needs identified in the needs assessment.

The heart and soul of a program plan are its mission, goals, and objectives. They're based on the needs assessment and serve as guideposts for every decision made about how the program will solve the problems and meet the needs.

The program mission is the big, broad overarching result to be accomplished that will meet the needs or solve the problem. The goals are how the mission will be accomplished.

The objectives are the specific actions that will enable the goals to be accomplished, which will enable the mission to be accomplished. They are all connected.

Think of these in terms of an umbrella—the mission is like the canopy or fabric part of the umbrella. It's the big, overarching part of the umbrella that meets the need of keeping you dry. Goals are like the ribs of the umbrella. They support the canopy so it can do its job of keeping you dry. Without the support of the ribs, the canopy doesn't work. Objectives are like the stretchers. They support the ribs that support the canopy. So, without the stretchers, the ribs don't stay up, and without them, the canopy doesn't work. (See **Figure 5-1**.) Think back to the last time you tried to use a broken umbrella in the rain. Did it work? (See **Figure 5-2**.)

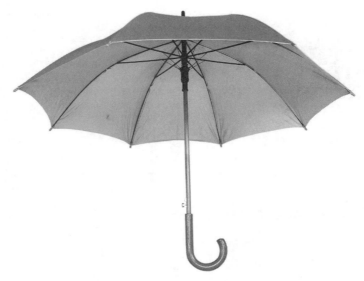

Figure 5-1 Mission, goals, and objectives umbrella
© Jantima14/Shutterstock

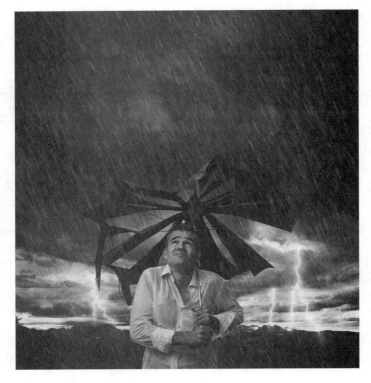

Figure 5-2 Broken umbrella in the rain
© Stock-Asso/Shutterstock

Develop Mission Statement, Goals, and Objectives

Before work begins on the tasks of developing the program mission, goals, and objectives, it's essential for the planning committee to review the priority health issue. While this may seem redundant, it ensures that everyone is on the same page in terms of what the program will address. In addition, it's critically important for all planning committee members to have a basic understanding of the priority health issue before they undertake these tasks.

Develop Mission Statement

A mission statement is just that—a one-sentence statement. It includes the name or title of the program, the health issue it addresses, the general means by which it addresses the health issue, and what it aims to accomplish (Koenig, 2013). It's clear, concise, and focused, preferably 20 words or less (Topnonprofits, n.d.) and written at a seventh- to eighth-grade reading level because this is the reading level of about half (48 percent) of the U.S. adult population (National Center for Education Statistics, 2013).

A simple, commonly used method for assessing readability and approximating corresponding grade level is the SMOG readability method (McLaughlin, 1969). (Note: SMOG is *not* an acronym but rather refers to the developer's birthplace, London.) To assess written material using SMOG:

1. Identify 10 consecutive sentences at the beginning of the material, 10 in the middle, and 10 at the end.
2. Count all the words in the 30 sentences that have three or more syllables, even if the same word is used over and over.
3. Add the number of polysyllabic words from all the sentences.

Table 5-1 SMOG conversion chart

Total number of polysyllabic words	Approximate reading grade level
1–6	5
7–12	6
13–20	7
21–30	8
31–42	9
43–56	10
57–72	11
73–90	12
91–110	13
111–132	14
133–156	15
157–182	16
183–210	17
211–240	18

Reproduced from: The SMOG readability formula. (n.d.). Retrieved from https://readabilityformulas.com/smog-readability-formula.php

4. Use the SMOG Conversion Chart in **Table 5-1** to estimate the reading level of the material based on the number of polysyllabic words counted.

As an example: The first 30 sentences of this chapter have a total of 58 polysyllabic words. According to the SMOG Conversion Chart, this equates to an 11th-grade reading level.

Reading level can also be assessed by using the reading level function in a word processing program or a free online readability analyzer. The ones listed next produce a SMOG grade level for individual sentences, such as a mission statement. They include

https://www.online-utility.org/english/readability_test_and_improve.jsp

https://www.webfx.com/tools/
read-able/
https://datayze.com/readability
-analyzer

Because readability grade level is an approximation, it's best to assess the statements or documents with more than one tool. For example, use the readability function in a word processing program as well as one of the online analyzers.

Components of a Mission Statement

A good way to start writing a mission statement is to answer the following question:

Who, will do what, how?

Who? Refers to the name or title of the program.

This is important because it conveys the topic, generates interest, and gives some information about its content or focus (Hairston & Keene, 2003). Following are a few examples:

New Vitality is a health and wellness program for seniors 65 and older (Atlantic Health Systems, 2020).

Healthy Living is a wellness program (Mayo Clinic, 2020).

Rock on Café improves the nutritional quality of school lunches (Johnston, Denniston, Morgan, & Bordeau, 2009).

Following are some suggestions for generating a good program name or title (Leahy, 1992):

– Write a title that begins with *Who, What, When, Where, How,* or *Why.*
– Write a title with a wording that ends in *ing.*
– Think of a familiar saying, song, movie, or book and change a word.

In addition, there are online resources for generating titles. One is Portent's content generator (www.portent.com) another is Tweak Your Biz (www.tweakyourbiz.com). While neither is specific to public health, they are good places to start brainstorming a title. There are also a myriad of sites that offer free

health slogans and taglines that may trigger an appropriate title.

Will do what?– Refers to the intended outcomes.

Use the results of the needs assessment as the basis for answering this question: What broad change does the program aim to accomplish relative to the problem or unmet need?

For example, if a needs assessment of high school athletes uncovered a problem with concussions, what will a program to address this aim to do? Will it minimize brain injury risk, improve safety of high school sports, reduce sport-related head injuries, or prevent concussion, specifically? This is a key question to answer because what the program aims to do drives "how" it will do it.

How? Refers to the means by which the outcomes will be accomplished.

The first task in determining how the health problem will be addressed is to search the professional literature. This is done to find out what others have done to address the issue and to find out how effective they were. Once this information is gathered, the planning committee can begin brainstorming the feasibility of how the program outcomes might be accomplished.

Continuing with the health issue of concussion in high school athletes, let's assume the planning committee decides that the program intends to minimize concussion risk. How might this be achieved? The literature search identified three ways: disseminate information about concussion prevention (Centers for Disease Control and Prevention [CDC], 2017), change policies (The Shipley School, n.d.), and concussion management training (Holtz et al., 2014). With this information, the planning committee can decide which of these is a feasible approach to minimize concussion risk in their community.

Once the planning committee answers the three questions—who, will do what, how—it can develop the mission statement. As an example, the three questions were used to dissect the following 17-word mission statement of the Utah Department of Health's Immunization Program which is to:

– improve the health of Utah's citizens through vaccinations to reduce illness, disability, and death from vaccine-preventable infections (Utah Department of Health, 2010).

Who? The Utah Department of Health Immunization Program

Will do **What**? Improve health and reduce illness disability and death from vaccine preventable infections

How? Through vaccination

While there is no one perfect format for a mission statement, using the following is a good way to start:

The mission of the (*Who?*) _____ is to (*do What?*)_____ , (*How?*)_____

Following are examples of mission statements that answer the questions of *who, what,* and *how,* and meet the criteria of brevity, clarity, and readability:

- The mission of the San Antonio Walks! program is to: increase the number of people getting physically active through walking (Fit City San Antonio, n.d.). *10 words, eighth-grade reading level (SMOG).*
- The mission of the Bicycle Recycling and Processing Program (BRPP) is to: promote sustainability on campus by breaking down barriers to cycling (Environmental Center, n.d.). *10 words, eighth-grade reading level (SMOG).*
- The mission of Charity:water is to: bring clean and safe *drinking water* to people in developing nations (Charity:water, 2020). *11 words, eighth-grade reading level (SMOG)*

Develop Goals

Once the mission statement is complete, goals are developed. Goals help establish the overall direction and focus of a program, define what it expects to achieve, and serve as the basis for developing objectives and strategies (CDC, 2008).

Following are five steps for developing goals:

Step 1—Brainstorm outcomes that support what the program will do to address the health problem.

Step 2—Identify the specific changes or results expected from the program.

Step 3—State the expected results in positive terms or as a reduction in the health problem.

The following verbs indicate a positive change or result: increase, grow, boost, enlarge, build up, add, raise, expand, widen, improve, strengthen, replace, redesign, adjust, convert, substitute, switch, trade, exchange, transform, alter, remodel, remake, modify, revamp, amend, develop, improve, enhance, perfect.

These verbs indicate a reduction in a health problem: reduce, decrease, eliminate, lessen, shrink, cut, minimize.

Step 4—Identify the intended audience in which the change or results are expected to occur.

Step 5—Write a goal that meets the following criteria:

– Identifies the intended audience.
– Describes the expected result/change in one declarative sentence
– Contains plain language that most people are likely to understand.
– Contains as few words as possible without unnecessary detail.
– Presents the expected change or results in positive terms or as a reduction in a health problem.
– Provides a focus for strategies and objectives for achieving the expected results (CDC, 2008).

Following are examples of short, concise goal statements written in plain language that identify the intended audience, the health issue, what the program will do to address the issue, and provide a focus for developing objectives and strategies.

- Improve influenza rates in those age 65 and older.
- Reduce substance use among university students.
- Decrease childhood obesity.

Although goals are written in a variety of formats, use the following one as a starting point:

The goal of the _____ program is to_____ (do what?) in, among, for _____ (intended audience).

Develop Objectives, Strategies, and Actions

While goals are broad statements that indicate the expected results, objectives are specific statements that describe the expected changes in behavior, skills, attitudes, policies, or other factors that will lead to the result. Given the diversity of factors associated with accom-

plishing a goal, at least two, and usually more, objectives are needed. Just as you can't have a team with only one player, you can't have a goal with only one objective. Objectives work together, just as teammates do, to make the desired result happen.

Objectives are critical to a program because they not only describe what is expected to happen, they also provide the criteria for evaluating whether it did happen. Going back to the team analogy, in order to know which team won a game depends on the criteria for winning. For example, in football or baseball, winning means getting the higher score, but in cross country or swimming, the team with the lowest score wins (they are the fastest runners or swimmers.) Objectives set the "criteria for winning," accomplishing the goal, getting the job done. They tell you what you must do and are the basis for the evaluation, which tells you if you did it. (See **Figure 5-3**.)

While the process of writing objectives may seem daunting and laborious, taking

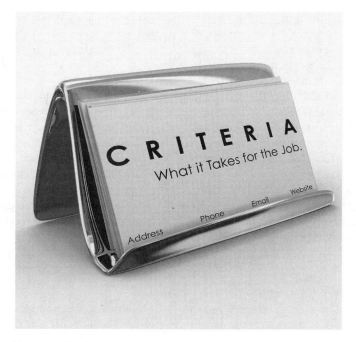

Figure 5-3 Objectives set criteria

the time to develop them is time well spent given their contribution to the success of a program. To expedite this, answering the following five questions will generate the information needed to write them.

1. *What will change?*
   This is the behavior, knowledge, attitude, skill, policy, or other factor that will change and contribute to meeting the goal. This is the "it" in the following questions.

2. *In what way will "it" change?*
   This is the type of change expected, defined in measurable terms by an action verb. For example: "it" will be increased, decreased, expanded, eliminated, prevented. (See **Table 5-2**.)

3. *By how much will "it" change?*
   This is the extent or degree to which "it" is expected to change as a result of the program when compared to conditions at baseline (before the program). The extent

Table 5-2 Action verbs

achieve	audit	compile	critique
acquire	authorize	complete	debate
activate	award	compose	decide
adapt	balance	compute	decrease
add	become	condense	defend
adjust	build	confer	define
administer	calculate	confirm	delegate
adopt	calibrate	connect	deliberate
advocate	carry out	consolidate	deliver
allocate	change	construct	demonstrate
allot	charge	consult	describe
analyze	check	contribute	design
answer	choose	control	designate
apply	circulate	convert	detect
appoint	classify	convey	determine
appraise	clean up	coordinate	develop
approve	climb	copy	devise
arrange	close	correct	diagnose
assemble	collaborate	correlate	diagram
assess	collect	counsel	differentiate
assign	combine	count	direct
assist	compare	create	disburse

(continues)

Table 5-2 Action verbs   *(continued)*

discharge	entertain	grasp	itemize
discipline	enumerate	group	join
disconnect	erect	guard	judge
discover	establish	guide	justify
discuss	estimate	hire	label
dismantle	evaluate	identify	launch
dispatch	examine	illustrate	lead
display	exchange	implement	locate
disseminate	execute	import	make
distinguish	exhibit	improve	manage
distribute	experiment	inaugurate	manipulate
diversify	explain	increase	manufacture
draft	extract	indicate	map
drive	fabricate	inform	match
dump	facilitate	initiate	maximize
duplicate	fashion	innovate	measure
edit	forecast	inspect	mediate
elaborate	forge	inspire	mend
elicit	form	install	mix
eliminate	formulate	institute	modernize
employ	fortify	instruct	modify
empower	foster	interpret	monitor
encourage	frame	interview	motivate
endorse	garner	invent	move
engineer	gather	inventory	multiply
enlist	gauge	investigate	name
enrich	generate	invigorate	negotiate
ensure	govern	involve	notify
enter	grade	issue	observe

(continues)

Table 5-2 Action verbs *(continued)*

obtain	propose	report	sort
open	provoke	represent	spearhead
operate	purchase	reproduce	specify
optimize	push	rescue	stack
order	quantify	research	start
organize	question	resolve	stimulate
originate	raise	respond	store
outline	rank	restore	strengthen
overhaul	rate	restructure	structure
oversee	rebuild	retrieve	study
package	recall	revamp	submit
perform	recite	review	succeed in
permit	recommend	revise	summarize
persuade	reconcile	revive	supply
pick up	record	revolutionize	survey
plan	reduce	reward	sustain
post	refer	salvage	synthesize
predict	refine	scan	systematize
prepare	reform	schedule	tabulate
prescribe	refresh	score	teach
present	register	screen	tend
preserve	regulate	search	test
prevent	reinforce	select	trace
procure	reiterate	send	trade
produce	reject	serve	train
program	release	service	transfer
promote	repair	shape	transform
prove	replace	solicit	turn around
provide	reply	solve	tutor

(continues)

Table 5-2 Action verbs   *(continued)*

update	verify		
use	weigh		
usher	write		
validate			

Reproduced from Lee, M. (n.d.). Active verbs for goal and objective statements. Retrieved January 28, 2019, from http://www.sbccd.org/~/media/Files/SBCCD/District/Research/Program%20Review/ActiveVerbs GandO.pdf

of change is expressed in numeric, quantifiable terms so it can be measured or calculated, for example, percent, counts, inches, pounds, hours, visits, admissions, to name a few. Because these are the criteria that will be used to evaluate the program and determine its success (or not), make sure it's realistic, attainable, and established using baseline data from the needs assessment or other data reflective of conditions *before* the program.

Setting the expectations for change too high is setting yourself up for failure, too low and the program may not have enough of an impact to solve the problem. However, surpassing an objective set too low is better than falling short of reaching an objective set too high. Like Goldilocks and the three bears, you're looking for that middle ground of "just right." To help in this quest, search the literature to find out the extent of change similar programs accomplished; review similar ones previously implemented (if there are any) in your department, agency, or community to determine past results; and solicit input from planning committee members who have experience working with the intended audience or the problem to get their insights.

4. *In whom or for whom will "it" change?*
   This is the intended program audience.
5. *By when will "it" change?*
   This is the specific time frame within which the change is expected to occur.

A variety of formats or sentence structures are used to write objectives. All are acceptable just as long as the statement contains the necessary information.

Following are two examples:

1. By the end of the fall semester 2024, alcohol-related incidents will decrease by 15% among

   (by when)   (what will change, in what way)   (how much)

XZY University students.

   (in whom)

2. Alcohol-related incidences will decrease by 15% among XYZ University undergraduates by

(what will change, in what way)   (how much)   (in whom)

the end of the fall 2024 semester.

(by when)

Types of Objectives

Objectives fall into one of two categories, process or outcome.

Process objectives focus on the tasks or activities associated with the processes or procedures of planning and implementing the program (National Cancer Institute, n.d.) organizationally, administratively, or logistically.

Following are examples of process objectives:

- Schedule flu and pneumonia vaccinations 2 hours per week at the Anytown senior center between October 1 and December 1 for those over 65.
- Install data management software for use by all 37 healthcare providers in the clinic by the second month of the 12-month project (Health Foundation of South Florida, n.d.).
- Develop a procedure to contact at least 10 obstetricians within the first month of the project to generate support for the program (National Cancer Institute, n.d.).

Outcome objectives focus on the changes expected as a result of the program at different lengths of time after it ends, that is, in the short, intermediate, or long term.

Short-term outcome objectives are the changes expected in the individual or personal attributes of the program participants, for example, knowledge, skills, beliefs immediately following the program or shortly thereafter.

Intermediate or medium-term outcome objectives are changes expected to occur in behavior results from the short-term changes.

Long-term outcome objectives, also called impact objectives, are those changes expected a year or more after the program ends. These reflect the broader program impact on mortality, morbidity, quality of life, or policies (Salabarria-Pena, Apt, & Walsh, 2007; The Pell Institute, 2019). Meeting these objectives is dependent on first meeting the short- and intermediate-term objectives.

For example, objectives for a neighborhood improvement program might be:

(Short-term objective) Homeowners will recognize that removing debris from around the outside of homes deters vermin.

(Intermediate objective) Twenty homeowners will remove the debris from their front and back yards within 6 months.

(Impact objective) Within 12 months, the number of vermin complaints made to the health department by neighborhood residents will decrease by 20 percent.

Smart Objectives. All objectives, regardless of whether they are process or outcome, are written as SMART objectives—specific, measurable, achievable, relevant, and time-bound. They clearly state who is going to do what, by when, and to what extent. They are doable with available resources and support accomplishing the goal. Objectives with these characteristics provide a structure for developing program strategies and actions, communicating the intended impact of the program to stakeholders, describing how goals will be met and progress toward them monitored and evaluated (Minnesota Department of Health, n.d.).

The following are CDC (2018a) guidelines for writing SMART objectives:

*An objective is **Specific** if it:*
Clearly states what is expected to change and in whom.

Contains only one action verb. (See **Table 5-2**.)

Does not contain vague verbs that are difficult to define and measure, such as appreciate, understand, know.

*An objective is **Measurable** if it:*
States the extent of change expected in quantifiable, countable terms—how much change is expected. For example, participants will lose 5 pounds.

*An objective is **Achievable** if it:*
Only includes changes or outcomes that are attainable, possible, or doable for the intended audience.

Only includes changes or outcomes that are attainable, possible, or doable with the available resources.

*An objective is **Relevant** if it:*
Contributes to achieving the goal and addressing the problem.

*An objective is **Timebound** if it:*
States how long it will take for the change to happen.

Use the "Write SMART Chart" in **Table 5-3** to write SMART objectives. Following is an example of a SMART objective written using the SMART Chart:

Paper recycling will increase 25 percent among residents of Bay Island Senior Complex within 6 months.

Table 5-3 Write SMART chart

Question	Answer (example)
What is expected to change and in whom?	Recycling in residents at Bay Island Senior Living Complex.
In what way will it change?	It will increase
How much will it change?	25 percent
Is it doable for the intended audience? Is it doable with the available resources?	Yes Yes
Does it contribute to achieving the goal and addressing the problem?	Yes
By when will it happen?	Within 6 months

Develop Strategies and Actions

While objectives specify *what* will change, strategies provide the directions for *how* the change will come about, and actions are the *ways* or activities that will lead to the change. Without realizing it, you use strategies and actions every day to meet your mission's goals and objectives. For example, if your mission is to have a career in public health, a goal that supports your mission is to earn a degree in a public health discipline. An objective that will enable you to meet your goal is to earn grades of C or better in your courses each semester. A strategy that will enable the goal and objective to be met is to attend class prepared. An action that will contribute to attending class prepared is reading the assigned pages in this textbook. Said another way—by reading this textbook (action), you'll be prepared for class (strategy), which will contribute to passing the course (objective), enabling you to earn a degree in a public health discipline (goal), leading to a career in public health (mission).

Following are six steps for developing program strategies and actions:

Step 1—Convene a meeting.
Meet with representatives from the intended audience, planning committee members, and others who are interested in or are in a position to contribute to solving the problem (Center for Community Health Development [CCHD], 2018a). Keep the size of the group manageable (10–12) to enable everyone's voice/opinion to be heard. Remember, program planning is a group effort. Giving the group a name—for example, strategy development committee or strategy group—can go a long way in making the members feel part of the program planning process and promote ownership of the program.

Step 2—Review the program mission, goals, and objectives.
To ensure everyone is on the same page, review the mission, goals, and objectives and clarify how each is related to the other before brainstorming strategies.

Step 3—Discuss each objective separately.
Discuss each objective individually and identify the behavior that's the focus of change or the behavior that's at the root of the problem. For example, if the objective is to increase flu vaccination of students living on-campus before winter break by 20 percent over the previous year, the problem behavior is that students are not getting vaccinated.

Step 4—Brainstorm strategies.
Ask members of the strategy group with the expertise to conduct a literature search to locate evidence-based programs that address the health issue and/or problem behavior. Ideally these programs will have the same intended audience as the program being planned.

An evidence-based program is one that has proof or evidence that it's effective. The evidence comes from research, both quantitative and qualitative, but sometimes from case reports and expert opinion (Titler et al., 2001). Its effectiveness is confirmed by publication of research and evaluation findings in peer-reviewed journals in the professional literature or reports (Brownson, Fielding, & Maylahn, 2009).

Evidence-based programs have the following common characteristics:

- Decision making based on the best available peer-reviewed evidence.
- Systematic use of data and information systems, that is, a mechanism for collecting, storing, and processing data (Zwass, n.d.).
- A program planning framework.
- Community input in assessing needs and decision making.
- A comprehensive evaluation.
- Dissemination of key findings to stakeholders and decision makers (Brownson et al., 2009).

While the public health literature is ripe with evidence-based programs to address almost any issue, doing a literature search to track them down can be time consuming. Fortunately, there are many resources available to make searching easier. **Table 5-4** contains a partial list of these resources.

The results of the literature search are shared with the strategy group. The applicability of the strategies found are discussed and other possible strategies brainstormed. To assist in brainstorming, **Table 5-5** contains a list of words for describing strategies.

Keep in mind that using multiple strategies to address an issue is more effective

Table 5-4 Evidence-based public health resources

Resource	Website	Annotation
Healthy People 2020	https://www.healthypeople.gov/2020/tools-resources/Evidence-Based-Resources	A database of evidence-based interventions searchable by strength of evidence, population, and intervention type.
Evidence-based Practices Resource Center-Substance Abuse and Mental Health Services Administration	https://www.samhsa.gov/ebp-resource-center	An online registry of evidence-based substance use and mental health interventions.
Innovations Exchange—Agency for Health Care Research and Quality	https://innovations.ahrq.gov/	A forum that provides the opportunity to share, learn about, and ultimately adopt evidence-based innovations in a range of healthcare settings and populations and searchable profiles of successful and attempted service delivery and policy innovations, tools, articles, and reports.
Research-tested Intervention Programs—National Cancer Institute	https://rtips.cancer.gov/rtips/index.do	A database of cancer control interventions and materials of research-tested resources.
The Community Preventive Services Taskforce Findings	https://www.thecommunityguide.org/task-force-findings	A collection of evidence-based findings and recommendations to improve health and prevent disease within states, communities, organizations, businesses, health systems, and schools.

Data from: NIH. (n.d.). Evidence based practices and programs. Retrieved January 2, 2019, from https://prevention.nih.gov/research-priorities/dissemination-implementation-research/evidence-based-practices-programs

Table 5-5 Descriptive words for strategies

administer	deliver	investigate	research
build	develop	manage	resource
celebrate	document	partner	review
collaborate	evaluate	promote	stimulate
consult	expand	provide	streamline
contract	extend	raise	subsidize
contribute	fund	recognize	support
coordinate	identify	report	survey

Reproduced from Department of Health & Human Services, State Government of Victoria, Australia (2010). Tip sheet: Municipal public health and wellbeing planning: Writing measurable objectives. Retrieved May 28, 2019, from http://www.health.vic.gov.au/regions/southern/downloads/Tip-sheet-writing-measurable-objectives.pdf than using one. For example, combining incentives for employee smoking cessation *and* policies for a smoke-free worksite is more effective than one or the other by itself (CDC, 2015).

> *Step 5—List the suggested strategies.*
> For each objective, the strategy group lists the potential strategies that came out of the brainstorming session and assesses them against the following criteria for a "good strategy."

A good strategy:

- Advances the mission by enabling the goals and objectives to be met.
  How does the potential strategy contribute to the goal and objectives?

- Aligns with available and emerging resources.
  What resources are needed to implement the strategy and are they available?
  If the necessary resources are not readily available, are there potential resource pools that can be explored?

- Deters opposition to the program and attracts allies.
  What is the potential for resistance to the strategy?
  Are there ways to minimize potential resistance?
  Who might be resistant?
  Is the strategy controversial; inconsistent with the cultural norms, expectations, or beliefs of the intended audience; or likely to cause opposition?
  Who would likely support the program?

- Reaches those affected by the problem who would benefit from the program.
  How does the strategy reach all of those affected by the problem?
  Does the strategy prevent the problem, reduce the problem, or reduce the risks (CCHD, 2018b)?

Another way to determine if a strategy is suitable for use is the PEARL test. This

entails considering each strategy in light of the following five criteria and eliminating or revising any that do not meet all five of them.

Propriety: The strategy is consistent with public health principles and essential services.

Economics: The strategy is financially possible and makes economic sense to implement.

Acceptability: The strategy is something the stakeholders and community will accept.

Resources: The strategy is supported by partner organizations with staff, expertise, and/or space needed for implementation.

Legality: The strategy is legal to implement (National Association of County and City Health Officials [NACCHO], 2013).

> *Step 6—Develop theory-based actions.*
> Once the planning committee agrees on the strategies, the next step is to develop actions—the specific activities or ways that will be used to implement the strategies to meet the objectives. Keep in mind that actions developed with a theoretical base are more likely to lead to accomplishing the goal than those developed without one (Bluethmann, Bartholomew, Murphy, & Vernon, 2016; Glanz & Bishop, 2010; Prestwich, Webb, & Connor, 2015; Tebb et al., 2016).

To develop theory-based actions:

1. Identify the problem behavior.
2. Brainstorm possible reasons or causes for the problem behavior.
3. Identify a theory that explains the reasons for the problem behavior. (See Chapter 2, Theories.)

4. Do a literature review for evidence of the theory's effectiveness in changing the problem behavior (Prestwich et al., 2015).
5. Use the theory constructs to develop actions for the strategy.

As an example, the goal for a community in Colorado was to better manage natural resources by restoring watershed areas, improving floodplain planning, and improving land use planning. A *strategy* chosen to accomplish this was to use green infrastructure to lessen storm water runoff. The *action* taken was the installation of rain gardens in the local park (Colorado Resiliency Resource Center, 2018). So, which theory might have guided this action?

A behavior contributing to the problem in this community was that permeable (soil) surfaces were being covered with impermeable materials, such as concrete and asphalt. One possible reason for this might have been industrial construction, which required paved streets and parking lots. Another might have been homeowner lack of knowledge about options for driveways, patios and walkways other than concrete and asphalt.

The possible reasons for the behavior are at the community and personal levels, which suggests an Ecological Model as the theoretical basis for developing actions. At the community level, the action was the installation of a rain garden in the local park. At the personal level, the actions might have focused on informing homeowners of permeable paving options for projects around their homes.

Going back to the flu example used previously, if the goal of the program is to decrease the incidence of flu on the campus of Any University by implementing a comprehensive flu vaccination program, and an objective is to increase flu vaccination rates of residential students before winter break by 20 percent over the previous year, then the problem behavior is that students are not getting vaccinated. Brainstorming reasons why students don't get vaccinated might reveal that students believe because they're young and healthy, and they therefore are not susceptible, or they have a fear of needles, or maybe they don't believe the vaccine works, or they think they'll get the flu from the vaccine (National Foundation for Infectious Disease, 2017). Which theory would explain the behavior? The Health Belief Model would explain that students don't believe they're susceptible to the flu because they are young and healthy their fear of needles and of getting the flu from the vaccine are perceived barriers to vaccination, and they don't see a benefit in getting the vaccine because they don't believe it works.

One strategy for addressing the problem behavior based on the Health Belief Model might be raising awareness of the different ways the flu vaccine is given. The action would be developing materials explaining that the vaccine is available by injection or a mist sprayed into the nose, thus eliminating the barrier of fear of needles.

Another strategy might be researching the incidence of flu among residential students on college campuses. The action would be writing an article for the student newspaper about the risk of students living in residence halls contracting flu to change perceived susceptibility.

Manage the Program

A major aspect of program planning is managing the many different "moving" parts that must work together for the program to be successful. Keeping things organized and everything and everyone on track can be challenging. Two tools that minimize disruption in program flow are a logic model and timeline.

Create a Logic Model

A logic model is a one-page road map, flowchart, or visual representation of how all the components of a program are related and work together (CDC, n.d., 2018b). It's a

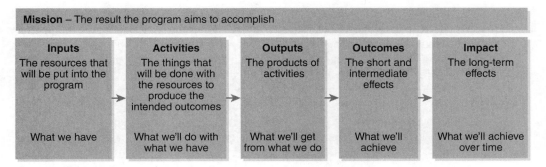

Figure 5-4 Sample logic model template

picture of the program that's worth a thousand words.

Logic models are used because they increase the likelihood of a program's success. They do this by:

- conveying the program's mission and expected results.
- describing the activities/actions expected to lead to the desired results.
- serving as a reference point for everyone involved in the program.
- involving stakeholders, enhancing the possibility of funding commitments and program ownership (CDC, n.d.).

There are no hard and fast rules for which program components to include in a logic model. However, the following are typically included:

- Mission—the result the program aims to accomplish.
- Inputs—the resources that will be used to implement program activities such as funding sources, staff, community partnerships.
- Activities—the things or events the program will do with the resources such as train community workers, develop a surveillance system, create a website.
- Outputs—the physical products or abilities that result from the activities such as

trained community workers, surveillance system in place, website online.

- Outcomes—the changes that occur in the people or conditions as a result of the outputs and activities in the short and intermediate terms. Impact—the long-term results of the activities and outputs such as decreased heart disease rates, elimination of infant mortality disparities, reduction of DWI-related fatalities (CCHD, 2020a; CDC, n.d., 2018b).

To understand how these components fit together, see **Figure 5-4** for an example of a logic model template.

Developing a logic model takes "logic," thinking through how one part of the program is connected to and works with another. In this way, the model explains why the program ought to work by showing how the activities correspond to the problem (CCHD, 2020a). It also takes the following six steps:

Step 1—Clarify the reason for developing the logic model.

For example, is the reason to talk with stakeholders about the program or to develop an evaluation plan?

Step 2—Convene a meeting with stakeholders, including the planning committee members, community members, representatives of the intended audience, partners, and any others with a stake in program outcomes.

Step 3—Determine if the focus of the logic model is a single program, a multiyear program or all the health department or agency's programs.

Step 4—Use the program objectives or goals as the basis for developing the logic model, setting priorities and clarify expectations.

Step 5—Search the literature to find out what others have done or are doing related to the program in terms of lessons learned, resources needed; discuss assumptions being made.

Step 6—Develop a set of linked activities and outcomes moving from "left-to-right" starting with the activities moving to outcomes

that the activities would produce, using "if, then" statements. For example, complete the following statement: If we have (input) and (input), we can (activity) and (activity), which will then result in (outcome) and (outcome).

If we have funding and participating animal control departments, we can inform our animal healthcare partners of the new animal health practice guidelines in public health and sponsor training for the providers, which will then increase the number of animal health providers who are aware of new animal health practice guidelines and who follow the new guidelines (CDC, n.d.).

Table 5-6 is an example of a logic model for an asthma program.

Table 5-6 Example of asthma program logic model

Program mission: To reduce the incidence of childhood asthma through a healthy homes initiative

| Inputs | Activities | Outputs | Outcomes | | |
			Short-Term	Intermediate	Impact
Health department staff	Educate families about environmental asthma triggers in home	Education sessions at schools Asthma management materials	Increase use of mattress and pillow covers Improvement in asthma knowledge, information and behavior scores	Reduction in number of days without symptoms after 3 months Reduction in asthma triggers	Long term improvement in family Reduction in ER visits and hospital admissions after 12 months.
Home inspectors	Conduct visual assessments for mold, moisture, and roaches.	Number of visual assessments for mold, moisture, and roaches.	Improvement in household cleaning skills	Reduction in asthma triggers	Reduction in mold, moisture, and roaches after 12 months
Rental property owners	Schedule regular pest management treatments	Number of pest management treatments completed	Reduction in roach infestation	Reduction in asthma triggers	Reduction in ER visits and hospital admissions after 12 months.

Data from: Murphy, A., Jacobs, D., Kawecki, C., Anderson, J., Jr., Akoto, J., Ashley, P., Nusum, M., & Pinzer, E. (2012, July). *The healthy homes program guidance manual.* Washington, DC: U.S. Department of Housing and Urban Development. Retrieved July 5, 2017, from https://portal.hud.gov/hudportal/HUD?src=/program_offices/healthy_homes/HHPGM

Create a Timeline

A timeline is a visual representation of the tasks associated with the program strategies and activities in the order they *will* happen. A commonly used timeline format for managing programs and projects is a Gantt chart.

The Gantt chart displays the program tasks, their start and completion dates, duration, and overlaps between them. It's helpful for communicating the program to stakeholders because they can see where they fit in the whole scheme of things and for monitoring progress and identifying tasks that are causing slowdowns (Boston University School of Public Health, 2016). See **Table 5-7** for an example of a Gantt chart.

To develop a Gantt chart:

1. Determine the program start and end dates.
2. List the major tasks to be completed.
3. Determine the start and end dates for each task.
4. Determine the order in which the tasks need to be completed.
5. Fill in the information using an Excel spreadsheet or a table in Word.

Develop a Budget

A budget is the only way to determine the cost of implementing a proposed program and if the resources needed are in line with the resources available. It's a tool for accurately showing what can and can't be done, for making decisions, and avoiding surprises after the program is in place (CCHD, 2020b).

Budgets have two parts, income and expenses. Income is funding that the program

Table 5-7 Sample Gantt chart for campus flu vaccination program

Task	9/1–9/15	9/16–9/30	10/1–10/15	10/16–10/30	11/01–11/15	11/16–11/30	12/1–12/15	12/16–12/30	1/1–1/15
Conduct focus groups	X								
Conduct online survey	X								
Analyze data		X							
Develop social media announcements			X						
Post social media announcements				X	X				
Implement vaccination sessions					X	X			
Conduct outcome evaluation							X		
Analyze evaluation results								X	
Write evaluation report									X

expects to generate for example, from grants, sale of items, or registration fees.

Expenses are the costs associated with implementing the program. They are of two types, direct and indirect. Direct expenses are those exclusively tied to a specific activity or program (National Institutes of Health [NIH], 2019). For example, direct expenses for a campus flu vaccination program would be the cost of the vaccine, syringes, alcohol swabs, adhesive bandages, and gloves (for the nurses administering the vaccine). Equipment, materials, supplies, and statistical and evaluation consultants needed exclusively for the specific program are other examples of direct expenses.

Indirect expenses are costs that support the overall organization that's implementing the program. While these are necessary for the program, they are not exclusive to it. They are expenses shared among all the programs the organization supports (NIH, 2019), for example, facility rent, heat, phones, insurance, and security guards. The expense to the program for indirect costs is proportional to the extent of program use. For example, if the program needs 50 percent of the office space, then its indirect cost for rent would be half the amount of the rent. For the hypothetical campus flu vaccination program, indirect costs would be health center staff salaries, phones, electricity, and any other resources that are shared by both the flu vaccination program and the other programs offered by the health center.

To get started, identify the direct expenses for each activity item such as:

– speaker fees.
– consultant fees (statistician, evaluator).
– materials specific to the program.
– transportation or travel expenses for staff, consultant, or speaker.
– program specific equipment.
– program/activity personnel salaries and benefits.

Once the direct costs for each activity item are determined, add the cost of each item across the activities. The sum is the amount needed for that item on the budget. For example, if three activities have material costs of $150, $400, and $1,200 each, the direct material cost for the program is $1,750.

List the direct expenses for the program in general, for example, program director salary and benefits, marketing and advertising, and evaluation consultants—which are typically underbudgeted. A rule of thumb is to budget between 15 and 20 percent of the total budget for evaluation (Corporation for National and Community Service, n.d.).

Table 5-8 is an example of a simple program budget.

Writing a Rationale

Once the program is planned, it's a good time to write a rationale. A rationale is a written document that clearly presents the reasoning behind a program. It's used to "sell" a program to people who have some vested interest in the problem or population the program addresses. These are the people who might control the finances, connections, permissions, dissemination pipelines, policy changes, visibility, staff, and any other needs of the program, in addition to representatives of the intended audience. A well-written rationale enables these important people to "see" how the proposed program tackles the problem.

A rationale is **not a description of** the program, but rather **a justification for** the program. It answers the question, "Why?"

For example, a son says, "Dad, I need the car keys." Dad responds, "Why?" The son replies, "I'm the designated driver tonight." The father didn't ask his son to describe what he was going to do with the keys, only *why* he needed them.

While there is no one right format or template for writing a rationale, all good rationales

Table 5-8 Sample budget for 300 person worksite exercise program

Category	Item	Subtotal	Total
Direct Costs			
Salary/benefits	Part-time (20 hrs/wk) wellness director Part-time personal trainer (20 hrs/wk)	$40,000 25,000	$65,000
Supplies	Brown bag lunches for "walk and talk" series	200	200
Printing	Fliers, posters, and recipe book	350	350
Materials	Exercise DVD and literature Walking/exercise logbooks	300 250	550
Equipment	Pedometers Treadmills Spin bikes	300 10,000 1,500	11,800
Incentives	Gift cards Gym membership reimbursement	500 1,000	1,500
Consultant	Evaluation specialist	15,000	14,300
Total Expenses			93,680
Income			
Promo items	Brown bag lunches—recipe book	200	200
Misc	Insurance reimbursement	36,000	36,000
Total Income			36,200
Total program cost			57,480

Data from: CDC, National Healthy Worksite. (2012). Worksite health: Sample budget. Retrieved March 9, 2020, from https://www.cdc.gov/workplacehealthpromotion/tools-resources/pdfs/NHWP_WH101_Implementation_Only_TAG508_1.pdf

are short (one page, if possible), concise, and well written and contain the following information:

– A program title and the names of the people or organization proposing the program.
– The problem the proposed program addresses.
– The existence of the problem within the intended audience, supported by data.
– A brief description of the proposed program.
– Reasons why the proposed program will succeed in addressing the problem compared to similar successful programs.

- The societal impact or benefits of solving the problem with the proposed program.
- The organization's strength or ability to address the problem with the proposed program.
- Reference list.

Imagine a rationale as a seven-layer cake (see **Figure 5-5**).

● Layer 1—What's the program title, and who developed it?

The top layer of a rationale is the title of the proposed program. Keep in mind that the title is important because it conveys the program topic, generates interest, and gives some information about its content or focus (Hairston & Keene, 2003).

● Layer 2—What problem does the program address?

The second layer introduces the health problem. In no more than two paragraphs, it describes the problem, explains why it's a

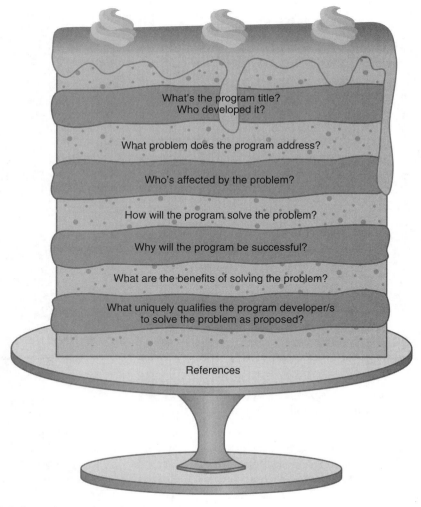

What's the program title?
Who developed it?

What problem does the program address?

Who's affected by the problem?

How will the program solve the problem?

Why will the program be successful?

What are the benefits of solving the problem?

What uniquely qualifies the program developer/s to solve the problem as proposed?

References

Figure 5-5 Seven-layer cake rationale

problem, tells why it should be addressed, and includes the data to back up the claims.

- Layer 3—Who is affected by the problem?

This layer is one paragraph that explains the problem in the intended audience and its negative consequences, and includes supporting data. Keep in mind that the aim of the rationale is to make a case for the proposed program to address the problem (McKenzie, Neiger, & Thackeray, 2017).

- Layer 4—How will the program solve the problem?

The fourth layer contains one or two paragraphs that explain how the proposed program intends to solve the problem in the intended audience (McKenzie et al., 2017).

- Layer 5—Why will the program be successful?

This paragraph contains an explanation of why the proposed program will work and how it compares to other successful programs (McKenzie et al., 2017).

- Layer 6—What are the benefits of solving the problem?

Layer six is one paragraph that explains the societal benefits of solving the problem and how this benefits the program participants.

- Layer 7—What uniquely qualifies the developers to solve the problem as proposed?

This layer is one paragraph that focuses on the strength and ability of the proposing organization to address the health problem. It includes documentation of the organization's past experiences with similar situations and makes a case as to why it's best suited to implement the proposed program (Nebiu, 2002).

- The icing on the cake

The icing on the "rationale" cake is concise, well-written prose. To this end, use the following plain language guidelines from the Plain Language Action and Information Network (PLAIN, 2011).

Write for the audience—Use words the people who will be reading the rationale understand. Don't "dumb it down" or use "big" words to impress.

Choose words carefully—Use simple, plain language words instead of unusual or complex ones. (See **Figure 5-6** and **Table 5-9** for examples. For a complete list, see https://www.plainlanguage.gov/guidelines/words/use-simple-words-phrases/.)

Avoid jargon—Jargon is unfamiliar or meaningless terminology used to impress

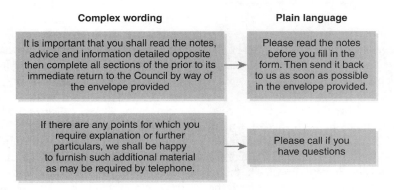

Complex wording

It is important that you shall read the notes, advice and information detailed opposite then complete all sections of the prior to its immediate return to the Council by way of the envelope provided

Plain language

Please read the notes before you fill in the form. Then send it back to us as soon as possible in the envelope provided.

If there are any points for which you require explanation or further particulars, we shall be happy to furnish such additional material as may be required by telephone.

Please call if you have questions

Figure 5-6 Examples of complex and plain language wording

Table 5-9 Examples of plain language alternatives

Complex wording	Plain language alternative
Acquaint yourself with	Find out about
Afford an opportunity	Let, allow
As a consequence of	Because
Despite the fact that	Though, although
Due to the fact that	Because
During which time	While
For the duration of	During, while
For the purpose of	To, for
Give consideration to	Consider, think about
In connection with	For, about
In the absence of	Without
In view of the fact that	Because
Irrespective of	Despite, even if
Relating to	About
Subsequent to	After
That being the case	If so,
To the extent that	If, when

Reproduced from Plain English Campaign (2020). http://www.plainenglish.co.uk/campaigning/examples/before-and-after.html

rather than inform the reader. Use everyday language whenever possible. For example, instead of saying "the patient is on positive pressure ventilatory support," use plain words—"the patient is on a respirator."

Minimize abbreviations—If abbreviations must be used, limit them to no more than three. Always define the abbreviation the first time it's used. For example, Centers for Disease Control and Prevention (CDC). Abbreviations should make it easier to read the document, not more difficult.

Be consistent—Using different terms to refer to the intended audience or the problem the program intends to address will cause confusion. If the problem is stroke, don't refer to it as cerebral vascular accident in one sentence, cardiovascular disease in another, and stroke in another.

The same is true for the intended audience—choose one term and use it consistently. Is it senior citizens, the aged, the elderly, or older adults?

Be concise—Write short sentences, and avoid using phrases with *of*, *to*, or *on*. Phrases with these words can usually be reduced to one word. For example:

> is able to = can
> on a monthly basis = monthly
> a number of = several, a few, or many
> on the grounds that = because

- The cake plate

The reference list is like the plate under a cake that supports it. It provides the sources of the information used to justify the claims presented in the rationale. All data and other information used in the rationale must be cited in the reference list following the appropriate style guide for writing citations.

Style guides are a set of rules for how and in what order the content of a citation in the reference list is written. For example, how the author's name is written, where the date of the publication is place in the citation, or which words in a title are capitalized. The American Psychological Association (APA) style is the one most commonly used in public health, but there are many others, including MLA (Modern Language Association), Chicago Style (*Chicago Manual of Style*), and AMA (American Medical Association), to name a few. If there is no preference, you won't go wrong using APA. See **Figure 5-7** for an example of a (seven-layer) rationale.

In practice, plans for implementation and evaluation are also developed in this step of the program planning process. However, a basic understanding of these is necessary before plans for them can be developed. This information is presented in Chapters 6—Implementing, and 7—Evaluating.

(Layer 1 – Program title and developers)

A Rationale for Food First: A Program to Address Hunger at Anywhere Community College

Developed by J. Doe and J. Smith

Anywhere Community College Office of Student Services

(Layer 2 – What problem does the program address?)

While most Americans (88%) have access to ample food every day, 12% or 15 million people do not. They are food insecure - unsure of having, or unable to get, enough food for their families every day because they lack the money or other resources. (United States Department of Agriculture [USDA], 2018)

(Layer 3 – Who is affected by the problem?)

Food insecurity is even a greater problem on campuses across the country where 36% of the general college population does not have enough food to eat on any given day. On community college campuses this number rises to more than 40%, with greater than 9% of students going without food for more than a day because they lack money. (Goldrick-Rab, Richardson, Schnieder, Cady, & Hernendez, 2018)

Insufficient food impacts students' ability to achieve academically. It affects their grades, test scores and chances of graduating. (Goldrick-Rab, 2018)

(Layer 4 – How will the program solve the problem?)

The proposed program, Food First, is designed to eliminate food insecurity on the Anywhere campus by establishing a campus food pantry. It will be stocked through a partnership with two local community food banks and by student donations of unused meals on their meal plan. Students in need will have the option of accessing food in the pantry or using the donated meal plan meals.

(Layer 5 – Why will it be successful?)

Anywhere Community College has applied for membership in the College and University Food Bank Alliance (CUFBA). As a member of CUFBA, we will have significant support from its more than 640 member campuses with established food pantries as we establish ours. Food pantries have been successful in decreasing food insecurity on the campuses where they exist.

(Layer 6 – What are the benefits of solving the problem?)

Being hungry, not knowing when your next meal will be or how you will get it undermines learning and academic success. Food First will remove the barrier of food insecurity enabling students to focus on learning and their academic endeavors.

(Layer 7 – What uniquely qualifies the developers to solve the problem?)

The Office of Student Services has experience setting up a similar program on campus, Nifty but Thrifty, a clothing thrift store where students can purchase gently used business clothing for job interviews. In addition, the Office of Student Services enjoys a congenial relationship with a variety of student organizations on campus and has a history of partnering with businesses and agencies in the community.

References:

Goldrick-Rab, S., Richardson, J., Schneider, J., Cady, C. & Hernandez, A. <u>Basic Needs Security Among Students Attending Georgia Colleges and Universities</u>. Hope Center for College, Community and Justice. (2018)

College and University Food Bank Alliance (2018). Our members. Retrieved March 3, 2019 from https://sites.temple.edu/cufba/members/

United States Department of Agriculture [USDA], 2018. Food security in the U.S: Key statistics and graphics. Retrieved March 3, 2019 from https://www.ers.usda.gov/topics/food-nutrition-assistance/food-security-in-the-us/key-statistics-graphics.aspx

Figure 5-7 Sample (seven-layer) rationale

Data from Goldrick-Rab, S., Richardson, J., Schneider, J., Cady, C. & Hernandez, A. (2018). Basic needs security among students attending Georgia colleges and universities. Hope Center for College, Community and Justice; College and University Food Bank Alliance. (2018). Our members. Retrieved March 3, 2019 from https://sites.temple.edu/cufba/members/; United States Department of Agriculture [USDA]. 2018. Food security in the U.S: Key statistics and graphics. Retrieved March 3, 2019 from https://www.ers.usda.gov/topics/food-nutrition-assistance/food-security-in-the-us/key-statistics-graphics.aspx

Chapter Summary

The planning stage of the planning process focuses on developing goals, objectives, strategies, and actions for a program to address the community's priority health issues that is feasible, well managed, and funded.

Planning in Practice Chapter Activity

Epidemic preparedness and control of communicable disease is subsumed under many of the essential public health functions. While each epidemic is different, whether it's Covid-19, HIV, or measles, the aim of public health programs developed to address the issue is the same—containment and prevention of disease spread. How this is accomplished depends on the disease.

Read the article below and answer the questions that follow.

Article: *Community-oriented epidemic preparedness and response to the Jerusalem 2018-2019 measles epidemic* (Stein-Zamir et al., 2019)

Link to article: https://www.ncbi.nlm.nih.gov/pmc/articles/PMC6836774/

Article Questions

1. Why was the program needed?
2. In which population did the outbreak occur?
3. Which determinants of health contributed to the outbreak?
4. Who served on the coalition (i.e., committee) that developed the program to address the outbreak?
5. What was the goal of the program?
6. What were the program objectives?
7. What strategy and actions did the committee plan to use to accomplish the goal?
8. Which components of the program were tailored to the meet the needs of the intended audience?
9. Although not identified in the article, which essential functions of public health were reflected in controlling this measles outbreak?
10. What aspects of this program would have differed if the disease was Covid-19?

References

Atlantic Health Systems. (2020). New vitality. Retrieved January 13, 2020, from https://www.atlantichealth.org/patients-visitors/education-support/community-resources-programs/new-vitality.html

Bluethmann, S. M., Bartholomew, L. K., Murphy, C. C., & Vernon, S. W. (2016). Use of theory in behavior change interventions: An analysis of programs to increase physical activity in posttreatment breast cancer survivors. *Health Education and Behavior.* Advanced online publication. doi:10.1177/1090198116647712

Boston University School of Public Health. (2016). Gantt charts as planning tools. Retrieved March 8, 2020, from http://sphweb.bumc.bu.edu/otlt/MPH-Modules/HPM/ProjectManagementTools/pmtools4.html

Brownson R. C., Fielding, J. E., & Maylahn, C. M. (2009). Evidence-based public health: A fundamental concept for public health practice. *Annual Review of Public Health, 30,* 175–201. doi: 10.1146/annurev.pu.30.031709.100001. https://www.ncbi.nlm.nih.gov/pubmed/19296775

Center for Community Health and Development (CCHD). (2020a). Chapter 2, Section 1: Developing a logic model or theory of change. Milstein, B., & Chapel, T.: University of Kansas. Retrieved March 7, 2020, from the Community Tool Box: https://ctb.ku.edu/en/table-of-contents/overview/models-for-community-health-and-development/logic-model-development/main

Center for Community Health and Development (CCHD). (2020b). Chapter 43, Section 1: Planning and writing an annual budget. Rabinowitz, P.: University of Kansas. Retrieved March 8, 2020 from Community Toolbox: https://ctb.ku.edu/en/table-of-contents/finances/managing-finances/annual-budget/main

Center for Community Health and Development, (CCHD). (2018a). Chapter 8, Section 4: Developing successful strategies: Plan to win. Naggy, J. & Fawcett, S. B.: University of Kansas. Retrieved February 12, 2019, from the Community Tool Box: https://ctb.ku.edu/en/table-of-contents/structure/strategic-planning/develop-strategies/main

Center for Community Health and Development (CCHD). (2018b). Chapter 8, Section 1: An overview of strategic planning or VMOSA. Naggy, J. & Fawcett, S. B.: University of Kansas. Retrieved February 12, 2019, from the Community Tool Box: https://ctb.ku.edu/en/table-of-contents/structure/strategic-planning/vmosa/main

Centers for Disease Control and Prevention, (CDC). (2017). Heads up. Retrieved January 20, 2019, from https://www.cdc.gov/headsup/index.html

Centers for Disease Control and Prevention (CDC), Adolescent and School Health. (2018). Evaluation briefs: Writing SMART objectives. Retrieved May 23, 2019, from https://www.google.com/url?sa=t&rct=j&q=&esrc=s&source=web&cd=2&ved=2ahUKEwiuh9_RxrLiAhRmuAKHQZrBugQFjABegQIGhAE&url=https%3A%2F%2Fwww.cdc.gov%2Fhealthyyouth%2Fevaluation%2Fpdf%2Fbrief3b.pdf&usg=AOvVaw0zhf49LENb8U-9n5Rr-ttJ

Centers for Disease Control and Prevention (CDC), Program Performance and Evaluation Office. (2018). Logic models. Retrieved March 7, 2020, from https://www.cdc.gov/eval/steps/step2/index.htm

Centers for Disease Control and Prevention (CDC), Workplace Health Promotion. (2015). Implementation. Retrieved March 21, 2019, from https://www.cdc.gov/workplacehealthpromotion/model/implementation/index.html

Centers for Disease Control and Prevention (CDC), Division of Adolescent and School Health. (2008). Healthy youth evaluation briefs: Writing good goals. Retrieved January 29, 2019, from https://www.cdc.gov/healthyyouth/evaluation/pdf/brief3a.pdf

Centers for Disease Control and Prevention (CDC), Division for Heart Disease and Stroke Prevention. (n.d.). Evaluation guide: Developing and using a logic model. Retrieved March 7, 2020, from https://www.cdc.gov/dhdsp/docs/logic_model.pdf

Charity:water. (2020). Mission statement. Retrieved April 23, 2020, from https://www.charitywater.org/about

Colorado Resiliency Resource Center. (2018). Actions to create resilient communities. Retrieved February 18, 2019, from https://www.coresiliency.com/actions-to-create-resilient-communities

Corporation for National and Community Service. (n.d.). Evaluation budgeting quick guide. Retrieved March 9, 2020, from https://www.nationalservice.gov/sites/default/files/documents/SIF%20Evaluation%20Budgeting%20Quick%20Guide.pdf

Environmental Center, University of Colorado, Boulder. (n.d.). Bicycle recycling and processing program. Retrieved January 6, 2019, from https://www.colorado.edu/ecenter/transportation/reference

Fit City San Antonio. (n.d.). San Antonio walks. Retrieved January 6, 2019, from https://www.fitcitysa.com/move-more/san-antonio-walks/)

Glanz, K., & Bishop, D. B. (2010). The role of behavioral science theory in development and implementation of public health interventions. *Annual Review of Public Health, 31,* 399–418. doi:10.1146/annurev.publhealth.012809.103604. Retrieved August 13, 2018, from https://www.annualreviews.org/doi/pdf/10.1146/annurev.publhealth.012809.103604

Hairston, M., & Keene, M. (2003). *Successful writing* (5th ed.). New York, NY: Norton. Retrieved September 17, 2018, from http://writing.umn.edu/sws/assets/pdf/quicktips/titles.pdf

Health Foundation of South Florida. (n.d.). Examples of process and outcome objectives. Retrieved February 27, 2019, from http://www.hfsf.org/wp-content/uploads/2017/02/objectives_examples.pdf

Holtz, G., Quintero, A., Crittenden, R., Baker, L., Goldstein, D., & Nedd, K. (2014). A countywide program to manage concussion in high school sports. *The Sport Journal, 20,* Retrieved January 20, 2019, from https://thesportjournal.org/article/a-countywide-program-to-manage-concussions-in-high-school-sports/

Johnston, Y., Denniston, R., Morgan, M., & Bordeau, M. (2009). Rock on café: Achieving sustainable system changes in school lunch programs. *Health Promotion Practice, 10*(2 suppl), 100s–108s. https://doi.org/10.1177/1524839908331272

Koenig, M. (2013). Non-profit mission statements—Good and bad examples. Retrieved December 31, 2018, from https://nonprofithub.org/starting-a-nonprofit/nonprofit-mission-statements-good-and-bad-examples/

Leahy, R. (1992). Twenty titles for the writer. *College Composition and Communication, 43*(4), 516–519. DOI: 10.2307/358644

Mayo Clinic. (2020). Healthy living program. Retrieved January 13, 2020, from https://healthyliving.mayoclinic.org/

McLaughlin, G. H. (1969). SMOG grading—A new readability formula. *Journal of Reading, 12*(8), 639–646.

McKenzie, J. F., Neiger, B. L., & Thackeray, R. (2017). *Planning, implementing & evaluating health promotion programs.* White Plains, NY: Pearson Education.

Minnesota Department of Health. (n.d.). Training and tools: SMART objectives. Retrieved May 23, 2019, from https://www.health.state.mn.us/communities/practice/resources/phqitoolbox/objectives.html

National Association of County and City Health Officials (NACCHO). (2013). Mobilizing action through planning and partnerships (MAPP): A users' handbook. Retrieved August 23, 2019, from https://www.naccho.org/

National Cancer Institute. (n.d.). Handout #2: Developing goals and objectives. Retrieved February 27, 2019, from https://cancercontrol.cancer.gov/use_what_works/mod3/Module_3_Handout_2.pdf

National Center for Education Statistics. (2013). Program for the international assessment of adult competencies. Retrieved April 22, 2020, from https://nces.ed.gov/pubsearch/pubsinfo.asp?pubid=2014008

National Foundation for Infectious Disease. (2017). Why aren't college students getting flu shots? Retrieved February 20, 2019, from https://nfid.wordpress.com/2017/12/06/why-arent-college-students-getting-flu-shots/

National Institutes of Health (NIH), Grants & Funding. (2019). Develop your budget. Retrieved March 9, 2020, from https://grants.nih.gov/grants/how-to-apply-application-guide/format-and-write/develop-your-budget.htm

Nebiu, B. (2002). Project proposal writing. Retrieved March 21, 2020, from http://documents.rec.org/publications/ProposalWriting.pdf

Plain Language Action and Information Network (PLAIN). (2011). Federal plain language guidelines. Retrieved March 1, 2019, from https://www.plainlanguage.gov/

Prestwich, A., Webb, T. L., & Connor, M. (2015). Using theory to develop and test interventions to promote changes in health related behavior: Evidence, issues, and recommendations. *Current Opinion in Psychology*, 5, 1–5. doi:10.1016/j.copsyc.2015.02.01

Salabarria-Pena, Y., Apt, B. S., & Walsh, C. M. (2007). Practical use of program evaluation among sexually transmitted disease (STD) programs. Department of Health and Human Services, National Center for HIV, STD, and TB Prevention, Division of STD Prevention. Retrieved June 27, 2019, from https://www.cdc.gov/std/program/pupestd.htm

The Pell Institute. (2019). Evaluation toolkit. Retrieved June 28, 2019, from http://toolkit.pellinstitute.org/evaluation-101/evaluation-approaches-types/

The Shipley School. (n.d.). Shipley policy on heading. Retrieved January 20, 2019, from https://www.shipleyschool.org/page/athletics/concussion-prevention-programs

Tebb, K. P., Erenrich, R. K., Jasik, C. B., Berna, M. S., Lester, J. C., & Ozer, E. M. (2016). Use of theory in computer-based interventions to reduce alcohol use among adolescents and young adults: A systemic review. *BMC Public Health, 16*(1), 517. doi:10.1186%2Fs12889-016-3183-x. Retrieved May 29, 2019, from https://www.ncbi.nlm.nih.gov/pmc/articles/PMC4912758/

Titler, M. G., Kleiber, C., Steelman, V. J., Rakel, B. A., Budreau, G., Everett, L. Q., ... & Goode, C. J. (2001). The Iowa model of evidence-based practice to promote quality care. *Critical Care Nursing Clinics of North America, 13*(4), 497–509. doi: 10.1188/14.CJON.157-159

Topnonprofits. (n.d.). 50 example mission statements. Retrieved December 31, 2018, from https://topnonprofits.com/examples/nonprofit-mission-statements/

Utah Department of Health. (2010). Immunize Utah. Retrieved January 6, 2019, from http://www.immunize-utah.org/about_us.html

Zwass, V. (n.d.). Information system. In *Britanica.com*. Retrieved December 19, 2018, from https://www.britannica.com/topic/information-system

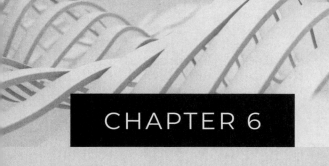

CHAPTER 6

Implementing

STUDENT LEARNING OUTCOMES

After reading this chapter, the student will be able to:

- Explain factors associated with successful program implementation.
- Identify challenges to successful program implementation.
- Discuss ethical challenges associated with program implementation.
- Develop an implementation plan.

Introduction

You're at the starting line for a race. The referee calls out "ready" and you focus, "set" and you get into position, "go" and you start running. The same is true in program planning. The needs assessment gets you focused, planning gets you into position, and implementation starts you running the program, putting the plan into action, setting it in motion … doing it.

But *how* you run the race is a key factor in whether you win or lose. If you don't start running at the right time, run at the right pace (is it a sprint, relay, or cross-country run), stay on course, control your breathing, chances are you're not going to win. In public health, it's how well the program is planned, and how effectively or efficiently it's implemented that can make the difference between success and failure.

Neither a poorly planned program well implemented, nor a well-planned program poorly implemented will result in a successful outcome. The difficulty with this is figuring out if the poor outcome is the result of an ineffective program or ineffective implementation (Durlak, 2013). When well-planned, evidence-based, community-supported programs fail, ineffective implementation is the likely culprit (Durlak & DuPre, 2008; Fixsen, Naoom, Blasé, Friedman, & Wallace. 2005; PEW, 2016).

When programs don't achieve their intended outcome, valuable resources are wasted, needed services are not delivered, and reluctance builds to try something new again (Saldana, 2014). More concerning is that some failed programs do more harm to the community than good. Consequently, the contribution implementation makes to the success of a program cannot be overstated.

Implementation Success

Going back to the previous running example, what factors would affect how you run the race, and consequently, its outcome? How would rain, high humidity or heat influence performance? What if the race were cross-country and there was a storm the night before that left debris in the road? And what if the thunder and lightning from that storm woke you up and you couldn't get back to sleep? How would an untied sneaker affect the outcome of the race?

Regardless of the type of program or the intended outcomes, a number of factors are known to affect program implementation and impact outcome. They include characteristics of the community, the organizations and providers, and the program itself (Durlak & DuPre, 2008; Stith et al., 2006).

Community Characteristics

Community characteristics are the unique aspects of the location where the intended audience lives that can either help or hinder program implementation. Given their potential impact, it's wise to consider them before implementation begins to minimize their effects. They include community readiness, capacity, politics, funding, and geography (Durlak & DuPre, 2008; Stith et al., 2006). (See **Figure 6-1**.)

Community Readiness. *Readiness* is the extent to which a community is prepared to put a program into action. It reflects the community's relationship with the problem, its level of recognition that the problem exists, and that something needs to be done about it (Edwards, Jumper-Thurman, Plested, Oetting, & Swanson, 2000).

Readiness is not instantaneous; rather, it evolves in the following nine stages.

Stage 1—No awareness
The community accepts, tolerates, or encourages the behavior related to the problem. It doesn't see the behavior as a problem but rather views it as a community norm. Readiness at this level can be improved by raising awareness of the problem through one-on-one meetings with community leaders, influential community members, community groups, and potential supporters to inform them of the situation (Edwards et al., 2000).

Stage 2—Denial
In the denial stage, the community sees the behavior as a problem but doesn't consider the behavior *its* problem or sees it as something that can't be changed. Denial can be improved by providing evidence that the problem does exist in the community through articles in religious, civic, or community bulletins or newsletters; on community websites; in local social media or other online venues; and sharing information about the problem at community group meetings (Edwards et al., 2000).

Stage 3—Vague awareness
Moving from denial to vague awareness, the community acknowledges a problem exists and that it needs to be addressed, but there's no motivation on the part of key leaders to do anything. The focus here is on motivating key leaders to begin doing something. Possible ways to accomplish this are by developing media messages related to the problem and publishing them in the local news outlets, either in print or online (Edwards et al., 2000).

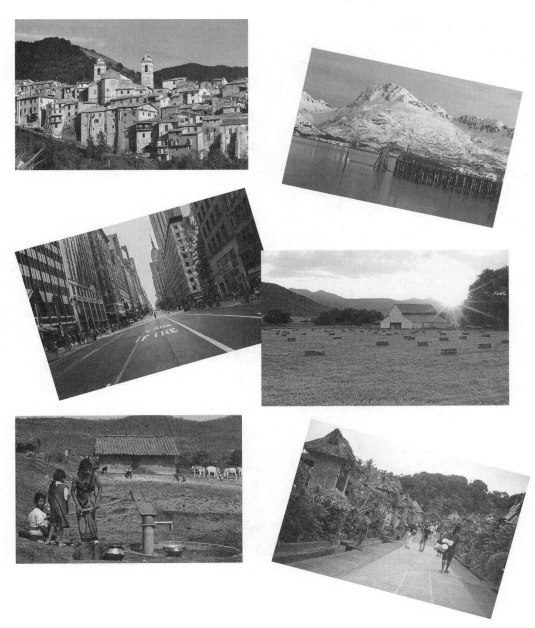

Figure 6-1 Community characteristics affect implementation

The top left photo -
© Franco Volpato/Shutterstock

Middle left photo
© Goran Bogicevic/Shutterstock

Bottom left photo
© Hari Mahidhar/Shutterstock

Top right photo-
© Olga Lyubochkina/Shutterstock

Middle right photo-
© Johnny Adolphson/Shutterstock

Bottom right photo -
© Poez/Shutterstock

Stage 4—Preplanning

A community is in the preplanning stage of readiness when it acknowledges the problem, has key leaders on board, and has formed committees in preparation for planning. Readiness in this stage can be improved by conducting focus groups to discuss the problem and begin formulating solutions (Edwards et al., 2000).

Stage 5—Preparation

When a community is in the preparation stage, it's actively planning ways to address the problem. It has secured funding, is discussing the pros and cons of programs, and is carrying out trials (Edwards et al., 2000).

Stage 6—Initiation

Initiation is the stage when implementation occurs. The community is ready, and the program is started (Edwards et al., 2000).

Stage 7—Stabilization

A community is in the stabilization stage when the program is underway, there is administrative support, and program issues become evident (Edwards et al., 2000).

Stage 8—Confirmation

When a community moves from the stabilization stage into the confirmation stage, it verifies the program's problems and makes adjustments to address them (Edwards et al., 2000).

Stage 9—Professionalization

During this last stage of readiness, efforts to prevent problems are detailed, staff are highly trained, and support of key authorities is secured (Edwards et al., 2000).

To minimize adverse effects of "unreadiness" on a program's success, at the least, a community should be in the preplanning stage before a program is implemented (Stith et al., 2006). If it isn't, strategies to improve its readiness should be used to get it to that level.

Community Capacity. Community capacity is the interaction of the skills, knowledge, and experiences of people with the resources and network of relationships in the community that can be used to solve problems and improve or maintain well-being (Chaskin, 2001). It reflects a sense of community through shared values, norms, and visions; the level of commitment to or responsibility for what happens in the community; and the ability to solve problems and access the resources needed to solve the problems (Chaskin, 2001; Durlak & DuPre, 2008; Stith et al., 2006).

Politics and Policies. Politics and policies are inherently intertwined with implementation for two reasons. First, they create the legal authority, funding, and functions needed to implement a program. Second, the implementation process itself is political because of the connections between government agencies, communities, and legislators (Lester, 2018).

It's through politics that elected officials are chosen. They, in turn, affect the adoption of policies and programs, create the capacity and infrastructure needed to implement them, and influence the choice of the people who oversee their implementation (Lester, 2018).

Funding. Without a reliable source of adequate funding, it's not possible for a program to go forward (Muthaura & Omwenga, 2017). Unfortunately, even though there is overwhelming evidence of the cost effectiveness of disease and injury prevention programs and emergency preparedness, public health is chronically underfunded (Trust for America's Health [TFAH], 2019).

As discussed earlier, funding is tied to political commitment (Frieden, 2014). Congress decides how much money each federal agency receives, what the funds can be used for, and how long the funds will be available (Centers for Disease Control and Prevention [CDC],

2013). About 75 percent of the appropriated federal dollars for the CDC and the U.S. Department of Health and Human Services are distributed to states and local programs (TFAH, 2017), which accounts for about 25 percent of local health department funding (National Association of Counties [NACo], 2019). In addition to federal and state monies, public health program funding sources include grants, contracts for specific services, private foundations, corporations, and charities.

Geography. Geography impacts implementation, especially in remote, rural locations with isolated or mobile populations (i.e., farm workers) and inadequate transportation. The effect of this can be significant if the program has multiple or lengthy sessions or is held during the winter, when weather becomes an added factor (Rural Health Information Hub [RHIhub], n.d.).

Provider Characteristics

Providers are the people responsible for delivering or presenting the program to the intended audience. They may be employees of the organization responsible for delivering the program (delivery organization), for example, the local health department, hospital, or nonprofit agency, or they might be freelance consultants hired for a specific program. Provider characteristics are traits or attributes that can impact implementation. They include the following:

- Beliefs and attitudes

  Providers who believe there is a need for the program and believe it will be effective in addressing the problem, are more likely to successfully implement it (Klimes-Dougan et al., 2009). Likewise, providers with a positive attitude toward the program tend to implement it more effectively (Payne & Eckert, 2010).

- Confidence (self-efficacy)

  Implementation is impacted by the level of confidence a provider has in his or her ability to deliver a program. Those who are confident in their ability are more likely to effectively deliver it (Klimes-Dougan et al., 2009) than are those who are not confident.

- Proficiency

  Providers with the skills and ability needed to implement a program are more likely to implement it effectively (Wanjiru, Kabara, & Milimo, 2016). Because training is key to developing provider proficiency (Durlak & DuPre, 2008), it should take place shortly before implementation begins, include hands-on practice, and be adapted when necessary to meet the provider's individual needs (Cresswell, Bates, & Shiekh, 2013). To support effective implementation over the course of the program, ongoing training and technical assistance should be available (Wandersman, Chien, & Katz, 2012).

Organizational Characteristics

Each organization, whether it's a health department, nonprofit agency, corporation, healthcare facility, or academic institution, is unique. Each has its own culture, history, expectations, strengths, and weaknesses, which can add to or detract from its ability to successfully implement a program. The specific organizational characteristics important to implementation are leadership support, resources availability, and shared decision making.

- Leadership support

  In order to successfully implement a program, proper oversight or management of all aspects of implementation are needed (Wanjiru et al., 2016). A supportive organization overall, and organizational leadership in particular, are among the greatest facilitators of evidence-based program implementation (Bach-Mortensen, Lange, & Montgomery, 2018).

- Resource Availability

  One of the greatest barriers to successful implementation is resources, specifically, sufficient and reliable funding secured before implementation begins (Bach-Mortensen et al., 2018) and staff.

When adequate funding is not available things can't get done. For example, more than half of local health departments rely on federal funds for preparedness activities. When funds are cut, it results in cuts in education and training initiatives to increase community resilience and preparedness (Bevington, 2014).

The importance of staff to successful implementation cannot be overstated. Untrained, inconsistent, and inadequate staff lead to unsuccessful or ineffective implementation. To prevent this, the requirements for each staff position in terms of skills, experience, and educational preparation should be determined before interviewing begins. People who don't meet the requirements should not be hired. This is a particular problem in rural locations, where qualified staff may not be readily available (RHIhub, n.d.).

Even with the most qualified staff, training is a must to facilitate successful program delivery. Training should be scheduled after all staff have been hired and immediately before initial program implementation. Because staff can make or break successful implementation, staff turnover should be anticipated and planned for (Elliot & Mihalic, 2004).

Other staffing resources that affect implementation are inadequate or poorly trained administrative/office support and technical assistance (Durlak & DuPre, 2008) for data analysis and evaluation. Nonstaffing resources that affect implementation include inadequate or inappropriate physical space or facilities (Winjiru et al., 2016).

- Shared decision making

When program decisions are made collaboratively with input from the delivery organization, community members, researchers/planners, and stakeholders, consistent with community-based participatory research principles, implementation is more likely to be successful. Top-down decision making by people far removed from the process of actually "putting the program into action" can be detrimental to program success.

The importance of recognizing and addressing organizational characteristics known to affect program implementation became apparent to a medical center administration intent on instituting a hospital-wide initiative for improving survival after an in-hospital "code" (cardiac arrest), when it didn't work. Implementation of the initiative was impeded by a lack of understanding by the staff of the institutional procedures or policies (policies and politics), incomplete staff training and certification in the basic skills needed during a code (provider skills), negative staff attitudes toward using new equipment (problem-solving belief), varying department cultures regarding defibrillation, i.e., shocking the heart (shared values), lack of empowerment for nurses to act independent from physicians in a code (shared decision making), and that implementing change takes more than a top-down command by administrators (shared decision making). Of all these impediments, the most important was a lack of understanding of the different department norms and cultures (Einav, Kaufman, & Varon, 2018). Had this been known, adjustments could have been made, which might have eased implementation.

Program Characteristics

As Diffusion of Innovation (Rogers, 2003) points out, an innovation's characteristics affect its adoption. Similarly, a program's characteristics can affect its implementation, specifically its compatibility and complexity.

- Compatibility

Compatibility is the extent to which a program is in sync with the delivery organization's practices, and the community's needs, values, and culture. The more compatible it is, the more likely it is to be implemented successfully (Durlak & DuPre, 2008).

- Complexity

Complexity refers to the intended audience's perception of how difficult the program is to understand or use. The more complex, the less likely it is to be successfully implemented (Day, Trotter, Donaldson, Hill, &

Finch, 2016). This doesn't mean to suggest that all programs should be simplistic. It means that complexity should be taken into consideration and adaptations made when feasible to make a difficult concept, behavior, or product as user friendly as possible.

Program characteristics can contribute in both positive and negative ways to successful implementation of the same program. This is what happened with the implementation of a fall prevention program for older community-dwelling adults. The program was compatible with the delivery organizations' practices, values, and other services, which contributed to its successful implementation. However, the program was too challenging (difficult) for some participants and too simplistic for others. As a result, the former group needed modifications, and the latter group dropped out (Day et al., 2016), which negatively impacted implementation.

Implementation Challenges

Putting a program into action is a complex undertaking wrought with many challenges whether it's an evidence-based program or one developed in the practice setting by staff. How challenges are approached can make a difference in the success of the program's implementation and its effectiveness in solving the problem it was developed to address.

Common implementation challenges include the following.

Fidelity

The effectiveness of an evidence-based program, that is, its ability to produce the expected results, is influenced by *fidelity*. Fidelity is the degree to which the program is delivered as it was designed by the original developers (Bonde, Stjernqvst, Sabinski, & Maindal, 2018). In other words, fidelity is how consistent program implementation is with the way it was meant to be implemented.

Low or weak implementation fidelity is one reason why evidence-based programs don't always produce the expected results when they're replicated. This is a problem because it can lead to the inaccurate conclusion that the program is ineffective (Breitenstein, et al., 2010) when in fact, the expected results didn't occur because of fidelity issues. (See **Figure 6-2**.)

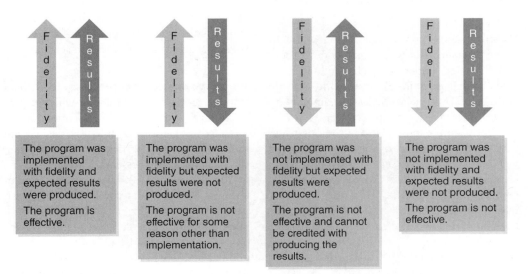

Figure 6-2 Fidelity of implementation and program results

Data from James Madison University, (2020). Assessment implementation fidelity. Retrieved March 18, 2020 from https://www.jmu.edu/assessment/sass/AC-step-four.shtml

Fidelity is a composite of the following factors or components: adherence, exposure or dose, delivery quality, participant responsiveness, program differentiation (Carroll et al., 2007; Dane & Schnieder, 1998) and adaptation (Carvalho, et al., 2013). Each alone or any combination of them can lead to less than desirable program results.

Adherence. Adherence is the extent to which the people delivering the program follow the implementation protocol, guidelines, and instructions or plans described and provided by the developers (Dane & Schnieder, 1998; Mihalic, 2002). In general, the greater the adherence to protocol, the greater the likelihood of effectiveness.

To help you understand adherence, let's say you're going on a picnic and you want to bring something for dessert. You call your grandmother and ask for her famous chocolate chip cookie recipe. If you follow (adhere to) the recipe and all the instructions *exactly,* the cookies should come out tasting *exactly* as they do when she makes them. But, if you're in a hurry and decide to bake them for less time than her instructions call for, you can rest assured those cookies will not be the same.

Dose. Dose or exposure refers to how much of the program, as it was originally developed and delivered under research conditions, is actually delivered in the real-world setting (Durlak & DuPre, 2008). It's the amount of services the intended audience receives

For example, how many of the originally developed and delivered activities were provided in the real-world setting? How long were classes or sessions held in the real-world setting compared to how long they were originally held by the developers? How much of the program content originally delivered was covered in the real-world setting? Given that dose impacts effectiveness (Wang et al., 2015), for greatest effectiveness, all activities should be delivered and delivered as they were developed.

Going back to those chocolate chip cookies, think of dose as amounts. How many cups of flour, how many eggs, how many teaspoons of vanilla does the recipe call for? If you want the cookies to come out tasting just like grandma's, you have to use the exact amounts listed in the recipe. If the recipe calls for two cups of flour but you use one, the end result is going to be mush.

Delivery Quality. Quality is a critical factor associated with successful program outcomes. It's the extent or degree to which the program is executed with excellence—that is, how well, clearly, and correctly the components are delivered by the provider. Quality is affected when an organization provides a program for the first time, offers it in a new setting, or is presented by new staff. These situations can result in major changes (Durlak, 2013), which impact delivery quality and, ultimately, effectiveness. When delivery is poor, it's the same as the intended audience not receiving the whole program (Pettigrew et al., 2015), which lessens the likelihood of an effective outcome.

Back to those cookies again. How well you carry out the instructions in the recipe will affect how the cookies come out. Over- or undermixing the ingredients, melting the butter too much, or not preheating the oven are all quality of execution issues common for a first-time cookie baker that affect the outcome of the cookie.

Participant Responsiveness. Participant responsiveness is the extent to which a program holds the interest or attention of the intended audience, their enthusiasm, and their willingness to participate in the program activities (Schaap, Bessems, Otten, Kremers, & van Nassau, 2018). Low or poor responsiveness, that is, inattention or lack of interest, occurs when participants don't find the program relevant (Carroll et al., 2007), don't enjoy it, are not satisfied with it, or don't appreciate it (Schaap et al., 2018). Lack of interest and inattention reduce program effectiveness.

How attentive you are while making those cookies will affect the way they come out. If you're not paying attention to what's going on when you put them in the oven, chances are you'll overbake them—which will make them hard as rocks and inedible. Grandma will not be happy.

Program Differentiation. Differentiation refers to the unique features of a program that are necessary for its success (Durlak & DuPre, 2008). When these features aren't replicated or retained during implementation in a real-world setting, effectiveness is negatively affected.

Program differentiation was not maintained in a program aimed at improving maternal and child health outcomes in Mexico, possibly reducing its impact. There were three distinct versions of the program being implemented at the same time. In the first version, the moms received health information text messages sent by program staff. In the second version, moms received health information text messages sent by community leaders and signed contracts with their community leader to commit to one of the following: taking folic acid supplements, attending all prenatal checkups, or responding to the text messages. In the third version moms received health information text messages from program staff and anonymous evaluations of the healthcare providers and the health care they provided (Gaitan-Rossi et al., 2019).

The first version was delivered as intended. However, the second and third versions were not. The program implementers were not able to recruit or train the number of community leaders needed for the second version. Consequently, it ended up being implemented in a similar way to the first, which was not intended (Gaitan-Rossi et al., 2019).

In the third version, the moms were supposed to complete evaluations of the healthcare providers and the care they received. The moms didn't complete these because they didn't receive an explanation as to why they should. Further, the health providers didn't encourage the moms to complete them because they had misconceptions about the program and didn't understand that the evaluations were intended as an incentive for them (Gaitan-Rossi et al., 2019).

Implementation fidelity, specifically dose and adherence, along with provider characteristics and training, affected the outcome of Focus on Youth in the Caribbean, an evidence-based HIV prevention program in the Bahamas. The program, integrated into the sixth-grade curriculum, consisted of 8 sessions and 46 activities, 30 of which were identified as core activities (Wang et al., 2015).

The more than 200 teachers participating in the program taught, on average, 24 of the 46 total program activities, 15.6 of the 30 core program activities, and slightly more than half (4.6) of the 8 required sessions. Only 2 teachers taught all the sessions and activities, and 6 didn't teach any (Wang et al., 2015).

Students in the classes of teachers who taught over 80 percent of the core activities and adhered to the format outlined in the program manual demonstrated greater levels of HIV/AIDS knowledge, reproductive health skills, self-efficacy, and intention to use condoms than did students in classes where teachers taught less than a third of the core activities and modified most of them. The results showed that implementation fidelity was significantly related to better results (Wang et al., 2015).

Adaptation. Because evidence-based programs are developed and implemented in controlled research environments, adjustments or adaptations are usually needed before they can be delivered in a real-world setting. Some adaptations are minor, for instance, translating materials from one language to another, but eliminating core elements is a major adaptation that can have major consequences. Core elements or activities are the essential components

High fidelity

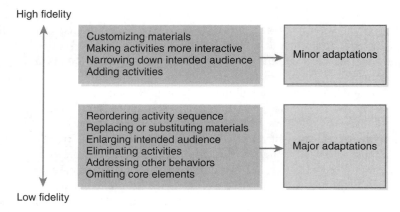

Figure 6-3 Adaptation affects fidelity

Data from Carvalho, M., Honeycutt, S., Escoffery, C., Glanz, K., Sabbs, D., & Kegler, M. (2013). Balancing fidelity and adaptation: Implementing evidence based chronic disease prevention programs. *Journal of Public Health Management and Practice 19*(4), 348–356.

that make an evidence-based program effective. They must be delivered as they were designed (Carvalho et al., 2013). (See **Figure 6-3**.)

Not knowing how to adapt a program and retain its effectiveness is a significant barrier to effective implementation (Bach-Mortensen et al., 2018). To avoid making ineffective or detrimental adaptations, it's best to consult and work collaboratively with the original developers (Durlak, 2013).

How much can you change the chocolate chip cookie recipe and still end up with cookies that taste like they're supposed to? Well, if the recipe calls for two large eggs, but you only have medium-size eggs, using them won't make much of a difference. However, if the recipe calls for sweet butter (unsalted) and ½ teaspoon of salt, but you figure butter is butter so use the regular butter (salted) in your refrigerator and the ½ teaspoon of salt, they won't taste the same—guaranteed! Lesson learned— Before making any changes to grandma's recipe, talk with her first. If you had, she would have told you to omit the salt in the recipe if you're using regular butter because it already has salt in it.

Contextual Fit

Programs are implemented at organizations by providers (implementers), who are generally either employees of the organization or consultants hired to put the program into action. Each organization's unique culture, structure, procedure, processes, resources, mission, and history along with characteristics of the community, audience, and stakeholders, shape the context within which implementation takes place.

Contextual fit, then, is the extent to which the characteristics of the setting are consistent with the program strategies, procedures, or elements. A good fit occurs when the implementers, intended audience, stakeholders, and other supporters determine the program is effective, doable, and sustainable in their setting (Hayes, O'Shea, Foley-Nolan, McCarthy, & Harrington, 2019), and there is a match between the values, skills, administrative support, and resources needed (Monzalve, 2016). Challenges arise when there is poor contextual fit or a mismatch between them (Horner, Blitz, & Ross, 2014).

Because contextual fit is important for successful program outcomes (Fixsen et al.

2005), mismatched aspects of contextual fit should be identified and addressed to minimize their negative impact on the outcomes. The most common mismatches are related to need, precision, evidence-base, efficiency, skills, cultural relevance, resource availability, and administrative support (Horner et al., 2014).

- Need

Every program should address an identified need, solve a problem, fill a gap, and produce results **valuable** to those delivering, receiving, and supporting its implementation (Horner et al., 2014). If the program doesn't do this, it doesn't fit. It should not be implemented and/or it should be replaced with one that does fit.

- Precision

The core program activities should be detailed, accurate, and clearly explained so their fit within the context of implementation can be determined. Activities that are not make it difficult to determine if what should be done fits the setting (Horner et al., 2014). In the case of evidence-based programs, challenges with inaccurate, unclear, or questionable activities can be rectified by consulting the developers to make a determination about fit.

- Evidence-base

There should be proof, verified by published outcomes, that the program produced the expected results (Horner et al., 2014) in a population and setting that shares the same characteristics as the real-world setting in which it will be delivered. If this is not available, evidence produced from a population and setting that functions in similar ways to the real-world setting is preferred over evidence from those that share fewer characteristics (Slocum et al., 2014). Implementing a program without proof that it works in a similar situation is likely to produce disappointing results.

- Efficiency

For contextual fit, there should be an efficient, practical use of the time, personnel, materials, and money for the program to produce the expected outcomes that match the time frames and budgets available. The challenge is knowing if there is. There should be a reasonable amount of time and effort allocated for initial program implementation. Once implemented, the use of time and effort to sustain the program needs to be as efficient or more efficient than the time and effort needed for other programs (Horner et al., 2014).

- Skills

Because contextual fit includes having the program implemented by people who have the skills necessary to implement it! When the implementers don't have the necessary skills, their shortfalls must be remedied to prevent a negative impact on program effectiveness. To address this challenge and improve contextual fit, there should be a clear understanding of the training, orientation, and other support to be provided (Horner et al., 2014).

- Cultural relevance

The program, its implementation, and intended outcomes should match the values of those implementing it, benefiting from it, and supporting it (Mwaria, Chen, Coppola, Maurice, & Phifer, 2016). When any of these are out of sync, adjustments or adaptations are needed. To avoid making changes that might jeopardize the integrity of the program, any changes should be made in consultation with the developers.

The impact of culture on implementation is not restricted to the culture of the intended audience or those benefiting from the program. The organization's culture also impacts implementation efforts. Organizational culture affects and guides what happens in the organization by defining what is appropriate behavior in various situations (Ravasi & Schultz, 2006). Consequently, organizational culture

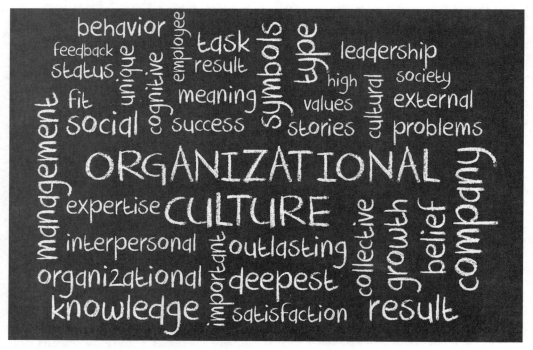

Figure 6-4 Organizational culture impacts implementation
© Grasko/Shutterstock

can either help or hinder implementation. Organizations with unclear values or beliefs, or where the culture encourages resistance to change, can be challenges to contextual fit and, ultimately, implementation success (Li, Jeffs, Barwick, & Stevens, 2018). (See **Figure 6-4**.)

- Organizational support

It's necessary for available resources to match those needed to implement the program (Horner et al., 2014), not only in terms of funding, but also staffing, space, time, and infrastructure (Rojatz, Merchant, & Nitch, 2017). Insufficient staff, difficulty recruiting staff (Kramer, Cote, Lee, Creekmur, & Saliba, 2017), heavy workloads, budget cuts, and lack of resources for training (Waller, Finch, Giles, & Newbury-Birch, 2017) can all impact contextual fit and delay or prevent implementation.

A mismatch between need and availability is a challenge that should be addressed before implementation begins. If the resources needed to implement the program as it was intended are not available, working with the developers to adapt it to better match what is available may be an option. Another option is to identify a program with resource requirements more in line with what is available.

Because implementation requires the support of an organization's key leaders, the program should respect their values and preferences (Sullivan et al., 2018). When it doesn't, support for implementation can be negatively impacted. This discrepancy might be addressed by working with the administrative decision makers and program developers to make adjustments that better align the two, without compromising the program's core components.

Having administrative support was key to implementing an in-school fruit and vegetable program in Australia. Schools were significantly more likely to implement the program if the principals believed the program was effective, easy to implement, important, and doable with available resources (Nathan et al., 2017).

Scaling

Taking a program from a research setting and implementing it in a real-world setting that reaches more people usually involves a change of size or scale (Milat, Newson, & King 2014). Scaling-up is the process of expanding a program to reach more people (World Health Organization [WHO], 2016). (See **Figure 6-5**.) Scalability is the potential for the program to be scaled while retaining fidelity and effectiveness (Milat, King, Bauman, & Redman, 2012).

The challenge of scaling is that the same controlled conditions and resources used in the research setting are usually not available in a real-world setting. It's more likely there will be fewer resources and multiple, pressing priorities. Under real-world conditions, scaling-up calls for balancing the desired outcomes

with the practical realities and constraints of the setting (WHO, 2010)

A number of frameworks are available to guide scaled program implementation. Two are outlined next—A Guide to Increasing the Scale of Population Health Interventions (Guide) (Milat, Newson, & King, 2014) and ExpandNet (WHO, 2010).

Guide to Increasing the Scale of Population Health Interventions (The Guide)

The Guide consists of a four-step process for scaling a program: assessing program scalability, developing a scale-up plan, preparing for scale-up, and scaling-up (Milat, Newson, & King, 2014).

Step 1—Assess Scalability. Since all programs are *not* appropriate for scaling, assessing scalability is the first step in the process (Milat, Newson, & King, 2014). Scalable programs are simple, clearly better than the available alternatives, and not reliant on a very specific

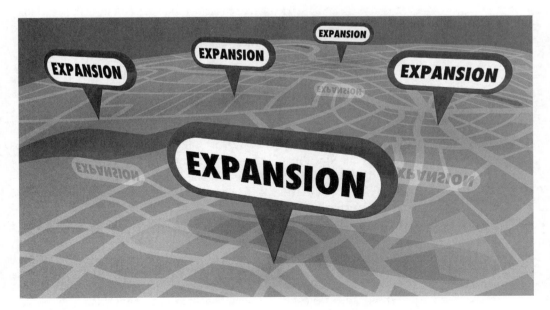

Figure 6-5 Scaling-up is expansion
© iQoncept/Shutterstock

context or people pushing them forward (Graham, 2018).

Scalability is determined by a program's effectiveness, reach and adoption, policy alignment, and acceptability and fit within the local context (Milat, Newson, Wolfenden, et al., 2014).

- Effectiveness

The most important characteristic of a scalable program is its effectiveness (WHO, 2010). An effective program is one that has demonstrated significant outcomes either through a highly controlled research study or an effectiveness study done in a diverse real-world setting (Milat et al., 2016).

Effectiveness is measured in terms of effect size, or how much difference there is between the results of people who participated in the program and those who did not (Sullivan & Feinn, 2012). This is important because scaling usually requires the program to be adapted in some way, which often reduces effectiveness. Therefore, a program with a greater effect size is more likely to retain effectiveness when it's scaled (Milat, Newson, & King, 2014).

Considering that scaling necessitates adaptation or adjustment to address contextual fit issues, assessing effectiveness includes understanding which core elements of the program are essential to maintain effectiveness (Milat, Newson, & King, 2014) and cannot be changed, and which are not essential and can be changed. If there is a mismatch between the resources needed for scaling-up core elements that cannot be adapted and the context within which the program is to be implemented, the likelihood of a successful outcome is reduced.

Knowing if the program is effective in different populations is also part of assessing its effectiveness (Milat et al., 2012). Some programs are very effective among populations that really don't need them, while not effective at all in those that do (Milat, Newson, & King, 2014).

The last part of the effectiveness assessment is determining if there are any unintended consequences or adverse outcomes associated with the program. If there are, actions should be taken to minimize them before the scale-up begins. If the adverse outcomes are extreme, the implementation might need to be abandoned altogether (Milat, Newson, & King, 2014).

The following questions are useful for assessing effectiveness:

- Is there proof of program effectiveness?
- What was the effect size of the original study that established effectiveness?
- Are the benefits likely to outweigh the costs?
- Can fidelity and the effect of the original program be maintained in the real-world setting within acceptable costs?
- Is it likely that the core elements of the program can be retained when scaled?
- Is effectiveness likely to differ with different audiences?
- Is it likely the program will have unintended or adverse outcomes (Milat, Newson, & King, 2014)?

- Reach and adoption

Reach refers to the likelihood of the program engaging, contacting, influencing, reaching as much of the intended audience as possible when it's scaled-up. Equally as important is the likelihood of as many settings (organizations, schools, worksites) as possible implementing the program (Milat, Newson, & King, 2014).

The following questions are useful for assessing reach and adoption:

- What is the likely reach of the program among those in the intended audience when scaled-up?
- What is the likely adoption rate in different settings or organizations?
- Is the likely reach and adoption great enough to have an impact on the intended audience?
- Is it likely that the program will have different levels of reach and adoption across audiences and settings (Milat, Newson, & King, 2014)?

- Policy Alignment

Programs with the best chance of scaling-up are those aligned with the priorities (WHO, 2010) of the delivery organization. Programs that don't address a pressing need or persistent problem of the delivering and/or funding organization are difficult to implement (Milat et al., 2012).

Alignment is also important in terms of the context or setting within which scaling will take place compared to the original research setting that established its effectiveness. This is particularly important to effectiveness if contextual factors, for example, income, culture, skills, and literacy were important to the successful outcomes produced by the original program (Milat, Newson, & King, 2014).

The program should also be compatible with other practices and programs already in place in the implementation setting (Milat et al., 2012). If the program to be scaled is similar to an existing program, there must be evidence that it's better than the existing program before it's even considered for scaling (Milat, Newson, & King, 2014).

The following questions are useful for assessing alignment:

- Is the program consistent with policy directions of the delivering and funding organizations?
- Does the program address an identified need of the organization responsible for funding?
- Is the context of the setting where scaling will take place comparable to the one in which the original research was carried out?
- Is the program compatible with similar programs in the same setting?
- Is there a similar program in place, and if so, is the new one better?

- Acceptability and fit

Simply put, is the program doable and acceptable to those who will be involved at all levels (stakeholders), and is scaling feasible? This is a judgment call made based on what is known about the stakeholders, the costs, staffing, and other resource needs (Milat, Newson, & King, 2014) and their availability.

The following questions are useful for accessing acceptability and feasibility:

- What resources were used to deliver the original program?
- How ready is the scale-up setting to provide these resources?
- Is the scaled-up program likely to be acceptable to the intended audience, funders, and other stakeholders?
- Are the potential scaled costs likely to fit within the available budget?

Step 2—Develop a Plan. The second step in the scaling process is to develop a plan. The plan comes together with the completion of eight tasks: writing a rationale, describing the program, conducting a contextual analysis, identifying potential partners, choosing the scale-up approach, considering evaluation options, estimating resources, and writing the plan (Milat, Newson, & King, 2014).

Task 1—Write a rationale

The information gathered to assess effectiveness in the first step is used to develop a rationale or justification for scaling the program in the second step (Milat, Newson, & King, 2014). Keep in mind that the rationale is a written document that clearly presents the reasoning behind a program.

Once the draft rationale is written, ask the following questions:

- Is there information missing that would add to building a case for scaling the program?
- Is there evidence from similar programs that can be used as part of the documentation?

Task 2—Describe the program

The description is a detailed explanation of the program that includes the key characteristics of the original program and the core elements essential to maintaining its effectiveness that must be retained. Because it's likely the original program will need adaptation to fit the setting in which it will be implemented, any changes that may impact its effectiveness should be carefully considered. Describing the program as simply as possible helps in communicating it to stakeholders (Milat, Newson, & King, 2014).

Once the draft description is completed, ask the following questions:

– Are the objectives clearly written?
– Is the intended audience clearly defined?
– Is the program described as simply as possible?
– Have the core elements necessary to maintain effectiveness been retained in light of the adaptations needed?

Task 3—Conduct contextual analysis

A contextual analysis is an examination of the political, social, and organizational environments. It's conducted to identify the contextual conditions, groups, or individuals likely to affect scaling-up in terms of their readiness or support (Milat, Newson, & King, 2014).

In completing the analysis, ask the following questions:

– Have the political, social, and organizational contexts in which the program will be scaled been outlined?
– Have key stakeholders been identified along with where they fit in the political, social, and organizational environments?
– Have potential stakeholders in support of scaling the program been identified?
– Have the individuals or organizations responsible for scale-up funding decisions been identified (Milat, Newson, & King, 2014)?

Task 4—Identify potential partners

Scaling-up involves getting a commitment from at least one other organization to take on the role of either the originating or delivery organization. The originating organization is responsible for developing the scale-up plan and occasionally oversight of implementation. The delivery organization is responsible for the direct implementation of the scale-up plan.

Sometimes, one organization can assume both roles; other times the originating organization does not have the capacity to also implement the plan. In this situation, the role of delivery organization can be shared by one or more other organizations. Sharing these responsibilities, however, involves establishing effective partnerships (Milat, Newson, & King, 2014).

To help identify organizations that might be good partners, and what their roles may be, takes knowing the key tasks or functions necessary for scale-up and then considering who might be best suited to complete them (Milat, Newson, & King, 2014).

To guide identification of potential partnerships:

– identify the tasks necessary for scaling up the program.
– define the role and outline the responsibilities of the originating organization.
– identify potential organizations with the capacity or the means to develop it to serve as a delivery organization.
– determine if more than one delivery organization is needed.
– assess the contextual fit between the potential delivery organization and the program.
– establish or strengthen partnerships to facilitate collaboration and coordination.

Task 5—Choose scaling approach

There are two main approaches to scaling, vertical and horizontal (WHO, 2010). They are not mutually exclusive and are oftentimes used together (Milat, Newson, & King, 2014).

• Vertical approach

A vertical scale-up approach involves implementing the program full-scale, all at once at all sites or across a whole system.

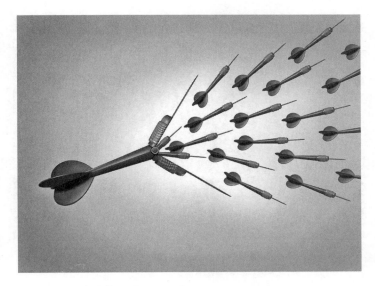

Figure 6-6 Vertical scale-up is full-scale expansion
© Lightspring/Shutterstock

(See **Figure 6-6**.) The advantage of a vertical approach is that compliance with the changes brought about by the program are generally mandatory and often accompanied by commitment from government with resources to support implementation. This means implementation can occur rapidly and cover a large area quickly. On the downside, this approach limits opportunities to adapt the program or respond to local contextual issues that arise during implementation, or to change or reverse the program if it's not working. Examples of vertical scale-up are mandatory seat belt laws, smoking bans (Milat, Newson, & King, 2014), and child immunization programs (Araya, Alvarado, Sepulveda, & Rojas, 2012).

- Horizontal approach

A horizontal approach entails implementing the program at different sites or to different groups in phases or stages, usually starting with a pilot program, followed by a step-by-step expansion. (See **Figure 6-7**.) The advantage of this approach is that lessons learned along the way can be used to improve the program or its implementation as it's delivered in different settings or with different populations. It's a good approach to use when there is concern about the scalability of a program or when resources are limited (Milat, Newson, & King. 2014).

An example of horizontal or phased scaling is the implementation of *Mobile for Reproductive Health (m4RH)*, an interactive text messaging system that provides simple, accurate, and globally relevant information on reproductive health (L'Engle, Plourde, & Zan, 2017). A controlled trial of this program in Kenya resulted in a 14 percent improvement in contraception knowledge among users of the system compared to a control group (Johnson et al., 2017). The outcome of a pilot study suggested it was one way to reach populations that are traditionally difficult to reach with family planning information. As a result, horizontal scale-up was used to expand the program into Rwanda, Uganda, and Tanzania along with content adaptations that were needed to reach key adolescent and youth audiences in those countries (WHO, 2011).

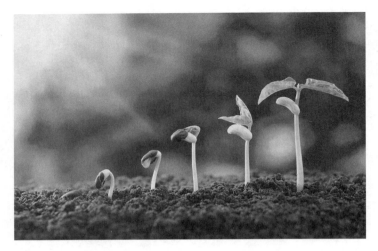

Figure 6-7 Horizontal scale-up is step-by-step expansion

© Lovelyday12/Shutterstock

The Goodwill-Nurse Family Partnership is an example of a collaborative effort of two programs that joined together and scaled their programs using both vertical and horizontal approaches. The goal of the collaboration was to scale horizontally to enable each service provider to reach additional families with their unique services, and vertically across programs to ensure easy access for families to a wider array of services (White, Delgado, & Severens, 2018).

Following are three steps for deciding which scale-up approach to use:

Step 1—Assess the merits of a horizontal approach by reviewing lessons learned from (similar, if available) programs that were scaled using a horizontal approach.

Step 2—Assess the merits of a vertical approach by reviewing lessons learned from (similar, if available) programs that were scaled using used a vertical approach.

Step 3—Choose the approach most efficient and appropriate for the program (Milat, Newson, & King, 2014).

Task 6—Consider evaluation and monitoring options

To ensure the scale-up is working as it should, it's important to evaluate and monitor the process as it's happening to determine if:

- the process is progressing as it was intended too.
- the program is effective, and whether its effectiveness is being maintained over time.
- the program's reach and adoption rates are having the intended impact.
- there are factors influencing reach and adoption, and what they are.
- the program remains acceptable to the intended audience and stakeholders over time.
- there is ongoing compatibility with other programs and the broader context (Milat et al., 2016; Milat et al., 2012).

In considering options for monitoring and evaluation:

- review literature to identify methods used to evaluate and monitor the scaling, outcomes, and impact of similar programs and/or those using a similar approach.

– based on the information reviewed, describe appropriate methods for evaluating and monitoring the scaling process being used, its outcomes, and impacts (Milat et al., 2012).

Task 7—Estimate resources needed

Critical to implementation of any program is the availability of adequate resources. Consequently, when preparing to scale-up a program, it's necessary to provide decision makers with as much information as possible about the estimated resource needs—human, technical, and financial—to enable a determination as to whether the program can be implemented given the resources and budget available (Milat et al., 2012).

In estimating resources:

– determine the human resources needed to scale the program, including those who will be responsible for delivering the program, and administrative and other support personnel. Estimate their associated costs, for example—recruitment expenses, salaries, benefits, training, travel.
– identify the technical resources needed, and estimate the cost of hardware (computers, printers, and the like) software, and other infrastructure needs.
– identify any other needed resources—educational materials, incentives, and so on, and estimate their costs.
– compile a summary of the resources and budgetary support needed to scale the program (Milat et al., 2012).

Task 8—Write the plan

Write a plan that presents a clear, concise case for scaling-up the program and an overview of how it will take place. The plan should be shared with the decision makers and other stakeholders in the originating organization, as well as potential delivery organizations, and consequently, written with this in mind (Milat, Newson, & King, 2014).

The written plan has six sections. The first section is the rationale, the second is the description of the program to be scaled, followed by a summary of the contextual situation in the third section. The fourth section identifies potential partners and their roles in the scale-up, the fifth describes how the scale-up will take place, and the final sixth section contains a realistic estimate of the resources needed to scale the program (Milat, Newson, & King, 2014).

Step 3—Prepare for Scaling-Up. This step concentrates on securing the resources needed to implement and sustain the program. Its focus is on consulting with stakeholders, establishing legitimacy, and securing resources. (Milat, Newson, & King, 2014).

• Consulting with stakeholders

Before scale-up begins, it's important to consult with key stakeholders to determine how acceptable and appropriate they find the program. This is done to identify those likely to support scale-up and those who may raise concerns that might need to be addressed (Milat, Newson, & King, 2014).

Consulting with stakeholders entails:

– sharing the scale-up plan with them.
– discussing their perceptions of the acceptability and appropriateness of the plan.
– identifying potential concerns they may have to the scale-up.
– identifying adaptations needed to address stakeholder concerns and eliminate barriers to implementation (Milat, Newson, & King, 2014).

• Establishing legitimacy for change

Before a scaled-up implementation can occur, stakeholders must agree there is a real or legitimate need for making a change to address a problem, and that the proposed program is a credible solution. To this end, it's necessary to promote or advocate for the proposed program's effectiveness and scale-up plan as both feasible and cost effective (Milat, Newson, & King, 2014).

The need for change will be legitimized once decision makers agree and state publicly that change is necessary (Milat et al., 2012), that the proposed program is effective, and that the plan for scaling is both feasible and financially sensible.

Strategies for establishing legitimacy for change include:

- determining the best ways to promote or advocate the merits of scaling-up to the decision makers, opinion leaders, and funders.
- identifying opinion leaders most likely to be successful in promoting the scale-up to the decision makers.
- securing support of opinion leaders to act as spokespersons for scaling-up the program.
- providing input into policy and budgetary processes, establishing advisory boards of key influencers (Milat, Newson, & King, 2014).

• Securing resources

Resources for implementation come from the reallocation of existing resources, through new resource streams or a combination of both. Keep in mind that resources are more than funding (Milat et al., 2012).

Resources also include the organizational skills and systems, staffing (Milat, Newson, & King, 2014), materials, and equipment needed to successfully implement the program on a larger scale. Because a single organization with all the necessary resources may not exist, partnerships between organizations with complementary resources and strengths is a good way to secure them (Milat et al., 2012; Norton & Mittman, 2010).

Securing resources includes:

- identifying the skill sets and staff needed for scaling.
- determining training needs and develop training workshops and materials.

- assessing if organizational infrastructure for scaling is in place.
- establishing partnerships necessary for scale-up.
- developing implementation guidelines and protocols.
- identifying funding sources and request funding (Milat, Newson, & King, 2014).

Step 4—Scaling-Up. The last step in the scaling process is putting the scale-up plan into action. Implementation is not an end, but rather an ongoing process of organizing, adjusting, and contingency planning. The focus of this step is strengthening organizational capacity, coordinating oversight, monitoring performance and ensuring sustainability. (Milat, Newson, & King, 2014).

• Strengthen partner organizational capacity

The organizations involved in the scale-up will undergo change as they take on new roles and responsibility associated with implementation that may strain their capacity. For instance, the originating organization may relinquish responsibility for program activities to the delivering organizations (Milat, Newson, & King, 2014), or there may be staff resentment because of increased responsibilities without corresponding compensation (Norton & Mittman, 2010).

Partner capacity can be strengthened by:

- identifying changes needed in the delivery organizations.
- determining what actions are needed to ensure the delivery organizations have the knowledge, skills, and systems in place for scaling-up and that they aligned with their values.
- determining which organization will be responsible for ensuring the above (Milat, Newson, & King, 2014).

• Coordinate oversight

Detailed agreements must be established across all organizations involved in the scale-up clarifying how, when, where, and by whom resources will be used (WHO, 2010). Organizations responsible for delivering the program need to determine how to accommodate these responsibilities along with their existing responsibilities. When more than one organization is involved in the scale-up, responsibilities need to be coordinated and information and resources shared across them all. Therefore, it's essential for systems to be in place so information can be shared (Milat, Newson, & King, 2014).

Coordinating oversight across partnering organizations can be supported by:

- setting up action plans and budgets for scale-up.
- allocating responsibilities to participating organizations.
- establishing mechanisms for coordinating scale-up activities.

- Monitor performance

It's important to monitor, evaluate, or track the program's progress and outcomes so adjustments can be made if the intended results are not produced (Milat et al., 2012; WHO, 2010). Evaluation methods should focus on the efficient delivery of the program measuring not only effectiveness, but also reach, fidelity, contextual fit, acceptability, and costs (Milat et al., 2012). It's also necessary to monitor or evaluate for quality improvement purposes and to provide information for key stakeholders, decision makers, and the public (Milat et al., 2012; WHO, 2010).

Evaluation is facilitated by:

- establishing an evaluation system for the scale-up during the planning step.
- establishing a timetable for periodic effectiveness reviews.
- conducting a cost-effectiveness analysis.
- allocating evaluation responsibilities to partnering organizations.
- establishing procedures for documenting progress, lessons learned, and the impact of scaling.

- Using the information gathered from evaluation for quality improvement and adaptations, and as the basis for reports shared with stakeholders and the public.

- Ensure sustainability

The aim of a program is a sustained policy, practice, or behavior change. Achieving this can be difficult when scale-up is confined to a horizontal approach. The expansion and replication of a horizontal scale-up ultimately need to be supported by vertical approaches, which are supported by policy, and realignment of budgets and resources (Milat et al., 2012).

Actions to support program sustainability include:

- identifying and implementing strategies to ensure the program will be sustained.
- using data collected through monitoring to support the case for continued funding and expansion (Milat et al., 2012).

ExpandNet

The ExpandNet framework is a nine-step process for scaling that assumes the feasibility and effectiveness of the program has been tested in the location context and found appropriate and successful in achieving the goals and objectives (WHO, 2010). It's based on four key principles that guide analysis, planning and decision making throughout the nine steps. They are systems thinking, sustainability, scalability and respect for human rights.

- **Systems thinking**

Systems thinking means keeping in mind that expansion and adoption of programs occur in a complex network of interactions and influences. It specifically refers to the interrelationships between the program, the delivery organization, the resource team, and the larger environment within which scaling-up takes place. Change in any one of these affects the others, which means balancing their relationships is a major task in scaling a program (WHO, 2010).

- **Sustainability** keeps attention focused on adoption and integration of the program in policies, program guidelines, budgets, and other aspects of the organization or health system (WHO, 2010).
- **Scalability** entails assessing the program's attributes for ease or difficulty based on the characteristics of the program related to success and through practical experience (WHO, 2010).
- **Respecting human rights** compels attention to human dignity, the needs and rights of vulnerable groups and gender perspectives, as well as promotion of equitable access for all to quality services (WHO, 2010).

Whether the program to be scaled is a new technology, product, practice, or a replacement for something already in use, the following steps can guide the scale-up process (WHO, 2010). The brief description below of the nine steps is summarized from *Nine Steps for Developing a Scaling-Up Strategy* (WHO, 2010). For an in-depth explanation, see http://expandnet.net/tools/

Step 1—Plan Action to Increase Scalability of the Program.
The very first action is to clarify what is going to be scaled-up. Identify exactly what the program is, including all actions or activities used during the initial pilot or research study.

Next, determine the likelihood that the program can be successfully scaled by assessing it against the following set of "CORRECT" characteristics. The more "yes" responses to these characteristics, the better.

Credible—The program is based on sound evidence from pilot testing in a comparable setting as the scale-up.

Observable—The results can be seen.

Relevant—The program addresses the problem.

Relative advantage—The program is better than existing practices and more cost effective.

Easy—The program is simple to set up at the delivery organization with existing resources.

Compatible—The program is compatible with the delivery organization's values and other services.

Testable—The delivery organization can test the program in stages without full adoption.

Step 2—Increase Capacity of Delivery Organization to Implement Scale-Up.
In this step, the delivery organization is identified and the extent of its capacity/resources for scaling is determined by using the following criteria:

- Perceived need

  Does the delivery organization see a need for the program and are people in the organization advocates of it?

- Implementation capacity

  Does the organization have the resources and capacity in terms of skills, training, supervision/leadership, monitoring progress, and human resources, and can it absorb the program without negatively impacting its other services?

- Timing and circumstance

  Are there changes underway at the organization that will impact scale-up either positively or negatively?

Step 3—Assess the Environment and Plan Actions for a Successful Scale-Up.
The environment in this step refers to conditions and organizations external to the delivery organization that affect the scale-up. These include contextual factors such as: the political system, the bureaucratic structure, socioeconomics, culture, healthcare system, human rights, and needs.

Determine what can be done to maximize environmental opportunities and minimize constraints using the following questions as a guide:

– Where are the external supports and constraints?
– Which informal and political connections might be helpful?
– How can advocates be recruited and opponents offset?
– What opportunities and constraints are likely to change with scale-up?
– Are there opportunities for collaboration with similar programs?
– How will the environmental conditions be monitored for changes?

Step 4—Increase Capacity of Resource Team. The resource team in this step refers to the people and organizations committed to implementing the program. Resource teams are more likely to be successful if they have:

effective leaders with authority at the delivery organization.

skills and experience in scale-up.

an understanding of the external environment within which scale-up will occur.

the ability to identify and generate funding.

in-depth understanding of the delivery organization's strengthens and weaknesses.

the capacity to conduct training at the delivery organization.

the capacity to assist the delivery organization with management issues.

the ability to advocate for the program

Availability to provide multiyear support.

To strengthen the resource team:

– include someone on the team who has credibility and authority at the delivery organization.
– identify gaps in needed skills and add members to the team with those skills.

– recruit experienced team members.
– bring the resource team to sites where scale-up has been successful.
– adjust the scope and pace of scaling to match available resources and support.

Step 5—Make Choices to Support Vertical Scaling-Up. Vertical scale-up support refers to the changes and choices related to program adoption at all sites or across a whole system. The following actions can help guide decision making for vertical scale-up:

– identify advocacy approaches appropriate for the changes needed.
– identify actions that can be taken to develop a sense of ownership to support its adoption as a part of routine operations.
– identify the person responsible for organizing the change processes.
– determine the technical support needed for the changes.
– identify ways to link support for the program to national health plans, for example, *Healthy People 2030*.
– determine and prioritize time frames for making needed changes.
– assess availability of resources for advocacy and dissemination initiatives.
– create ways to monitor scale-up.
– select monitoring criteria.

Step 6—Make Choices to Support Horizontal Scale-Up. Horizontal scale-up support refers to changes and choices needed to replicate a program in different sites or in a larger or different population group. The following actions can help guide decision making for horizontal scale-up:

– identify informal channels and relationships useful for garnering support for introducing the program into a new area.
– decide on how information about the program will be shared/communicated.
– ensure communication about the program is clear, concise, and tailored to the intended audience.

- determine the number of sites expected to adopt the program.
- select the expansion period and method—phased in or rapid implementation over what time frame.
- analyze differences between sites, and determine if adaptations are needed.
- decide if partners are needed for scale-up.
- analyze the cost of scale-up for each site, and decide on partnering to defray costs.
- determine if resources are readily available or if they need to be mobilized.
- choose monitoring criteria for establishing the process, outcomes, and impact of implementing the program.

Steps 7 and 8—Determine the Role of Diversification and Plan Actions to Address Spontaneous Scale-Up. These steps are beyond the scope of this chapter. For more information about them, see http://expandnet.net/tools/.

Step 9— Finalize the Scale-Up Strategy and Identify the Next Steps. Creating a plan for scaling takes more than just summing up the various recommendations from the previous steps. It also takes creativity and a vision of what's most important in the setting in the near future, what actions can wait, and what would be ideal, but cannot be accomplished.

To finalize the scale-up plan:

- review the recommended actions under each step, make necessary revisions, and prioritize the actions.
- prepare a table for presentation to the larger group of stakeholders that contains the recommended actions and conveys their priority.
- develop a more specific operational plan, once the basic scale-up plan is agreed upon, that details the activities to be undertaken, by whom, and in what time frame.

The previous steps reflect a process for scaling a program. In working through the steps, challenges to implementation/scaling of the program in the setting should become apparent. The recommended actions in **Table 6-1** may help in overcoming them.

Table 6-1 ExpandNet framework scale-up challenges and recommended actions

Challenge Category	Actions
Program credibility	Bring stakeholders to the pilot site. Test program in settings that differ from the pilot site to assess the feasibility of large-scale expansion.
Program complexity	Consult with developers and key stakeholders to determine if the core elements of the program can be simplified to facilitate expansion.
Delivery organization strengths and weaknesses	Plan initial expansion with a delivery organization that has the advocates, resources, and willingness needed for adoption.
Environmental constraints	Organize workshops and other forums to address concerns of contextual fit within the community.
Resource team	Identify weaknesses, and recruit members with appropriate expertise.
Resource availability	Collaborate with other organizations implementing similar initiatives to benefit from lower costs of buying supplies in quantity.

Data from World Health Organization (WHO). (2010). Nine steps for developing a scale-up strategy. Retrieved from https://www.who.int/reproductive health/publications/strategic_approach/9789241500319/en/

Ethical Challenges

Ethical challenges are dilemmas or situations that require hard choices to be made, of which there are no lack in public health. For example, resource allocation can trigger a dilemma between funding a program that results in small improvements in quality of life for a large portion of the population or a lifesaving program that benefits a few. Efforts to contain the spread of infectious diseases raise difficult questions about using isolation and quarantine for tuberculosis, pandemic Covid-19, and the appropriateness of restricting individual choices to safeguard the welfare of many. The public health threats of noncommunicable diseases, including those caused in part by unhealthy behaviors such as smoking, poor diet, or lack of exercise, raise questions about the extent to which public health authorities should interfere with personal health choices (Coleman, Bouesseau, & Reis, 2008).

When faced with an ethical challenge, decision making is not black and white, but gray. Decisions are neither right nor wrong, but a degree of rightness and wrongness. They're arrived at by utilizing core ethical principles as a framework to guide the decision-making process and provide a way to justify the decisions made (CDC, 2017). (See **Figure 6-8**.)

Ethical or moral principles are the fundamental truths of right or wrong that serve as the foundation for beliefs, behaviors, or reasoning (principle, 2020). Ethical challenges require decisions that balance the actions needed to resolve the dilemma based on reasoning grounded in the core principles of medical ethics (Leadbeater et al., 2018), beneficence, nonmaleficence, autonomy, and justice (Beauchamp & Childress, 2012). (See **Figure 6-9**.)

- Beneficence

Beneficence is the principle concerned with maximizing potential benefits to individuals and society and minimizing potential harms. It entails a moral obligation to help or provide benefits to others (Beauchamp & Childress, 2012) by acting in ways that protect individual welfare and promote the common good (Coughlin, 2008).

- Nonmaleficence

The moral obligation to "do no harm" is the principle of nonmaleficence (Beauchamp, 2003). Whether it's done intentionally or unintentionally because of negligence, disregard,

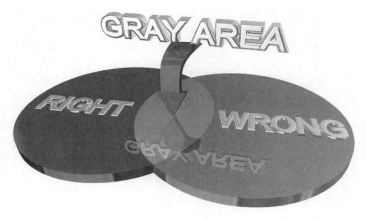

Figure 6-8 Ethical challenges require hard choices
© iQoncept/Shutterstock

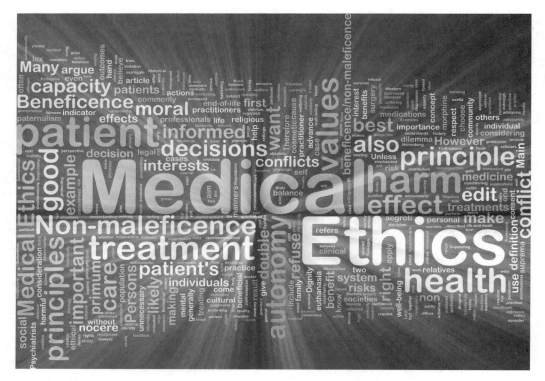

Figure 6-9 Ethical principles
© Kheng Guan Toh/Shutterstock

neglect, or inattention, doing harm is a fundamental moral wrong (Beauchamp, 2003; Beauchamp & Childress, 2012).

- Respect for autonomy

  Respect for autonomy is the ethical principle that focuses on an individual's right of self-determination. It's the obligation to respect the right of others to make their own voluntary decisions (Coughlin, 2008).

- Justice

  The principle of justice is the obligation of fairness in the distribution or sharing of benefits and risks (Beauchamp, 2003). A fair sharing of benefits from a public health program means the program is useful to all those affected by it and that each person has an equal share of its potential benefits. Justice also holds society responsible for correcting inequalities in the distribution of resources, in that those who are least well off should benefit most from what is available (Coughlin, 2008).

The central ethical challenge in public health is balancing respect for autonomy with the responsibility of government to provide citizens with some degree of protection in relation to health (Krebs, 2008). Given this, health promotion programs by their very nature present ethical challenges related to autonomy— freedom of choice and informed consent— because their ultimate aim is to change behavior. This is of special concern in multicultural settings where diverse populations believe in or engage in practices considered "unhealthy" by public health professionals. This can lead to the inadvertent idealization of a particular lifestyle (Guttman, 2017) and unintentional harm.

Ethical Challenges of Scale-Up

When programs are adapted for real-world settings with diverse populations, they present a whole host of ethical challenges that call for balancing activities essential to implementation with the core ethical principles. These challenges are likely to emerge during seven distinct activities related to implementation scale-up, including

- Consulting with stakeholders in selecting a program for implementation.

Ethical challenges can emerge during consultative activities related to balancing the potential for promoting the common good with the interests of the consultant. The ethical principles that come into play here are beneficence, nonmaleficence, autonomy, and conflicts of interest (Leadbeater et al., 2018).

While avoiding conflicts of interest is not cited as an ethical principle, per se, it can be subsumed under the principle of beneficence. Any time decisions are made in an official capacity that are influenced by potential personal gain rather than by what's best for the common good, it's unethical.

- Forming contractual or collaborative relationships for program implementation.

Ethical challenges can emerge in the process of developing relationships with delivery organizations related to balancing the potential for improving public welfare with equitable distribution of resources. The ethical principles that come into play are justice, autonomy, and conflict of interest (Leadbeater et al., 2018).

- Implementing programs that involve vulnerable populations

When working with vulnerable populations (youth, disadvantaged groups, minorities, immigrants, native peoples) the ethical chal-

lenges that can emerge are related to balancing the need for fidelity and access to the population with the need to promote and respect self-determination. The relevant core ethical principles in this situation are autonomy, beneficence, and justice (Leadbeater et al., 2018).

- Adapting programs

When programs are adapted, the ethical challenge is to balance the need for fidelity with the community's needs and resources. The core ethical principles in this situation are justice and autonomy (Leadbeater et al., 2018).

- Accessing publicly available data

Using publicly available sources in the absence of consent presents an ethical challenge of balancing public welfare and access to benefits of research with confidentiality, and self-determination. The applicable core ethical principles in this situation are autonomy and conflict of interest (beneficence) (Leadbeater et al., 2018).

- Building capacity through commercialization

The challenge in building capacity to support implementation and scale-up through profit-making endeavors is balancing the associated activities with the interests of communities, institutions, and public agencies. The relevant ethical principles in these situations are beneficence, conflict of interest, and justice (Leadbeater et al., 2018).

- Facilitating program replication

The ethical challenge of helping groups replicate a program is to balance the interests of the program developers with the public's benefits of replication. In addition to challenges raised by fidelity issues, the applicable core ethical principles in this situation are autonomy and beneficence/conflict of interest (Leadbeater et al., 2018).

Developing an Implementation Plan

Implementation is a complex process that exerts a considerable influence on program outcomes. It involves anticipating, recognizing, and acting in ways to ensure the program is carried out successfully, effectively, and ethically in all settings and populations. This takes planning.

Planning for implementation entails developing an implementation plan, a written document that details the *who, what,* and *when* of the program. Following are three tasks that when completed, produce the information needed for the plan (Johns Hopkins, 2018).

Task 1—Identify Who Is Responsible for What. This first task is to identify *who* among the program partners will take on what roles and responsibilities. To complete this task, the planning committee or the implementation subcommittee does the following:

Reviews the program plan and identify the skills or competencies needed to implement the program, for example, materials development, training, interviewing, and data analysis.

Identifies partners whose staff/employees have the needed skill sets.

Outlines how implementation will be coordinated among the partners by answering the following questions:

- Who will serve as the lead or coordinating agency?
- Who will be the lead person?

- Who will provide oversight of the different aspects of implementation (Johns Hopkins, 2018)?

Task 2—Outline What Tasks are Necessary. The purpose of this task is to outline *what* must be done to implement the program activities. The outline answers the following questions:

- What activities need to be implemented?
- What preliminary steps are needed to ensure the activities can be implemented?
- What is the sequence of the activities?
- What activity will be the responsibility of which partner (Johns Hopkins, 2018)?

Task 3—Determine When Activities Will Occur. With the activities identified and assigned to the partners, this task focuses on establishing a timeline for *when* they'll be implemented. The timeline is established by answering the following questions:

- When is implementation of each activity planned?
- When do activities linked to others in the sequence of activities have to be implemented (Johns Hopkins, 2018)?

Task 4—Create the Plan. Once all the implementation information is gathered, the final task is putting it together to create the implementation plan. **Figure 6-10** is an example of an implementation plan.

Oral Health Awareness Program Implementation Plan	
Lead agency: Office of Dental Health, Anywhere County Health Department	
Lead person: Flossie Dailie, DDS, MPH	
Implementation approach: Vertical scale-up implementation in all dental health clinics in the county.	

Implementation Partners	Expertise
Agency: Department of Public Health, Anywhere State University **Contact person: Heath Proe, PhD** **Department Chairperson**	**Data analysis Strategy development Evaluation Literature review**
Agency: County Dental Association **Contact person: Carrie Toth, DDS** **President**	**Message design Materials development**

Agency: Local health departments
 	
Contact person: Alfie Rogers, Spartaville
       Cooper Janson, Greentree
       Maddie Pettori, Fayette
       Ellie King, Lakeford
       Beth Jamlin, Wickerton
	Data collection Marketing

Activity	Responsible partner	Timeline
Activity 1: **Design potential awareness messages**	**County Dental Association**	**March 1–March 31, 2021**
Preliminary steps/linked activities		
Assess oral health behaviors	Local health departments	October 1–October 31, 2020
Analyze assessment data	Department of Public Health, Anywhere State University	November 1–November 30, 2020
Identify intended audience	All partners	December 10–December 15, 2020
Search literature for successful oral health awareness messages	Department of Public Health, Anywhere State University.	January 15–February 15, 2021
Convey literature search results to County Dental Association	Department of Public Health, Anywhere State University.	February 22–February 28, 2021

Figure 6-10 Sample implementation plan

Data from Johns Hopkins, Center for Communication Programs. (2018). Implementation plan. Retrieved March 13, 2020, from https://sbccimplementationkits.org/lessons/step-6-implementation-plan/
American Association for Community Dental Programs. (n.d.). A guide for developing and enhancing community oral health programs. Retrieved March 15, 2020, from https://www.aacdp.com/Guide/step4_1.html

(continues)

Activity 2: Conduct focus groups with intended audience to test potential messages.	Local health departments	April 15–May 15, 2021
Preliminary steps/linked activities		
Identify potential focus group members in each municipality	Local health departments	March 1–March 22, 2021
Locate and secure sites to conduct focus groups	Local health departments	March 1–March 22, 2021
Invite potential focus group members	Local health departments	March 23–April 1, 2021
Activity 3: Select awareness message	All partners	June 25–June 30, 2021
Preliminary steps/linked activities		
Analyze focus group data	Department of Public Health, Anywhere State University	May 15–June 15, 2021
Prepare analysis report for partners	Department of Public Health, Anywhere State University	June 15–June 22, 2021

Figure 6-10 (Continued)

Chapter Summary

Successful implementation depends on modifying impeding characteristics of the program, community, organizations, and providers; addressing ethical and other challenges related to fidelity, contextual fit, and scaling; and having a plan to carry out the program actions and activities.

Planning in Practice Chapter Activity

A well-planned, poorly implemented program is destined to fail. A poorly planned, poorly implemented program is certain to fail. Identifying and addressing planning weaknesses and implementation challenges is critical for program success.

To demonstrate this, read the following article and answer the questions below.

Article: *Going to scale: Design and implementation challenges of a program to increase access to skilled birth attendants in Nigeria* (Okeke et al., 2017).

Link to article: https://www.ncbi.nlm.nih.gov/pmc/articles/PMC5437674/

Article Questions

1. What needs assessment data indicated there was a need for this program in Nigeria?

2. What was the main objective (goal) of the Midwives Service Scheme?

3. What were the programmatic strategies for addressing the issue?
4. How was the program funded?
5. What criteria did a primary (local) health clinic (PHC) have to meet to participate in the implementation of this program and have midwives assigned to it?
6. What program and implementation weaknesses contributed to the program's failure?
7. Choose one of the implementation issues you identified in question 6, and suggest what might have been done to prevent it from negatively impacting the program.
8. What recommendations did the authors make for improving this program?
9. Although not explicitly stated in the article, which scale-up approach was used to implement this program? Provide evidence to support your response.
10. How might the use of a different scaling approach have benefited the implementation of this program?

References

Araya, R., Alvarado, R., Sepulveda, R., & Rojas, G. (2012). Lessons from scaling up a depression treatment program in primary care in Chile. *Pan American Journal of Public Health*, 32(3), 234–240. Retrieved April 17, 2019, from https://scielosp.org/article/rpsp/2012.v32n3/234-240/en/

Bach-Mortensen, A. M., Lange, B. C. L., & Montgomery, P. (2018). Barrier and facilitators to implementing evidence-based programs among third sector organizations: A systematic review. *Implementation Science*, 13(103).

Beauchamp, T. L. (2003). Methods and principles in biomedical ethics. *Journal of Medical Ethics*, 29(5), 269–274. doi: 10.1136/jme.29.5.269. Retrieved April 28, 2019, from https://www.ncbi.nlm.nih.gov/pmc/articles/PMC1733784/

Beauchamp, T. L., & Childress, J. F. (2012). *Principles of biomedical ethics* (7th ed.). New York, NY: Oxford University Press.

Bevington, F. (2014). NACCHO's 2013 national profile of local health departments show continued funding cuts for preparedness. Retrieved March 16, 2020, from http://nacchopreparedness.org/nacchos-2013-national-profile-of-local-health-departments-shows-continued-funding-cuts-for-preparedness/

Bonde, A. H., Stjernqvst, N. W., Sabinski, M. S., & Maindal, H. T. (2018). Process evaluation of implementation fidelity in a Danish health-promoting school program. *BMC Public Health*, 18. https://doi.org/10.1186/s12889-018-6289-5. Retrieved March 21, 2019, from https://bmcpublichealth.biomedcentral.com/articles/10.1186/s12889-018-6289-5

Breitenstein, S.M., Gross, D., Garvey, C.A., Hill, C., Fogg, L., & Resnick, B. (2010). Implementation fidelity in community-based interventions. *Research in Nursing & Health*, 33(2), 164–173. https://doi.org/10.1002/nur.20373

Carroll, C., Patterson, M., Wood, S., Booth, A., Rick, J., & Balain, S. (2007). A conceptual framework for implementation fidelity. *Implementation Science*, 2(40). doi: 10.1186/1748-5908-2-40. Retrieved March 26, 2019, from http://www.implementationscience.com/content/2/1/40

Carvalho, M., Honeycutt, S., Escoffery, C., Glanz, K., Sabbs, D., & Kegler, M. C. (2013). Balancing fidelity and adaptation: Implementing evidence-based chronic disease prevention programs. *Journal of Public Health Management Practice*, 19(4), 348–356. doi: 10.1097/PHH.0b013e31826d80eb

Centers for Disease Control and Prevention (CDC). (2013). Public health financing. Retrieved March 16, 2020, from https://www.cdc.gov/publichealthgateway/docs/finance/Public_Health_Financing-6-17-13.pdf

Centers for Disease Control and Prevention (CDC), Office of Science. (2017). Public health ethics. Retrieved March 17, 2020, from https://www.cdc.gov/os/integrity/phethics/index.htm

Chaskin, R. J. (2001). Building community capacity: A definitional framework and case studies from a comprehensive community initiative. *Urban Affairs Review* 36(3), 291–323. https://doi-org.ezproxy.wpunj.edu/10.1177%2F10780870122184876

Coleman, C. H., Bouesseau, M. C., & Reis, H. (2008). The contribution of ethics to public health. *Bulletin of the World Health Organization*, 86(8), 577–656. Retrieved May 6, 2019, from https://www.who.int/bulletin/volumes/86/8/08-055954/en/

Coughlin, S. S. (2008). How many principles for public health ethics? *Open Public Health*, 1(1), 8–16. doi: 10.2174/1874944500801010008. Retrieved April 28, 2019, from https://www.ncbi.nlm.nih.gov/pmc/articles/PMC2804997/

Cresswell, K. M., Bates, D. W., & Sheikh, A. (2013). Ten key considerations for the successful implementation and adoption of large-scale health information technology. *Journal of the American Medical Information Association*, 20(e 1), e 9–e 13. doi: 10.1136/amiajnl-2013-001684 Retrieved March 20, 2019, from https://www.ncbi.nlm.nih.gov/pmc/articles/PMC3715363/

Dane, A. V., & Schneider, B. H. (1998). Program integrity in primary and early secondary prevention: Are implementation effects out of control? *Clinical Psychological Review*, 18(1), 23–45. https://doi.org/10.1016/S0272-7358(97)00043-3

Day, L., Trotter, M. J., Donaldson, A., Hill, K. D., & Finch, C. F. (2016). Key factors influencing implementation of falls prevention exercise programs in the community. *Journal of Aging and Physical Activity*, 24, 45–52. http://dx.doi.org/10.1123/japa.2014-0143

Durlak, J. A. (2013). The importance of quality implementation for research, practice and policy. Office of Human Services Policy, U.S. Department of Health and Human Services, *ASPE Research Brief*. Retrieved March 7, 2019, from https://www.researchgate.net/publication/239950487_Why_Program_Implementation_is_Important

Durlak, J. A., & DuPre, E. A. (2008). Implementation matters: A review of research on the influence of implementation on program outcomes and the factors affecting implementation. *American Journal of Community Psychology*, 41, 327–350. doi: 10.1007/s10464-008-9165-0

Edwards, R. W., Jumper-Thurman, P., Plested, B. A., Oetting, E. R., & Swanson, L. (2000). Community readiness: Research to practice. *Journal of Community Psychology*, 28(3), 291–307. doi: https://doi.org/10.1002/(SICI)1520-6629(200005)28:3<291::AID-JCOP5>3.0.CO;2-9

Einav, S., Kaufman, N., & Varon, J. (2018). Barriers to effective in-hospital resuscitation: Lessons learned during implementation of a hospital wide code system. *Critical Care & Shock*, 21(3), 128–139. Retrieved March 18, 2019, from http://criticalcareshock.org/2018/08/barriers-effective-hospital-resuscitation-lessons-learned-implementation-hospital-wide-code-system/

Elliot, D. S., & Mihalic, S. (2004). Issues in disseminating and replicating effective prevention programs. *Prevention Science*, 5(1), 47–53. Retrieved March 18, 2019, from https://link.springer.com/article/10.1023/B:PREV.0000013981.28071.52

Fixsen, D. L., Naoom, S. F., Blasé, K. A., Friedmann, R. M., & Wallace, F. (2005). *Implementation research: A synthesis of the literature*. Tampa, FL: University of South Florida, Louis de la Parte Florida Mental Health Institute, The National Implementation Research Network (FMHI Publication #231). Retrieved March 8, 2019, from https://nirn.fpg.unc.edu/resources/implementation-research-synthesis-literature

Frieden, T. R. (2014). Six components necessary for effective public health program implementation. *American Journal of Public Health* 104(1), 17–22. https://dx.doi.org/10.2105%2FAJPH.2013.301608

Gaitan-Rossi, P., Lobato, S. D. C., Navarro, A. C. P., Esteva, A. A., Garcia, M. R. V., & Vilar-Compte, M. (2019). Fidelity of implementation of Prospera Digital: Evaluation of a multi-site *mHealth* program aimed at improving maternal health outcomes in Mexico. *Current Development in Nutrition*, 3(10). Retrieved from https://doi.org/10.1093/cdn/nzz107

Graham, T. (2018). How to scale up social impact—the challenge of the 21st century. Apolitical Group Limited. Retrieved April 19, 2019, from https://apolitical.co/solution_article/how-to-scale-up-social-impact/

Guttman, N. (2017). Ethical issues in health promotion and communication programs. *Oxford Research Encyclopedias*, doi: 10.1093/acrefore/9780190228613.013.11. Retrieved April 25, 2019, from http://oxfordre.com/communication/view/10.1093/acrefore/9780190228613.001.0001/acrefore-9780190228613-e-118

Hayes, C. B., O'Shea, M. P., Foley-Nolan, C., McCarthy, M., & Harrington, J. M. (2019). Barriers and facilitators to adoption, implementation and sustainment of obesity prevention programs in school children. *BMC Public Health*, 19(198), https://doi.org/10.1186/s12889-018-6368-7. Retrieved April 3, 2019, from https://bmcpublichealth.biomedcentral.com/articles/10.1186/s12889-018-6368-7

Horner, R., Blitz, C., , & Ross, S. W. (2014). The importance of contextual fit when implementing evidence-based programs. *U.S. Department of Health and Human Services, Office of Human Service Policies, ASPE Brief*. Retrieved April 3, 2019, from https://aspe.hhs.gov/report/importance-contextual-fit-when-implementing-evidence-based-programs/what-contextual-fit

Johns Hopkins, Center for Communication Programs. (2018). Implementation plan. Retrieved March 13, 2020, from https://sbccimplementationkits.org/lessons/step-6-implementation-plan/

Johnson, D., Juras, R., Riley, P., Chatterji, M., Sloane, P., Choi, S. K., … Johns, B. (2017). A randomized controlled trial of the impact of a family planning mHealth service on knowledge and use of contraception. *Contraception*, 95(1), 90–97. doi: 10.1016/j.contraception.2016.07.009.

Klimes-Dougan, B., August, G. J., Lee, S. C., Realmuto, G. M., Bloomquist, M. L., Horowitz, J. L., & Eisenberg, T. L. (2009). Practitioner and site characteristics that relate to fidelity of implementation: The earlier riser prevention program in a going-to-scale program trial. *Professional Psychology: Research and Practice*, 40(5), 467–475. doi: 10.1037/a0014623

Kramer, B. J., Cote, S. D., Lee, D. I., Creekmur, B., & Sal-iba, D. (2017). Barriers and facilitators to implemen-tation of VA home-based primary care on American Indian reservations: A qualitative multi-case study. *Implementation Science, 12*(109). doi: 10.1186/s13012 -017-0632-6. Retrieved April 8, 2019, from https:// www.ncbi.nlm.nih.gov/pmc/articles/PMC5581481/

Krebs, J. (2008). The importance of public health ethics. *Bulletin of the World Health Organization, 86*(8). Retrieved April 26, 2019, from https://www.who.int /bulletin/volumes/86/8/08-052431/en/

Leadbeater, B. J., Dishion, T., Sandler, I., Bradshaw, C. P., Dodge, K., Gottfredson, D., … Smith, E. P. (2018). Ethical challenges in promoting the implementation of preventive programs: Report of the SPR Task Force. *Prevention Science, 19*(7), 853–865. doi: 10.1007/ s11121-018-0912-7. Retrieved April 26, 2019, from https://www.ncbi.nlm.nih.gov/pubmed/29936579

L'Engle, K., Plourde, K. F., & Zan, T. (2017). Evi-dence-based adaptation and scale-up of a mobile phone health information service. *mHealth, 3*(11), doi: 10.21037/mhealth.2017.02.06. Retrieved April 18, 2019, from https://www.ncbi.nlm.nih.gov/pmc /articles/PMC5427190/

Lester, P. (2018). Policy drivers: Putting the politics back in implementation. Retrieved March 11, 2020, from http://www.socialinnovationcenter.org/archives /3012

Li, S. A., Jeffs, L., Barwick, M., & Stevens, B. (2018). Organizational contextual features that influence the implementation of evidence-based practices across health care settings: A systematic integrative review. *Systematic Reviews, 7*(72), https://doi.org/10.1186/s13 643-018-0734-5

Mihalic, S. (2002). *The importance of implementation fidel-ity.* Center for the Prevention of Violence. Retrieved March 19, 2020, from http://www.incredibleyears .com/wp-content/uploads/fidelity-importance.pdf

Milat, A. J., King, L., Bauman, A. E., & Redman, S. (2012). The concept of scalability: Increasing the potential adoption of health promotion into policy and prac-tice. *Health Promotion International, 28*(3), 285–298. doi: 10.1093/heapro/dar097. Retrieved April 11, 2019, from https://academic.oup.com/heapro/article/28 /3/285/633262

Milat, A. J., Newson, R., & King, L. (2014). Increasing the scale of population health programs: A guide. Sydney: New South Wales Ministry of Health. Retrieved April 11, 2019, from http://www.health. nsw.gov.au/research/Publications/scalability-guide.pdf

Milat, A. J., Newson, R., King, L., Rissel, C., Wolfenden, C., Bauman, A., Redman, S., & Griffin, M. (2016). A guide to scaling up population health programs. *Public Health Research Practice, 26*(1). http://dx.doi. org/10.17061/phrp261. Retrieved April 17, 2019,

from http://www.phrp.com.au/issues/January-2016 -volume-26-issue-1/a-guide-to-scaling-up-popula tion-health-interventions/

Milat A. J., Newson, R., Wolfenden, L., Rissel, C., Bau-man, A., & Redman, S. (2014). Increasing the scale and adoption of population health program: Experi-ences and perspectives of policy makers, practitioners and researchers. *Health Research Policy and Systems, 12*(18). doi: 10.1186/1478-4505-12-18

Monzalve, M. (2016). *Examining the relationship between contextual fit and implementation fidelity on behavior support plans and student outcomes.* (Unpublished doc-toral dissertation). University of Oregon, Eugene, OR. Retrieved April 3, 2019, from https://scholarsbank .uoregon.edu/xmlui/handle/1794/20684

Muthaura, M. K., & Omwenga, J. (2017). Factors influ-encing implementation of projects in community based organizations in Kenya: A case of child regional education support services. *International Journal of Scientific and Research Publications, 7*(6), 576–587. Retrieved March 13, 2019, from http://www.ijsrp.org /research-paper-0617.php?rp=P666526

Mwaria, M., Chen, C. C., Coppola, N., Maurice, I., & Phifer, M. (2016). A culturally responsive approach to improving replication of a youth sexual health pro-gram. *Health Promotion Practice, 17*(6), 781–792. https://doi.org/10.1177%2F1524839916667382

Nathan, N., Wiggers, J., Wyse, R., Williams, C. M., Sutherland, R., Yoong, S. L., … Wolfenden, L. (2017). Factors associated with the implementation of a vege-table and fruit program in a population of Australian elementary schools. *Health Education Research, 32*(2), 194–205. https://doi.org/10.1093/her/cyx038

National Association of Counties (NACo). (2019). Protect funding for core public health services and prevention programs. Retrieved March 16, 2020, from https:// www.naco.org/resources/protect-funding-core-local -public-health-services-and-prevention-programs

Norton, W. E., & Mittman, B. S. (2010). Scaling-up health promotion/disease prevention programs in community settings: Barriers, facilitators, and initial recommenda-tions. Report submitted to Patrick and Catherine Wel-don Donaghue Medical Research Foundation. Retrieved April 22, 2019, from https://www.donaghue.org/wp-content/uploads/Final-Scaling-Up-Report.pdf

Payne, A. A., & Eckert, R. (2010). The relative importance of provider, program, school, and community predic-tors of implementation quality of school based pre-vention programs. *Prevention Science, 11*(2), 126–141. doi: 10.1007/s11121-009-0157-6

PEW Charitable Trust. (2016). Implementation oversight for evidence-based programs. Retrieved March 8, 2019, from https://www.pewtrusts.org/en/research -and-analysis/issue-briefs/2016/05/implemen tation-oversight-for-evidence-based-programs

Pettigrew, J., Graham, J.W., Miller-Day, M., Hecht, M.L., Krieger, J.L., & Shin, Y.J. (2015). Adherence and delivery: Implementation quality and program outcomes for the 7th grade keepin it REAL program. *Prevention Science, 16*(1), 90–99. https://dx.doi.org/10.1007%2Fs11121-014-0459-1

principle. (2020). in Lexico.com. Retrieved March 17, 2020, from https://www.lexico.com/en/definition/principle

Ravasi, D., & Schultz, M. (2006). Responding to organizational identity threats: Exploring the role of organizational culture. *Academy of Management Journal, 49*(3), 433–458. doi: 10.2307/20159775

Rogers, E. M. (2003). *Diffusion of innovation.* New York, NY: Free Press.

Rojatz, D., Merchant, A., & Nitsch, M. (2017). Factors influencing workplace health promotion intervention: A qualitative systematic review. *Health Promotion International 32*(5), https://doi.org/10.1093/heapro/daw015

Rural Health Information Hub (RHIhub). (n.d.). Common implementation challenges. Retrieved March 22, 2019, from https://www.ruralhealthinfo.org/toolkits/rural-toolkit/3/implementation-challenges

Saldana, l. (2014). The stages of implementation completion for evidence-based practice: Protocol for a mixed methods study. *Implementation Science 9*(43). Retrieved March 12, 2019, from http://www.implementationscience.com/content/9/1/43

Schaap, R., Bessems, K., Otten, R., Kremers, S., & van Nassau, F. (2018). Measuring implementation fidelity of school-based obesity prevention programmes: A systematic review. *International Journal of Behavioral Nutrition and Physical Activity, 15*(1). https://doi.org/10.1186/s12966-018-0709-x. Retrieved March 26, 2019, from https://ijbnpa.biomedcentral.com/articles/10.1186/s12966-018-0709-x

Slocum, T. A., Detrich, R., Wilczynski, S. M., Spencer, T. D., Lewis, T., & Wolfe, K. (2014). The evidence-based practice of applied behavior analysis. *Behavioral Analysis, 37*(1), 412–56. doi: 10.1007/s40614-014-0005-2. Retrieved April 4, 2019, from https://www.ncbi.nlm.nih.gov/pmc/articles/PMC4883454/

Stith, S., Pruitt, I., Dees, J., Fronce, M., Green, N., Som, A., & Linkh, D. (2006). Implementing community based prevention programing: A review of the literature. *The Journal of Primary Prevention, 27*(6), 599–617. doi: 10.1007/s10935-006-0062-8.

Sullivan, G. M., & Feinn, R. (2012). Using effect size—or why the P value is not enough. *Journal of Graduate Medical Education, 4*(3), 279–282. doi: 10.4300/JGME-D-12-00156.1 Retrieved April 15, 2019, from https://www.ncbi.nlm.nih.gov/pmc/articles/PMC3444174/

Sullivan, J. L., Adjognon, O. L., Engle, R. L., Shin, M. H., Afable, M. K., Rudin, W., White, B., ... VanDusen Lukas, C. (2018). Identifying and overcoming implementation challenges: Experience of 59 non-institutional long term care services and support pilot programs in the Veterans Health Administration. *Health Care Management Review, 43*(3), 193–205. doi: 10.1097/HMR.0000000000000152. Retrieved April 8, 2019, from https://www.ncbi.nlm.nih.gov/pmc/articles/PMC5991173/

Trust for America's Health (TFAH). (2017). A funding crisis for public health and safety: State by state public health funding and key health facts. Retrieved March 14, 2020, from https://www.tfah.org/report-details/a-funding-crisis-for-public-health-and-safety-state-by-state-public-health-funding-and-key-health-facts-2017/

Trust for America's Health (TFAH). (2019). The impact of chronic underfunding of America's public health system: Trends, risks and recommendations. Retrieved March 16, 2020, from https://www.tfah.org/report-details/2019-funding-report/

Waller, G., Finch, T., Giles, E. L., & Newbury-Birch, D. (2017). Exploring the factors affecting the implementation of tobacco and substance abuse use interventions within a secondary school setting: A systematic review. *Implementation Science 12*(130). https://doi.org/10.1186/s13012-017-0659-8

Wandersman, A., Chien, A. H., & Katz, J. (2012). Toward an evidence-based system for innovation support for implementing innovations with quality: Tools, training, technical assistance, and quality assurance/quality improvement. *American Journal of Community Psychology 50.* 445–459. Retrieved from http://dx.doi.org.ezproxy.wpunj.edu/10.1007/s10464-012-9530-x

Wang, B. A., Stanton, B., Deveaux, L., Poitier, M., Lunn, S., Koci, V., ... Rolle, G. (2015). Factors influencing implementation dose and fidelity thereof and related student outcomes of an evidence-based national HIV prevention program. *Implementation Science, 10*(44). doi: 10.1186/s13012-015-0236-y. Retrieved March 21, 2019, from https://implementationscience.biomedcentral.com/articles/10.1186/s13012-015-0236-y

Wanjiru, N., Kabara, S., & Milimo, J. (2016). Factors affecting implementation of evidence based practice among physiotherapists in MOI teaching referral hospital, Kenya. *International Journal of Physiotherapy, 3*(3), 267–272. doi: 10.15621/ijphy/2016/v3i3/100825

White, R., Delgado, B., & Severens, L. (2018). Scaling up, scaling out: Lessons from Goodwill of Central and

Southern Indiana and nurse-family partnership. Retrieved April 17, 2019, from https://community actionpartnership.com/external_resources/scaling -up-scaling-out-lessons-from-goodwill-of-central- and-southern-indiana-and-nurse-family-partnership/

World Health Organization (WHO). (2010). *Nine steps for developing a scaling-up strategy.* Geneva, Switzerland: World Health Organization. Retrieved April 12, 2019, from https://www.who.int /reproductivehealth/publications/strategic_approach /9789241500319/en/

World Health Organization (WHO). (2011). ExpandNet. Beginning with the end in mind: Planning pilot projects and other programmatic research for successful scaling up. Geneva, Switzerland: World Health Organization. Retrieved April 18, 2019, from https://www .who.int/reproductivehealth/publications/strategic _approach/9789241502320/en/

CHAPTER 7

Evaluating

STUDENT LEARNING OUTCOMES

As a result of reading this chapter, the student will be able to:

- Differentiate between formative and summative evaluation.
- Discuss the different evaluation designs.
- Explain sampling methods.
- Develop an evaluation plan and timeline.
- Write an evaluation report

Introduction

If the thought of evaluation is daunting, keep in mind that you've had years of experience with it. In every grade in grammar school, middle school, and high school, you took quizzes, tests, exams, and completed assignments. At the end of every school year, you received grades based on how well you performed on those quizzes, tests, exams, and assignments. Those grades reflected the extent to which you met the goals of the course. They were "evaluations."

What Is Evaluation?

Evaluation is *"an assessment, as systematic and impartial as possible, of an activity, project, program, strategy, policy, topic, theme, sector, operational area, or institutional performance. It analyses* the level of achievement of both expected and unexpected results by examining the results chain, processes, contextual factors and causality using appropriate criteria such as relevance, effectiveness, efficiency, impact and sustainability" (United Nations Evaluation Group [UNEG], 2016, p. 7). Evaluation is a process for collecting, analyzing, and interpreting data to determine the effectiveness and efficiency of a program (Centers for Disease Control and Prevention [CDC], 2019) used to find out if a program did what it was intended to do, and if resources were used wisely (CDC, 2012a).

In addition, evaluation is used to:

- Detect unexpected program outcomes.
- Judge if what was done, was supposed to be done.
- Ascertain how the program can be improved.
- Document behavior changes over time.

- Resolve implementation barriers and refine delivery, if needed.
- Meet accountability requirements of funders and other stakeholders.
- Contribute to the scientific basis of public health programs.
- Shape future resource allocation.
- Advise policy decisions.
- Judge a program's merit, worth, and significance (Capwell, Butterfloss, & Francisco, 2000; Center for Community Health and Development [CCHD] 2018a; CDC, 2012a, 2019; Gargani & Miller, 2016; Metz, 2007; Murray, Aylward, Cooke, Martin, & Sidford, n.d.; Spiegelman, 2016; Substance Abuse and Mental Health Services Administration [SAMHSA] 2012; UNEG, 2016; World Health Organization [WHO], 2013).

Evaluation is an essential part of public health program planning. Without it we run the risk of either wasting valuable resources on ineffective programs or, perhaps even worse, continue practices that do more harm than good, sometimes for years (Vaughan, 2004). Case in point is abstinence only education.

In 1981 the U.S. federal government began funding programs that promoted abstinence, specifically chastity and self-discipline, to reduce teen pregnancy rates (Santelli et al., 2017). In 1996, there was a major expansion in federal support to states for establishing abstinence only education programs. Abstinence only education was defined as an educational or motivational program with the *exclusive* purpose of teaching the social, psychological, and health gains to be realized by abstaining from sexual activity specifically that:

- abstinence from sexual activity outside marriage is the expected standard for all school-aged children,
- abstinence from sexual activity is the only certain way to avoid out-of-wedlock pregnancy, sexually transmitted diseases, and other associated health problems,

- a mutually faithful monogamous relationship in the context of marriage is the expected standard of human sexual activity,
- sexual activity outside of marriage is likely to have harmful psychological and physical effects,
- bearing children out-of-wedlock is likely to have harmful consequences for the child, the child's parents, and society (Social Security Administration, 1996).

Multiple evaluations of these programs over decades found they were ineffective; they just didn't work. They didn't prevent pregnancy, and they didn't prevent sexually transmitted infections. Despite this, they continue to have considerable political support from some groups (Santelli et al., 2017) and financial support from the federal government of over $2.1 billion between 1982 and 2019 (Sexuality Information and Education Council of the United States [SIECUS], 2018). However, by 2009 nearly half the states in the United States stopped applying for funding for these programs precisely because evaluation findings showed they didn't work (SIECUS, 2018).

The evaluation process serves four other functions: accountability, organizational learning, knowledge generation, and relationship building (United Nations Office on Drugs and Crime [UNODC], 2017).

Accountability

Evaluation provides evidence to demonstrate fiscally responsible management of funds, goal attainment, and service delivery, as promised, and quantifies the "return on investment" or program impact relative to the use of public resources (U.S. Department of Energy, n.d.) and establishes the extent of program compliance with polices and plans (UNODC, 2017).

It also provides answers to the following accountability-related questions:

– *What are the planners trying to accomplish with the program?*

- *Are the planners taking the right actions to accomplish it?*
- *How will the planners know if/when they accomplish it?*
- *Do the results of the program justify the cost?*
- *Are there ways to reduce costs (SAMHSA, 2012)?*

Organizational Learning

Evaluation provides evidence for determining whether the delivery organization is doing the right things and doing them the right way in order to establish what works, what doesn't work, and why; verify the extent to which intended and unintended results occurred and their impact on stakeholders; and make recommendations and compile lessons learned for improving program effectiveness and efficiency (UNODC, 2017; U.S. Department of Energy, n.d.).

It also provides answers to the following questions related to organizational learning:

- *Is the program working as it was intended?*
- *Is it the right program to address the problem?*
- *Are any changes needed before the program can continue or be replicated elsewhere?*
- *Are the planners doing what they said they would do?*
- *Are there program effects that were neither intended nor anticipated (SAMHSA, 2012)?*

Knowledge Generation

Evaluation produces information about innovative practices and specific topics that is shared with stakeholders and the organization(s) involved (UNODC, 2017).

It answers the following questions related to knowledge generation:

- *Would other organizations be able to implement the program?*
- *Does the information generated and lessons learned contribute to the body of knowledge about what works and what doesn't work (SAMHSA, 2012)?*

Relationship Building

By providing opportunities for stakeholders to discuss the evaluation with each other, it helps build relationships between stakeholders, which increases their understanding of each other's needs. This fosters chances for future collaboration (UNODC, 2017), provides stakeholders with a better understanding of the program and its outcomes, and energizes program supporters and wins over program critics (SAMHSA, 2012).

Types of Evaluation

Evaluation is an umbrella term for the process of data collection, analysis, and interpretation done throughout the course of a program to assess different aspects of its efficiency and effectiveness. Under the evaluation umbrella are two general types, formative and summative.

As the name implies, formative evaluations are done while the program is being formed. Summative evaluation is done after the program is implemented, as in a summary of its effects.

Formative Evaluation

Formative evaluations are done early in the planning and implementation stages. They focus on determining the feasibility and appropriateness of the program, materials and procedures (Salabarria-Pina, Apt, & Walsh, 2007; Smith & Ory, 2014). Two formative evaluation are needs assessment and process evaluation.

Needs Assessment

A needs assessment is a systematic way of finding the gaps between "what is" and "what should be" (Kaufman, 1988) and prioritizing what can be done to fill the gap and meet the need. It's a method for collecting information that's crucial for identifying what the most pressing problems are and for whom, guiding decision making in the course of developing a program, and then serving as baseline data for determining how effective the program was in meeting the needs and solving the problem (Watkins, West Meiers, & Visser, 2012). This topic is discussed further in Chapter 4.

Process Evaluation

Process evaluation, also called implementation evaluation, is done during the implementation stage of a program. It focuses on *how* the program is being implemented, the process, the nuts and bolts of putting it into action, and the effects of this on the overall success of the program.

Think of the program as a bookcase. Imagine the bookcase came in pieces and you put it together. How you put it together determined if your efforts were successful when you were done, that is—if it held your books. So, you opened the box, took out the pieces, read the instruction sheet, and sprang into action. Did you follow the instructions exactly? Did you put it together the way it was intended to be put together? Did you use the right screwdriver? Did you use all the screws? Did you put the support brackets in the right place? Did you use a level to make sure the shelves were straight? When you finished putting the bookcase together, did it hold your books as you expected? If not, why not? Is it that the bookcase was poorly designed, or is it that you have a few loose screws, or maybe a missing support bracket, or the shelves are slanted? *How* you put the bookcase together is the problem, not the bookcase itself. This is what process evaluation is all about—how a program is put into action and how it affects the program results.

Conducting a Process Evaluation. Just as a needs assessment takes planning, so does a process evaluation. Following are six general steps to guide this endeavor.

- Step 1—Form a committee

The first task in a process evaluation is to form a committee that consists of stakeholders as well as staff, preferably with some evaluation experience. The first order of business for the committee is to decide who will conduct the evaluation, an internal staff person or an external consultant (Bowie & Bronte-Tinkew, 2008). There are pros and cons to each of these. **Table 7-1** presents some of them. (See Chapter 3—Preparing to Plan.)

If the committee decides to conduct the evaluation using internal staff, hiring an external evaluation consultant should be considered to serve in an advisory capacity. While this is an added expense, it's less than if the consultant has full control over the evaluation. For example, in an advisory capacity, the consultant might make recommendations on data collection methods and instruments, interpreting statistics, and proofing reports (Health Assessment and Research for Communities [HARC], 2016), but not be involved in doing any of the work.

- Step 2—Describe the program

The process evaluation begins with a complete description of the program, including the purpose, underlying theory, objectives, and strategies that together are expected to produce the intended outcomes (Bertrand, 2006; Moore et al., 2014; Saunders, Evans, & Joshi, 2005).

Although this information may seem redundant, it's essential that everyone involved in the evaluation understands what is being done, how, and why. This is especially important if an outside consultant is conducting the evaluation. (See **Figure 7-1**.)

- Step 3—Describe acceptable program delivery

In this step, how each strategy and activity should be delivered is described in detail regarding fidelity, dose (delivered and received), and reach (Linnan & Steckler, 2002; Saunders et al., 2005). Also described are acceptable staff performance associated with the program and required for delivering program-related products.

Table 7-1 Pros and cons of internal staff versus external consultants

	Internal Staff		External Consultant	
	Pro	**Con**	**Pro**	**Con**
Cost	Less expensive No commuting, travel, parking fees			More expensive Commuting/travel/ parking fees extra
Learning curve	No learning curve No orientation or time needed for program explanation			Learning curve Needs orientation and explanation of program
Collaboration	Doesn't require developing working relationship with another team of people Decreased chance of miscommunication			Requires developing a working, collaborative relationship with a new group of people Increased chance of miscommunication
Expertise		Subject matter expert, not evaluation expert Increased risk of making basic mistakes	Evaluation expert from years of experience and educational preparation	
Objectivity		Perceived lack of objectivity or impartiality Results seen as biased not objective	Results seen as objective, impartial and taken more seriously	
Perspective		Too close to the program to see emerging issues or changes	Outside perspective allows for changes and issues to be seen	

Data from: Heath Assessment and Research for Communities. (2016). Internal vs external evaluation—pros and cons. Retrieved June 25, 2019, from https://harcdata.org/internal-vs-external-evaluation/

Media Matters is a school-based program developed to reduce adolescent risk behaviors through enabling understanding of how media work to construct reality, create meaning, and influence behavior. Based on Bandura's (1986) Social Cognitive Theory (SCT), the Media Matters curriculum focuses on self-efficacy, behavioral capability, and observational learning to increase student self-efficacy in their ability to deconstruct media messages to become more critically aware of and resistant to the unhealthy behaviors often reinforces. The primary objectives of Media Matters are to increase self-efficacy for abstaining from alcohol and tobacco use and to influence the social norms within the school environment so that alcohol and tobacco consumption are viewed as unhealthy choices. To this end, the program provides a venue for students to create their own messages to influence the social norms for behaviors and issues with which they are directly involved. The classroom strategies include small group work, demonstration and feedback, problem solving, and role playing.

Figure 7-1 Example of process evaluation program description

Reproduced from: Saunders, R.P., Evans. M. H., & Joshi, P. (2005) Developing a process evaluation plan for assessing health program implementation: A how to guide. *Health Promotion Practice*, 6(2), 134–147. doi: 10.1177/1524839904273387

- Step 4—Develop questions

Since a process evaluation provides insight into a program's implementation, in this step the committee clarifies the aim of the evaluation and develops questions about context, fidelity, dose, delivery, reach, and recruitment (Linnan & Steckler, 2002).

Clarifying the purpose of the evaluation is important. Not only will it determine the evaluation questions, but also the type of data needed and the methods used to collect them (Bowie & Bronte-Tinkew, 2008).

Considering that it's easy to get carried away with developing questions, and usually not possible to answer all of them, it's best to identify and prioritize the most important ones (Moore et al., 2014), specifically those that address reach, dose, and fidelity. See examples of process evaluation questions in **Table 7-2**. (See Chapter 4, Assessing, for details on a process for prioritizing.)

- Step 5—Determine data collection methods

Process evaluations are primarily conducted using qualitative methods (Boor & Woods, 2006), although sometimes quantitative methods are, too (Schneider et al., 2009). When both methods are used, it's referred to as mixed methods.

Qualitative methods used for process evaluation include observations, structured interviews, and focus groups. Quantitative methods include surveys, reports, checklists, attendance logs, self-administered questionnaires, project archives, and community profiles (Linnan & Steckler, 2002).

Unfortunately, it's not always apparent when it's best to use qualitative versus quantitative methods. Sometimes the method used is determined by the availability of resources. In this situation, the method used is the most cost-effective one that can generate the data needed to answer the evaluation questions (Linnan & Stickler 2002).

When resources are not a determining factor for deciding which method to use, answering questions about the intent of the process evaluation can point the committee in the right direction. "Yes" answers to the following questions suggest the use of *qualitative* methods.

Is the intent of the process evaluation to:

- identify elements of the program that are likely to be effective?
- get feedback while the program is in its early stages?
- determine why an aspect of the program isn't working?
- understand the implementation facilitators and barriers of one aspect of the program (CDC, 2011)?

Table 7-2 Implementation concern and process evaluation questions

Implementation concern	Process evaluation questions
Context	What community, social/political, or other situational issues could potentially affect intervention implementation?
Fidelity	To what extent was implementation consistent with the underlying theory? To what extent was staff training provided as intended by the developers?
Dose (delivered)	To what extent were all units of the program (classes, presentations, demonstrations, etc.) provided? To what extent was all intended content delivered?
Dose (received)	To what extent were participants engaged in the activities? To what extent did participants engage in follow-up behaviors?
Reach	What proportion of the intended audience participated in each session delivered? How many participants attended at least half of the sessions delivered?
Recruitment	What were the barriers to recruiting participants from the intended audience? What planned recruitment activities were used?

Reproduced from: Saunders, R.P., Evans. M. H., & Joshi, P. (2005). Developing a process evaluation plan for assessing health program implementation: A how to guide. *Health Promotion Practice*, *6*(2), 134–147. doi: 10.1177/1524839904273387

"Yes" answers to the following questions point in the direction of using *quantitative* methods (CDC, 2011).

Is the intent of process evaluation to:

- document how much change occurred in some characteristic addressed by the program?
- reveal the costs associated with the implementation of program component?

If there are "yes" answers under both sets of questions, it suggests that a mix of both methods (mixed methods) is the best approach. This is the approach that was used in the process evaluation of HEALTHY, a 3-year school-based primary prevention program designed to reduce type 2 diabetes risk factors in middle school children (Schneider et al., 2009).

The four distinct, but integrated components of HEALTHY were physical activity, nutrition, behavior change, and social marketing. The physical activity component introduced a curriculum of HEALTHY PE (physical education) lesson plans and classroom management to increase student participation in moderate-to-vigorous physical activity. The nutrition component addressed the quantity and quality of food and beverages offered throughout the school food environment, including cafeteria meals, after-school snacks, and a la carte and vending machines.

The behavior education component provided students with knowledge and skills to facilitate healthy lifestyle choices both inside and outside the school environment. The communications campaign used social marketing to design and place promotional materials in the schools to motivate students, build excitement around each semester's behavior goals, and integrate the components into a cohesive program (Schneider et al., 2009).

Qualitative methods used to conduct the process evaluation included observation, interviews, and focus groups. The quantitative methods were feedback forms and logs (Schneider et al., 2009).

Physical education classes were observed to assess if classes were delivered in a manner consistent with the intent and design of the HEALTHY lesson plans, a majority of students engaged in activity quickly at the beginning of the class, the teaching assistant from the HEALTHY staff was present during the class, and whether there were any barriers that might have prevented or discouraged the students from engaging in moderate-to-vigorous physical activity (Schneider et al., 2009).

Observation was also used to evaluate the nutrition component, which included all food and beverage points of service, that is, breakfast, lunch, a la carte, vending machines, school stores, and menu reviews. The purpose of these observations was to determine if the school was meeting the food service and nutritional goals of the HEALTHY program and to determine which of the 12 unique core strategies were being met at the time of the observation (Schneider et al., 2009).

Classes in which the behavior education component of the program took place were observed as well. These observations were done to determine if the session was delivered as intended, to see if the majority of students were able to follow the instructions, and to detect any barriers to implementation (Schneider et al., 2009).

Interviews were conducted with HEALTHY staff responsible for training school personnel. These were done to explore staff perceptions of the degree to which each program component was being implemented as planned within each school, as well as to identify barriers to and facilitators of the program (Schneider et al., 2009).

Interviews were also used to obtain information from the student participants, with parental consent. Students provided information about their recollection of program components, perceptions of specific study activities and their overall opinions of the HEALTHY program (Schneider et al., 2009).

School administrator interviews were conducted to gather information about if and how the program affected the regular functioning of the school. For example, scheduling, student conduct, and school employee morale. These interviews also provided insight into how the program was perceived by the school administration (Schneider et al., 2009).

Interviews of school staff were designed to not only learn about their perceptions of the overall program, but also to prompt their opinions about the parts of the program with which they were most familiar. Staff were also asked for suggestions to improve future implementation of similar programs (Schneider et al., 2009).

Focus groups were used to generate feedback from students who participated in the communications campaign as communication liaisons between their peers and the program delivery team. The focus group discussions shed light on student perception of the HEALTHY program, and their role in it and provided suggestions for the next semester (Schneider et al., 2009).

Feedback forms were completed by classroom teachers each time a HEALTHY educational session was delivered. The form was used to collect data on the date and time of each session and whether any barriers to its implementation were encountered (Schneider et al., 2009).

Student-peer liaison training sessions were tracked using logs. The logs provided a way to ensure that students were not missing more than 1 hour of class per week for program-related activities (Schneider et al., 2009). (See **Table 7-3** for an example of process evaluation questions, information, and methods.)

Once the data collection methods are determined, exactly how the data will be collected is clarified in terms of the following:

- The instruments to be used.
- The processes or procedures to be followed.
- The frequency of collection.

Table 7-3 Process evaluation questions, information, and methods

Process questions	Information to collect	Methods
To what extent was the project implemented as planned?	How well did program staff follow procedures in the plan?	Focused staff feedback sessions
	What factors helped or hindered delivery quality?	Observations of activities
To what extent were core element activities conducted as planned?	The number of promotional items distributed to participants	Counts of promotional materials
	The number of training sessions delivered	Counts of training sessions
	The number of support hours provided to participants	Total hours of support provided in project period
	The number of core elements delivered	Checklists for staff to report the core elements that they demonstrated
How much community interest and activity did the projects generate?	The number of people who attended the activities	Attendance counts for activities
	The number of people who completed activities (i.e., attended all sessions of a multiday training)	Participant feedback forms asking them to evaluate their experience
	The number of people who requested assistance	Reference desk usage counts
	The number of people who used the equipment or websites made available through your project	Visitor counts for computer labs, kiosks, etc. Website traffic statistics
To what extent was the intended audience reached?	The proportion of all program participants who were from the intended audience	Demographic data from program or activity registration forms
How effective were recruitment strategies for attracting members of the intended audience?	The strategies that worked well to attract participants from the intended audience	Written participants' feedback forms asking what attracted them to the program or activity Counts of participants who completed all activities (e.g., all sessions of a multiday training)
	The barriers that hindered recruitment	Feedback sessions with project staff
	The strategies that helped maintain participant involvement	Participant interviews

(continues)

Table 7-3 Process evaluation questions, information, and methods   (continued)

Process questions	Information to collect	Methods
What contextual factors in affected project implementation?	Factors that helped or hindered program staff ability to implement the project	Program staff focus groups Participant focus groups
	Factors that influenced participants' ability to participate in program activities?	Participant interviews

Data from: National Institutes of Health, National Network of Libraries of Medicine. (n.d.). Booklet 2—figures. Retrieved June 18, 2019, from https://nnlm.gov/neo/guides/booklet2figures#fig10

- The persons responsible for collecting the data.
- The cost associated with collecting the data.
- Any potential burden to the participants and staff (Linnan & Steckler, 2002).

- Step 6—Analyze the data and write a report

In general, quantitative data analysis typically begins with descriptive statistics which include frequencies, central tendencies (mean, median, and mode), and variability or ranges. The results of the data analyses answer questions related to fidelity, dose, and reach (Moore et al., 2014).

Qualitative data analysis provides for a more in-depth understanding of the how and why of implementation. For instance, how context affects implementation, or why participants engage in some program activities and not others. However, analyzing qualitative data is time intensive and complex in comparison to analyzing quantitative data. Because of this, qualitative data collection should ideally be done before or at least at the same time as quantitative data are collected to avoid having an abundance of data and no time for analysis (Moore et al., 2014).

Once the data are analyzed, the next step is to create a report in which the results are interpreted and put into a form the committee members can understand and use. If key stakeholders are involved in crafting and prioritizing the process evaluation questions, it makes sense to get their input on the type of reports they would like to see generated (Linnan & Steckler, 2002).

Sometimes, even though programs look great on paper, they just don't work, and the planning committee is left wondering why. If a process evaluation had been done, they would know why.

This is what happened with a stress management program in a department of a large utility company in the United Kingdom (UK). The program was developed in response to a legal requirement for employers to assess the risk of stress-related illness from work activities. To comply, the company implemented a program that involved having the department managers use the results of an employee stress risk assessment (SRA) tool to develop action plans to reduce stress (Biron, Gatrell, & Cooper, 2010).

The program activities included a workshop for department managers to learn about the SRA, managers distributing a login code to each employee in his/her department to access the SRA, employees completing the SRA, managers closing access to the SRA once 60 percent of the department completed it, managers receiving a report containing their department's grouped SRA results, managers meeting with their department employees to discuss problems identified by the SRA and agree on an action plan to address the issues, and implementing the action plan. The intended outcome of the program was a reduction in exposure to stressors, which would lead to improved health and well-being and improved performance indicators such as absenteeism (Biron et al., 2010).

The implementation of this program depended on expectations about three key groups, the human resource staff, department managers, and department employees.

- It was expected that the human resource staff responsible for conducting the managers' workshop were themselves trained to teach the workshops, and that they would correctly deliver the workshop information (Biron et al., 2010).
- It was expected that the managers would be available and willing to attend the workshop, would be more knowledgeable about the stress response after their training workshop, would see a need for change and be committed to using the SRA to facilitate change, would print the group SRA report and correctly interpret the results, would hold meaningful, constructive department discussions, and would have the skills and resources to implement the action plans (Biron et al., 2010).
- It was expected that the department employees' perceptions, expectations, and beliefs about the program improving work conditions would compel them to complete the SRA, that a high level of trust existed between the department employees and their manager, and that the department compositions would remain stable and contain no less than six employees at all times to maintain the confidentiality of the group SRA results (Biron et al., 2010).
- It was expected that department employees would be supportive and involved in the process, that consensus would be reached on the priority stress issues and how they would be addressed, that the

actions decided on would be implemented with fidelity, and that accomplishments and changes would be communicated to everyone. The program did not work (Biron et al., 2010).

To determine why the program failed, a mixed methods process evaluation was conducted. Quantitative data were collected through surveys to evaluate the level of implementation and its effects. Qualitative data were collected through interviews and observation notes to evaluate the implementation processes (Biron et al., 2010).

Department manager interviews revealed that although most agreed preventing stress at work was a corporate responsibility, they felt that one workshop was not enough to make them use the SRA, that stress-related issues were sensitive topics that should not be discussed in a group with strangers, that although stress is an important topic, it occurs more at the senior level, and that department employees were laid back, and while their work was tedious, it was not stressful. In addition, many of the departments lost managers to job change, lost employees to department changes, or had a reduction in employees to less than six, which automatically excluded them from using the assessment (Biron et al., 2010).

The takeaway from the process evaluation interviews revealed that department stress was low and the stress assessment wasn't needed (Biron et al., 2010). This did not bode well for successful implementation of the program.

Because the program assumed managers were experts on employee sources of stress, it relied on them to translate the risk assessment results into feasible action plans without having the infrastructure or expertise support needed. Other contextual issues included the lack of stability within the departments, which was a necessary condition for program success, and the use of a department-based approach, which assumed the managers were not the cause of the employee stress. And finally, although the program appeared to receive a commitment from top management, the lack of resources allocated to it—no steering committee, support for managers, or budget to implement specific actions, did not reflect a true commitment to its success (Biron, 2010).

Summative Evaluation

Summative evaluation measures program effectiveness or its ability to produce the desired outcomes in a real-world setting (Spiegelman, 2016). It provides answers to questions such as:

— Were the program objectives met?
— Does the overall program structure need improvement or modification?
— What was the overall impact of the program?
— What resources are needed to address the program's weaknesses (The Pell Institute, 2019)?

There are two types of summative evaluation, outcome and impact. The differences between the two are when in the course of the program they are done and what they measure. Outcome evaluation, also called short-term outcome evaluation, is done immediately at the end of the program or anytime within the following six months. It measures if the outcome or short-term objectives were met. Impact evaluation, also called long-term outcome evaluation, is done a year or more after the program ends. It measures the effects of the program in terms of its long-term goals and objectives and broader societal, policy, or organizational structure changes. Together, outcome and impact evaluations enable decisions to be made about specific aspects of the program and its future direction.

Outcome Evaluation (Short-Term Outcome Evaluation)

An outcome evaluation measures the short-term changes in personal attributes—knowledge, attitudes, skills, and beliefs—expected in the intended audience as a result of participating in the program. For example, the short-term changes expected from participating in a sexually transmitted infection (STI) prevention program might be increased knowledge about disease transmission, or improved condom negotiating skills (Salaberria-Pena et al., 2007).

Determining short-term changes takes two data points, the degree of the personal attribute at baseline or *before* participating in the program and the degree of the attribute *after* participation. The degree of the attribute at baseline is pretest data; after participation it's posttest data. The difference between the two is the extent of change.

For example, to measure the change in knowledge about preventing STI transmission, participants at an STI prevention program would answer a set of written questions before the program began, participate in the program, then answer the same questions again after the program. The difference between the number of correct answers before and after (pre and post) would be analyzed to determine if there was any significant change.

Similarly, baseline condom negotiation skills might be evaluated by observing two participants' role play at the beginning of an STI prevention program using a predetermined set of criteria to establish their baseline skill level. They would be observed again role-playing at the end of the program using the same set of criteria to determine their skill level. The extent of change is the difference between their skill level before and after the program.

Data for outcome evaluations are generally collected by quantitative methods. For instance, changes in participant knowledge, attitudes, and beliefs are almost always measured by a survey using a questionnaire with closed-ended questions (Tobacco Technical Assistance Consortium, n.d.). Changes in skills might be measured by observation using an observation guide.

Following are some tips for getting started with a short-term outcome evaluation (Tobacco Technical Assistance Consortium, n.d.).

TIP 1 <u>Focus</u> on one aspect of the program at a time, preferably the most critical one, especially if funding for the evaluation is limited.

TIP 2 <u>Identify</u> each short-term outcome objective associated with the aspect of the program being evaluated.

TIP 3 <u>Decide</u> how each outcome objective can/will be measured.

TIP 4 <u>Develop</u> a set of guidelines for collecting the data (e.g., where and when it will be collected, and by whom).

TIP 5 <u>Collect</u> baseline data before starting any program activities associated with the outcome.

TIP 6 <u>Collect</u> data again after participants complete the program to collect postprogram data.

For the outcome evaluation of the G.R.E.A.T. (Gang Resistance Education and Training) program, students completed a questionnaire prior to participating in the program to collect pretest (baseline) data and then again shortly after completion of the program to collect posttest data. The program's goals were to help youth avoid gang membership, reduce their involvement in violence and criminal activity, and develop positive relationships with law enforcement. Posttest data were used to determine if participation in the program changed gang membership, self-reported delinquency, attitudes toward the police, and the presence of risk and protective factors associated with problem behaviors (Esbensen et al., 2013).

Pre- and posttest data analysis showed lower rates of gang affiliation and membership among students who completed the G.R.E.A.T. program, more-positive attitudes toward the police, less-positive attitudes about gangs, more use of refusal skills, more peer pressure resistance, fewer associations with delinquent peers, more prosocial peers, less self-centeredness, and less anger. These outcomes indicated the program's short-term effectiveness in reducing

gang affiliation, improved law enforcement relationships, and protective factors (Esbensen et al., 2013). Had the process evaluation not been done, these positive changes would not have been known.

Impact Evaluation (Long-Term Outcome Evaluation)

An impact or long-term outcome evaluation is used to determine the effects or changes a program caused that would not have happened without the program (Gertler, Martinez, Premand, Rawlings, & Vermeersch, 2011). It's used to determine how effective a program is at reaching its goals and at bringing about wide-reaching changes such as those in disease risk, morbidity, and mortality that persist over time (CDC, 2012a; SAMHSA, 2012; UNEG, 2013).

An impact evaluation is most appropriate when:

– a program has been in place for a while (at least 12 months) (International Rescue Committee, 2018).
– the intended outcomes occurred, and evidence is needed to verify that the program caused them (International Rescue Committee, 2018).
– impact is not evident (Organization for Economic Cooperation and Development [OECD], 2006).
– the program is a pilot that's planned to be scaled-up (OECD, 2006).

In addition to determining effectiveness, impact evaluation also answers questions about which aspects of a program work and which don't work (OECD, 2006). With resources always in short supply, impact evaluation provides the evidence needed for accountability and decision making about whether a program should be continued as is, redesigned, discontinued, expanded, or replicated (OECD, 2006; UNEG, 2013).

Specifically, an impact evaluation provides answers to the following key questions:

- Was the program effective in producing its impact/long-term outcomes?
- Were there any unexpected, unintended, or unanticipated effects (positive or negative), and if so, are they the result of implementation failure or some aspect of the program itself?
- Did the program make a difference?
- What part of the difference can be attributed to the program?
- What aspect of the program made the difference?
- Can the program be expected to produce similar results in a different setting (SAMHSA, 2012, UNEG, 2013)?

An example of the value of an impact evaluation is seen in the Comprehensive Rural Health Project (CRHP) in India. The CRHP began as a way to deliver curative and preventative care to a predominately poor, rural population with high child mortality and notoriously inadequate public health care and education. Since its inception in 1970, the project has grown from serving a single village to serving approximately 300 villages and half million people (Mann, Eble, Frost, Premkumar, & Boone, 2010).

The CRHP services are provided by mobile health teams, a local hospital, and village health workers who are the heart of the project. The health workers are women selected by members of their village to receive intensive training in primary health care and health promotion, which includes family planning, women and child health, and home birth. Their role is to disseminate health information in their villages through discussion groups and household visits, administer basic remedies and medications, perform safe deliveries, and detect and refer high-risk pregnancies and deliveries to more qualified healthcare providers (Mann et al., 2010).

The mobile health teams are comprised of a nurse, a physician, a social worker, and paramedics. The team visits project villages monthly to support and mentor the villages' health workers and to refer complicated cases to the hospital. The hospital provides emergency, medical, surgical, and outpatient care to project village residents and those from the surrounding areas (Mann et al., 2010).

Although overall child survival improved in some project villages over the four decades the CRHP was in place, no evidence was available showing that the improvement was the result of the project. To remedy this situation, an impact evaluation was done (Mann et al., 2010).

The primary purpose of the evaluation was to establish the project's long-term impact on the mortality rates among children under age 5 in CRHP villages by comparing them to the rates of children in similar villages that were not participating in the CRHP. The secondary aims were to compare sanitation, health knowledge, number of children per woman, place and type of delivery and type of birth attendant; indicators of antenatal, delivery, and postnatal care; and child morbidity of households and women in those households in CRHP villages and non-CRHP villages (Mann et al., 2010).

Data were collected through a survey of households and interviews with the women in those households. The household survey consisted of a questionnaire to collect information on household-level factors such as wealth, sanitation, and water supply. Information collected through the interviews included a full birth history, history of pregnancy-related care, healthcare expenditure, health knowledge, and morbidity of children under 5 years of age (Mann et al., 2010).

Results of the impact evaluation revealed a 30 percent reduction in child mortality and greater health knowledge of the women (mothers) in the CRHP villages when compared to non-CRHP villages (Mann et al., 2010). The evaluation data supported what was assumed—that the program was effective.

Table 7-4 Comparison of formative and summative evaluation

Formative Evaluation		
Evaluation type	**Why is it done?**	**When is it done?**
Needs assessment	To identify needs To maximize the likelihood of program success	At the beginning of the planning process
Process evaluation	To determine the extent of consistency between implementation and the way it was intended to be implemented To determine if the program is acceptable and accessible to the intended audience To document how well the program is working	At the beginning of implementation During operation of an existing program.
Summative Evaluation		
Outcome/ Short-term outcome	To determine the degree to which the program objectives were met	At the end of the program or program component
Impact/ Long-term outcome	To determine changes caused by the program	After the program ends

Data from: Salabarria-Pena, Y., Apt, B. S., & Walsh, C. M. (2007). Practical use of program evaluation among sexually transmitted disease (STD) programs. Department of Health and Human Services, National Center for HIV, STD, and TB Prevention, Division of STD Prevention. Retrieved June 27, 2019, from https://www.cdc.gov/std/program/pupestd.htm

Table 7-4 provides a comparison of process, outcome, and impact evaluation.

Evaluation Designs

Evaluation designs are the procedures or methods used to guide data collection and analysis. They are the same or similar to those used in research studies to collect and analyze data (CDC, 2019). Consequently, summative evaluation is often called "evaluation research" or an "evaluation study." While the designs may be the same, there are important fundamental differences between research and evaluation.

Evaluation is done to determine the effectiveness of a specific program, understand why it may or may not have worked, and improve it. Research, on the other hand, is done to test a theory and produce generalizable information that can be applied to the population at large and to contribute to the knowledge base (CDC, 2019).

The three designs used for evaluations are experimental, quasi-experimental, and non-experimental. In order to understand how they differ, it's necessary to first understand sampling and control groups.

Sampling

A sample is a subset of all the program participants selected when it's not feasible to include all of them in the evaluation. We know that if a sample is representative of a population, then the results from the sample reflect the results that would have been generated if the entire population had been included.

In an evaluation, the sample is selected from among all the program participants using a sampling method. Sampling methods are of two types, random (probability) or nonrandom (nonprobability), with different techniques for each. The sampling method used depends on the evaluation questions, the level of data accuracy needed, available resources, and the evaluation design (The Pell Institute, 2019).

Random (Probability) Sampling. Random sampling, also called probability sampling or random assignment, is the method that gives every person in the intended audience an equal chance of being included in a sample. In an evaluation, random sampling means every person participating in the program would have an equal chance of being included in the evaluation sample. In this way, random sampling is the most reliable method of ensuring sample results accurately reflect the results that would have occurred if data had been collected from the entire intended audience.

Random sampling also eliminates sampling bias or the situation when some participants are more likely than others to be selected for the sample. Sample bias is a problem to be avoided because it can affect the accuracy of

the sample results, as they may not reflect the results that would have been obtained had all the program participants completed the evaluation. For example, if program participants are asked to volunteer to be in the evaluation sample the evaluation results may not be accurate because people who volunteer tend to be more health conscious than people in general (Shantikumar, 2018) and tend to have strong opinions (Smith, 2012).

Imagine conducting an impact evaluation for a weight-loss program and asking for volunteers to complete the evaluation. Now, imagine the people who volunteered were those who lost weight. Chances are the evaluation results would be positive, indicating the program was effective. Now imagine the volunteers were the people who didn't lose weight. Chances are the evaluation results would be negative, indicating the program was ineffective. Neither would be an accurate reflection of the results of all the program participants. If the participants had been randomly selected to the sample, there would have been a mix of those who lost weight and those who didn't, and the results would be reflective of the results if all the program participants had competed the evaluation.

Two random sampling techniques often used to select those program participants who will take part in the evaluation from among all the program participants are simple random sampling and stratified random sampling. Simple random sampling techniques are the easiest to use. They include drawing names from a hat and assigning those people to the sample (The Pell Institute, 2019) or tossing a coin for each person where heads means inclusion in the sample, and tails not. Other simple random sampling methods include using a shuffled deck of cards where a card is pulled for each participant. If the number on the card is even, the assignment is the sample. Dice can be used as well. Using one die, if the throw equals a number below or equal to 3, the assignment is the sample (Suresh, 2011).

Stratified random sampling is used when program participants need to be divided into groups based on some characteristic that is meaningful to the evaluation before they are randomly assigned to the sample. For example, in evaluating the effectiveness of a program to reduce undergraduate alcohol use by year, the program participants would first be divided into groups by their academic year—freshman, sophomore, junior, and senior—and then an equal number from each year would be randomly assigned to the sample (The Pell Institute, 2019).

Nonrandom (Nonprobability) Sampling. As the name suggests, nonrandom sampling is not random, which means all participants do not have an equal chance at being in the sample. Rather, participants in a nonrandom sample are selected by those conducting the evaluation, referred by others, or because of convenience (The Pell Institute, 2019) by being in the right place at the right time. There are five commonly used methods for establishing a nonrandom sample: convenience, purposive, quota, snowball, and self-selection (The Pell Institute, 2019).

- Convenience sampling

In convenience sampling, the sample consists of whoever happens to be in a given place at a given time. For example, a convenience sample for a school-based childhood obesity prevention program evaluation would be the parents/guardians attending a Parents Teachers Association (PTA) meeting on a particular evening. A convenience sample of participants in a diabetes management program would be all the participants attending the final session of the program. College and university students in a classroom are often used as a convenience sample. Think about how many times you were sitting in a class and asked to complete a questionnaire or take part in a study. It's convenient for a researcher to ask a classroom full of students to take part in a survey as compared to contacting the same number of students individually.

- Purposive sampling

In purposive sampling, those conducting the evaluation select people for the sample whom they believe are representative of all the program participants (The Pell Institute, 2019). The sample participants are chosen "on purpose" by the evaluators.

- Quota sampling

Similar to stratified random sampling, quota sampling also separates program participants into groups based on some characteristic first, and then chooses from among the groups those to be included in the sample. The difference between quota and stratified random sampling is that quota sampling does not randomly select who will be in the groups. Instead, the evaluators choose who will be in each group (The Pell Institute, 2019).

- Snowball sampling

As the name implies, snowball sampling relies on referral to form the sample. It begins with the evaluator identifying a few people to include in the sample. These key people are then asked to refer others who might want to participate in the sample (The Pell Institute, 2019).

- Self-selection sampling

Self-selection sampling is just as it sounds. Program participants self-select or volunteer to be part of the evaluation sample (The Pell Institute, 2019).

Sample Size

The process of establishing a sample begs the question—How many people should be in the sample? The simple answer is that there is no one simple answer or standard sample size. Sample size is based on confidence level, margin of error, and population size.

Confidence Level. Confidence level is a percent that reflects how often the results from a sample would fall within a certain range of the results from all program participants, if the evaluation was repeated over and over again (Baker & Bruner, 2012; Statistics How To, 2014). Said another way, if the evaluation was done over and over using different samples from the entire population of program participants, the confidence level is the percent of time the sample results would match the results from the entire population of program participants (Statistics How To, 2014). Because there can never be 100 percent confidence in the accuracy of sample results, the standard confidence levels are 90, 95, and 99 percent.

Margin of Error. Margin of error is also a percent, but it reflects how off the sample results might be from the true results from the entire population of program participants. Standard margins of error are 3, 5, and 10 percent (Baker & Bruner, 2012; Statistics How To, 2014).

The standard confidence level for evaluations is 95 percent with a 5 percent margin of error. What this means is—if the evaluation was repeated over and over with different samples from the entire population of program participants, 95 percent of the time the sample results would differ by no more than 5 percent (+ or −) of what the true results are for the entire population of participants (Baker & Bruner, 2012).

In order for the sample results to reflect the results of the entire population of program participants as accurately as possible, a certain number of people are needed in the sample. Here's why—Imagine for a moment that 100 people attended a program, and 3 people were randomly selected for the evaluation sample. How confident would you be that sample results based on 3 people reflect the results you would have gotten if the other 97 people participated in the evaluation? Not very.

Now imagine if the sample had 80 people randomly selected from the 100 program

Table 7-5 Sample sizes at 95 percent confidence and 5 percent margin of error

Total intervention population	Sample size
100	80
150	109
200	132
250	152
300	169
350	184
400	197
450	208
500	218
750	255
1000	278
5000	357

participants. How confident would you be that the sample results reflect the results you would have gotten if the other 20 participants also completed the evaluation? (See **Table 7-5** for examples of sample sizes for a given population size at the 95 percent confidence level with a 5 percent margin of error.)

The following formula can be used to calculate a sample size for any size population at 95 percent confidence with a 5 percent margin of error:

$n = 385 \div ((1 + (385/N))$
(Baker & Bruner, 2012).

Example: If the entire population of program participants consisted of 472 people, then the sample needed for a 95 percent confidence level and a 5 percent margin of error is 212.

$n = 385 \div ((1 + (385/472))$
$n = 212$

Sample size can also be calculated using one of the many free online calculators including those at the following sites:

Survey Monkey—https://www.survey monkey.com/mp/sample-size-calculator/

Survey Systems—https://www .surveysystem.com/sscalc.htm

Qualtrics—https://www.qualtrics. com/blog/calculating-sample-size/

UCLA—http://statistics.ucla.edu/

Following are three rules of thumb for determining sample size:

First rule of thumb—If less than 100 people participated in the program, a sample isn't used or needed. All the participants are included in the evaluation. If 100 or more people participated, a sample is needed (Baker & Bruner, 2012).

Second rule of thumb—The proper size of the sample depends on the total number of program participants, the confidence level, and margin of error.

Third rule of thumb—A sample that's larger than what's necessary is needed to compensate for people refusing to participate in the evaluation. To calculate a sample size that compensates for refusals, first estimate a refusal rate (Baker & Brunner, 2012), then use it in the following formula:

Desired sample size $\div (1 - \text{refusal rate})$ = sample size compensating for refusals.

For example: If the desired sample size is 122, and you estimate that 30 percent of the sample will refuse to complete the evaluation, the sample needs to contain 174 people to compensate for the refusals.

Estimated refusal rate = 30%
$$122 \div (1 - 0.30) = 174$$

Control Group

A control group is a group of people as similar to the program participants as possible, but who don't participate in the program. The control group is used for comparison purposes to validate program effectiveness. It's critical for an impact evaluation.

When changes occur in the program participant group (usually called the intervention group), that don't occur in the control group, this is evidence that the changes were caused by the program and would not have happened otherwise. It's a way to document what the outcome would have been for program participants if they had not participated in the program (Gertler et al., 2011).

The decision to use or not use a control group is made while the program is being planned. Waiting until the time of the evaluation to decide to use a control group doesn't work. Random sampling is used to select who from the intended audience will participate in the program and who will serve as the control group *before* implementation of the program.

For example, a control group was used to determine the effectiveness of a program to improve immunization rates of 2-year-old children at seven WIC (Women, Infants, and Children) sites in Chicago. Of the seven sites, four were randomly assigned to participate in the program and three to the control group (Hutchins et al., 1999), ensuring the two groups were as alike as possible since any one site had the same chance as all the others of being assigned to either the control or program group.

At the four WIC sites where the program was implemented, all children under age 5 were screened by an immunization assistant at every visit to determine their vaccination status. The parents or guardians received a printout of the vaccination screening results, and children in need of immunizations were referred to the appropriate service provider or clinic. As an incentive, parents/guardians of children who were up-to-date with their immunizations received a three-month supply of food vouchers instead of the standard one month supply (Hutchins et al., 1999). No part of the immunization program was offered at the three control group sites. Children and their parents just received the usual care, which included nutritional counseling, food vouchers for 1 month, and referrals to the usual healthcare services (Hutchins et al., 1999).

To determine the effectiveness of the immunization program, changes in immunization rates at the program sites and the control group sites were compared at the end of the first and second years of the program. After 1 year, the immunization rates at program sites increased 23 percent compared with a 9 percent decrease in the rates at the control sites. After two years of implementation, the rates at the program sites increased 52 percent, from 37 percent at baseline to 89 percent, while there was no significant change in the rates at control group sites (Hutchins et al., 1999).

Although the increase in immunization rates at the program sites would still have been known even if a control group wasn't used, what would not have been known with certainty is if the program accounted for the improvement. By using a control group, that uncertainty was eliminated.

As useful as random sampling and control groups are for providing evidence of cause and effect, using them in a community setting sometimes isn't ethical or feasible (CDC, 2012b; Rural Health Information Hub [RHIhub], 2019). It may not be ethical because it means offering a program to one group but not another group (CDC, 2012d; RHIhub, 2019). It may not be feasible because of spillover or the inadvertent exposure of the control group to the program, or a lack of resources (Knowledge for Health, 2017).

For instance, a public health program in India aimed at raising the childhood immunization rates in villages with rates of 2 percent compared to the overall country rate of 38 percent that used control groups was called out as being unethical. In villages where the program was implemented, monthly village "immunization camps" were held, and incentives were given (small portions of lentils and a plate) to parents when their children completed a full course of immunizations. In the control villages either the immunizations camps were held but no incentive was given, or neither the camp was held, nor the incentive given. As a result, the immunization rate of children in the program villages rose from 2 percent to 39 percent, to 18 percent in the control villages that only received the camps, and to only 6 percent in control villages that did not receive either the camp or the incentive (Banerjee, Duflo, Glennerster, & Kothari, 2010).

Using control groups in this program was considered unethical. Since the rate of vaccine coverage was so low in all the villages, children in the control villages could have been at risk of dying from a vaccine-preventable disease (Deepak, 2010).

Experimental Design

Experimental design entails using a control group established by random sampling of the intended audience. This is considered the gold standard in research and evaluation (RHIhub, 2019) because it eliminates the problems of selection bias and any issues that might occur from differences in culture, race, or other factors (CCHD, 2018b).

Once the control and program participant groups are formed, everyone in each group completes a pretest (questionnaire) to collect baseline data on the factors the program addresses (knowledge, attitudes, skills, behaviors, etc.), *before* the program begins. After baseline data collection is completed, the program is implemented for the participant group only. The control group does not take part in any aspect of the program.

At the end of the program, both groups are posttested using the same questionnaire that was used for the pretest. Each group's pre- and posttest results are compared for differences. If the posttest results for the program participant group differs from the control group, the differences (changes) are attributed to the program (Knowledge for Health, 2017).

When the control group is randomly assigned from the intended audience and the two groups start off equivalent with the program, the only difference between them from pretest to posttest, then any changes in the participant group are caused by the program. Being able to determine that the program caused the outcome with as much certainty as possible is a major advantage of this design.

The steps for conducting an evaluation using an experimental design include

Step 1—Form the participant and control groups by randomly assigning members of the intended audience to the one of the groups.

Step 2—Collect baseline (pretest) data from both groups.

Step 3—Compare the pretest data from the control group and participant group against each other to identify any baseline differences.

Step 4—Implement the program for the program participant group.

Step 5—Posttest both groups at the end of the program using the same questionnaire that was used for the pretest.

Step 6—Compare the pretest results with the posttest results for each group separately to determine if anything changed.

Step 7—Compare the posttest results for both groups against each other to identify differences attributable to the program.

Quasi-Experimental Design

A quasi-experimental evaluation design is a "sort of" experimental design. While it uses a control group, the group is not randomly selected (CDC, 2012b). Instead, it's created either by individuals from the intended audience self-selecting which group they want to be part of, or by the program planners assigning or matching individuals to the control group based on characteristics relevant to the program and/or present in the program participant group, or a combination of both (White & Sabarwal, 2014).

When the control group is formed in these ways, it can't be assumed that it's equivalent to the program participant group, which is critical for any differences in outcomes between the groups at the end of the program to be attributed to the program (White & Sabarwal, 2014). To address this, both groups are pretested and their results compared so any differences between them are identified *before* the program is implemented. This allows for any posttest differences between the groups, other than those previously identified, to be attributed to the program.

The steps for conducting a quasi-experimental design evaluation include:

Step 1—Assign members from the intended audience to the control or program participant groups or have them self-select their group.

Step 2—Pretest the control and program participant groups using the same questionnaire.

Step 3—Compare the pretest results of both groups to identify baseline differences.

Step 4—Implement the program for the program participant group.

Step 5—Posttest both groups at the end of the program using the same questionnaire that was used for the pretest.

Step 6—Compare the posttest results from both groups to identify differences other than those established at pretest that may be attributed to the program.

A quasi-experimental design was used to evaluate the effectiveness of a smoking prevention program for 10- to 15-year-olds attending eight different secondary schools in Germany.

Although the program implementers wanted to randomly assign students to the control and program participant groups, the schools refused to participate if this was done. Instead, the schools split their students into the two groups, with half in the control group and half in the program group (Brinker, Stamm-Balderjahn, Seeger, Klingelhofer, & Groneberg, 2015).

Baseline (pretest) sociodemographic and smoking status data were collected confidentially from the control groups and the program groups in each school by the classroom teachers using paper-and-pencil questionnaires prior to the start of the program. Once baseline data collection was completed, the program began (Brinker et al., 2015).

The program consisted of two 60-minute sessions presented by medical students on strategies used by tobacco companies to get them to smoke. The aim was to influence student decision-making skills. Six months after the end of program, posttest data were collected confidentially by the classroom teachers using the same paper-and-pencil questionnaire as the pretest (Brinker et al., 2015).

At baseline, 6.4 percent of the students overall reported smoking with no significant differences between the percent of smokers in the control group versus the program group. Six months after the program, 4.6 percent of the smokers in the program group reported quitting, compared to only 1.1 percent in the control group (Brinker et al., 2015).

Nonexperimental Evaluation Design

The nonexperimental or single group design, also called pretest/posttest design, doesn't use a control group or random sampling. Instead, data are only collected from the program participants (CCHD, 2018b; RHIhub, 2019). This design is the easiest to do and the one traditionally used for program evaluation, although it's the least accurate (CCHD, 2018b; CDC, 2012b).

In nonexperimental design, the program participants complete a pretest, participate in the program, and complete a posttest. The pretest data are compared to the posttest data to determine if there are differences. If differences are found, this design assumes they were caused by the program (CCHD, 2018b; SAMHSA, 2012). Causation cannot be attributed to the program because there is no control group to confirm what would have happened without the program. The *cause* of the differences (changes) can't be established, only that something happened. Despite this, taking measures before and after a program is far better than taking no measurements at all (CCHD, 2018b).

Another nonexperimental design is posttest only. This is exactly what it sounds like—data are only collected from participants at the end of the program; pretest data are not collected. Similar to the pretest–posttest design, causation of the posttest results cannot be attributed to the program. However, when the purpose of the evaluation is to determine if participants know the information or have the skill a program addressed, this design is appropriate (SAMHSA, 2012).

A test in a course is a typical example of a posttest design. Students attend a course and are tested at the end to determine if they know the information taught during the course. Without a pretest, it can't be assumed that the course was responsible for their knowledge. It's possible they knew the information before they took the course.

Steps for conducting an evaluation using a nonexperimental pretest/posttest design include:

Step 1—Pretest program participants before starting the program.

Step 2—Conduct the program.

Step 3—Posttest program participants at the end of the program.

Step 4—Compare pretest and posttest results to identify any differences.

A pretest/posttest design was used to evaluate the General Awareness Training (GAT) component of a suicide prevention program for the construction industry in Australia. The program consisted of a 1-hour training session for construction workers at their worksites to engage and motivate them in suicide prevention. It aimed to increase awareness and understanding of mental health and suicide, reduce stigma associated with suicide, and encourage helping behaviors—both in terms of help-seeking (for oneself) and help-offering (to coworkers in distress) (King et al., 2018).

The aim of the evaluation was to determine the effectiveness of GAT to change suicide attitudes and beliefs. Pretest data were collected before GAT began, and posttest data immediately afterwards. No control group was used (King et al., 2018).

Using an Evaluation Framework

An evaluation framework is a guide or set of steps for conducting an evaluation. Of the many available, a commonly used one is the CDC's Framework for Program Evaluation in Public Health, summarized next (CDC, 2017a).

Which framework the committee chooses to use is less important than *using* the framework chosen. Just as with behavior change theory, frameworks work best when used in totality, rather than in a piecemeal fashion. Following the steps of a framework, whichever one selected, will keep the things on track and focused.

CDC Framework for Program Evaluation

The CDC Framework for Program Evaluation in Public Health (Framework) entails completing 6 steps and meeting 30 standards.

The 6 steps include engaging stakeholders, describing the program, focusing the evaluation design, gathering credible evidence, justifying conclusions, and ensuring use of the results and sharing lessons learned (CDC, 1999).

The 30 standards are organized into the following four groups that ensure specific aspects of the evaluation are met: *utility standards* ensure an evaluation will serve the information needs of the intended users; *feasibility standards* ensure an evaluation will be realistic, prudent, diplomatic, and frugal; *propriety standards* ensure an evaluation will be conducted legally, ethically, and with regard for the welfare of those involved and those affected by its results; *accuracy standards* ensure an evaluation will convey technically adequate information about the program's merit (CDC, 1999).

In addition to serving as a structure for conducting an evaluation, the Framework also serves as the basis for planning an evaluation and, once the evaluation is completed, writing an evaluation report. While logically a discussion of how to plan an evaluation should precede a discussion of how to conduct an evaluation, in this case, understanding the steps and standards of the Framework are necessary before it can be used to guide planning. (See **Figure 7-2**.)

CDC Framework Steps

The following six steps of the Framework are carried out in sequence with the earlier steps setting the foundation for those that follow (CDC, 1999, 2017a).

Step 1—Engage Stakeholders. Stakeholders are the individuals or organizations with an investment in what will be learned from and done with the evaluation results. In general, stakeholders fall into one of three groups:

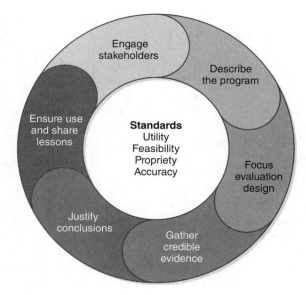

Figure 7-2 CDC framework for program evaluation steps and standards

Centers for Disease Control and Prevention (1999) Framework for program evaluation in public health. *Morbidity and Mortality Weekly Report 48*(RR-11)

- Those involved in the program such as sponsors, coalition partners administrators, staff.
- Those served or affected by the program such as clients, neighborhoods, advocacy groups.
- Those interested in the program and who would use the results such as community groups, clients, elected officials.

Stakeholders are involved in the evaluation process to ensure their perspectives are understood and their concerns and values are addressed. When stakeholders are engaged, it increases the likelihood that the evaluation results will be useful, improves the evaluation's credibility, helps to clarify roles and responsibilities, enhances cultural competence, helps protect human subjects, and averts real or perceived conflicts of interest. When stakeholders are not engaged, you run the risk of the evaluation results being ignored, criticized, or resisted (Joint Committee on Standards for Education Evaluation, 1994).

To engage stakeholders, consult with and include them in designing and conducting the evaluation. Make a concerted effort to include less-powerful groups or individuals in the evaluation process to avoid conflicts and overemphasizing the values of any specific person or group. Coordinate their input throughout the evaluation process. Keep them abreast of progress through periodic meetings and reports.

Step 2—Describe Program. The program description sets the frame of reference for all evaluation decisions that follow. It enables comparisons to be made with similar programs and facilitates the connection of program components to their effects (Joint Committee on Standards for Education Evaluation, 1994). Consequently, the program description should convey the mission, goals, objectives, and strategies of the program in sufficient detail to:

- ensure they can be understood.
- discuss the program's capacity to effect change.
- convey its stage of development.

– explain how it fits into the larger organization and community.

Work with stakeholders to formulate a clear and logical description because evaluations done without agreement on the program description tend to be less useful. Include the following in the description:

- Statement of need

Describe the problem the program addresses and the people affected. This information is contained in the needs assessment.

- Expected effects

Describe what is expected to happen or change as a result of the program for it to be considered a success. Since program effects unfold over time, this description should be arranged by time—from the immediate effects, intermediate and long-term. Additionally, mention should be made of anticipated potential unintended effects of the program.

- Activities

Describe, in sequence, what the program does to enable the changes to happen. Doing this demonstrates how each activity relates to another and how the underlying change theory was used. Distinguish between activities that are the direct responsibility of the implementing organization and those of related programs or partners (U.S. General Accounting Office [U.S. GAO], 1998). It helps to also make note of any external factors that might affect the program's success.

- Resources

Describe program resources—time, talent technology, equipment, money, and other assets—available for program activities. These descriptions should convey the amount and extent of the service the resource is used for and point out where there is a mismatch between what's needed and what's available (U.S. GAO, 1992).

- Stage of development

Describe the program's stage of development—planning, implementation, or effects/maintenance stage. Considering a program's stage of development reflects its maturity, programs recently implemented differ from those that have been operating for years. For example, programs in the planning stage are untested, so the purpose of evaluation is to refine the plans. Programs in the implementation stage are being field-tested and modified, so the purpose of evaluation is to identify how they work in a real-life setting as opposed to an ideal research setting. Programs in the last stage have had enough time pass for their effects to emerge, so the purpose of evaluation is to identify and account for both intended and unintended effects.

- Context

Describe the program's context, including the setting, environmental influences such as history, politics, geography, social and economic condition, and any efforts of organizations related to or competing with the program. It's important to understand the context within which the program is implemented so the evaluation designed is sensitive to the contextual issues. It also helps in accurately interpreting evaluation results and assessing the generalizability of the findings.

- Logic model

Create a logic model to show how the program is supposed to work, how the strategies lead to the program results, and in what sequence. Include the following elements: inputs, activities, outputs, and results (immediate, intermediate, and long-term effects) (Lipsey, 1993).

Step 3—Focus Evaluation Design. Deciding how to best conduct the evaluation is a must because not all designs will produce information that meets the needs of the stakeholders and/or use resources wisely. The evaluation method or design should be selected based on its ability to provide the evidence needed to answer the stakeholders' questions. The design chosen has implications for what will count as evidence, how that evidence will be gathered, and what kind of claims can be made as a result of that evidence (U.S. GAO, 1992).

The aim is to create an evaluation strategy with the greatest potential of being useful, feasible, ethical, and accurate. To this end, the following are considered.

- The purpose of the evaluation

In general, evaluations are done for the following purposes:

To gain insight—An evaluation conducted to gain insight provides information in the early planning stages about the practicality of a new approach or an innovative method to address the need.

To change practice—An evaluation to change practice is appropriate in the implementation stage of an established program to describe what it has done and to what extent. The information can be used to improve program processes, operations, or strategies to improve the quality, effectiveness, or efficiency of program activities.

To assess effects—An evaluation conducted to assess effects examines the relationship between program activities and consequences. This evaluation is appropriate for mature programs for identifying effects and ensuring that significant consequences are not overlooked.

- Who will use the evaluation results.

Since the evaluation findings are the direct consequences of the design used, the people who will be using the results should have a role in choosing the evaluation focus. Their involvement is key to clarifying the

intended uses of the findings, prioritizing the evaluation questions, and preventing the evaluation from becoming irrelevant.

- How the results will be used.

Vague uses for the evaluation results decrease the chances that the evaluation will address any one user's needs. Consequently, stakeholders should have input into planning and prioritizing the uses for the evaluation results with all uses linked to one or more specific user.

- What questions the evaluation will answer.

Evaluation questions set the boundaries of the evaluation by stating what aspects of the program will be addressed. Having stakeholders create questions reveals what's important to them and what they believe the evaluation should answer (U.S. GAO, 1992).

Following are questions to guide design selection:

What's being evaluated?

Is the entire program being evaluated or one component (Education Development Center, 2018)? An evaluation of one aspect of a program may call for a different design than an evaluation of an entire program. For example, a pretest–posttest design may be appropriate to evaluate the effect of a specific educational activity on participant knowledge, but a quasi-experimental design is needed to evaluate if the overall program met its outcome objectives.

What questions need answering?

Are answers needed for questions about the long-term impact of the program or short-term outcomes (SAMHSA, 2012)? For example, is the evaluation expected to answer whether any change took place in participants' knowledge (pretest–posttest design), or is evidence needed to document that participating in the program *caused* a change (experimental or quasi-experimental design)?

How feasible is the design that will answer the questions?

Are the resources available in terms of budget, time, and staff, to conduct an evaluation using the design that will best answer the questions? If an experimental design is best, is it ethical to randomly assign participants to a control group (SAMHSA, 2012)?

In going through the process of selecting an evaluation design, keep the following in mind:

— Complex evaluation designs (experimental and quasi-experimental) are more costly, but their findings are more accurate.
— Complex evaluation designs are more difficult to implement and require greater expertise in research methods and analysis.
— As the complexity of an evaluation increases, so does the chance that something will go wrong, especially if there is not enough evaluation expertise involved in the effort.
— No evaluation design is safe from having its results questioned.
— Some evaluation is better than no evaluation. Even though the resources to use the most rigorous evaluation design may not be available, it's important to do something even if that means using the least rigorous design (posttest only) (National Center for Mental Health and Youth Violence Prevention, 2004).

• What, if any, agreements are in place?

These might be legal contracts, detailed protocols, or memoranda of understanding that summarize the procedures and clarify roles and responsibilities among those who will carry out the evaluation plan (Joint Committee on Standards for Education Evaluation, 1994). They include statements describing what has been agreed upon concerning the purpose of the evaluation, how it will be implemented using the available resources, the users, uses, questions, design, deliverables, a timeline, and budget.

Step 4—Gather Credible Evidence.

An evaluation should strive to collect information that stakeholders see as credible, believable, relevant, and able to answer their questions (Basch, Silepcevich, Gold, Duncan, & Kolbe, 1985). When stakeholders are involved in defining and gathering data they find credible, they are more likely to accept the evaluation's conclusions and to act on its recommendations (Fetterman, Kaftarian, & Wandersman, 1996). When stakeholders have concerns about the quality of the data or when serious consequences are associated with concluding that program effects exist when in fact none do, or vice versa, it may be best to consult with specialists in evaluation methodology (Basch et al., 1985).

The aspects of data collection that typically affect perceptions of credibility include indicators, sources, quality, quantity, and logistics.

• Indicators

These are the specific measures that provide the basis for the data collected and the criteria for judging the program. They are developed from the general program concepts, context, and expected effects. For example, measures of program activities such as participation rate, levels of client satisfaction, the efficient use of resources; measures of program effects such as changes in participant behavior, community norms, policies or practices, health status, and quality of life.

• Sources

People, documents, and observations are the sources of evidence or data that are needed to measure the indicators. Collecting data from more than one source for an indicator allows for different perspectives. This provides a more comprehensive view of the program and enhances the evaluation's credibility. Using both quantitative and qualitative data increases the likelihood that the data will be balanced and meet the needs and expectations of the users.

- Quality

High-quality data are reliable, valid, and useful. Data quality is affected by the design of the data collection instrument, procedures, training of data collectors, data sources, data management, and error checking. The level of quality for any one evaluation is the level that meets the stakeholders' baseline for credibility.

- Quantity

The quantity of data collected in an evaluation affects the confidence level or accuracy of the conclusions drawn from the evaluation. How much data are collected is determined by the number of people participating in the evaluation or the sample size. The confidence level and the sample size should be decided in advance.

- Logistics

Logistics entail the procedures, timing, and infrastructure needed for collecting and handling the data. Each procedure must align with the cultural context of the setting and ensure privacy and confidentiality of the data and the source are protected.

One way to minimize the potential for data credibility issues is by having an evaluator with the skills and expertise needed to carry out high-quality evaluations. Following are guidelines developed by the United Nations Evaluation Group (UNEG, 2008) and used by the WHO (2013) to identify evaluators with the necessary skill set. They include the following:

1. Knowledge of the program context.
2. Technical and professional skills in evaluation design, data collection, analysis, and reporting.
3. Interpersonal skills including those needed for communication (written and oral), negotiation, facilitation, and cultural sensitivity.

4. Personal attributes including ethical behavior, judgment capacity, education, and experience in evaluation and research.
5. Management skills for evaluation projects, teams, resources, and training.

Step 5—Justify Conclusions. Before stakeholders use the evaluation findings, they must agree that the conclusions are justified. This is accomplished by linking the conclusions to the supporting evidence and standards (criteria) against which they were judged. Conclusions are justified based on standards, analysis and synthesis, interpretation, judgment, and recommendations.

- *Standards* reflect the stakeholders' values and provide the foundation for making comparisons and judgments about the program's performance (Scriven, 1998).
- *Analysis and synthesis* are the processes used to decipher facts from the data collected. The procedures used to examine and summarize involve deciding how the data will be organized, classified, compared, and ultimately, displayed. These decisions are guided by the evaluation questions, the type of data (qualitative or quantitative) you've collected, and input from stakeholders and users of the results.
- *Interpretation* is the process of understanding and determining the meaning of the findings. Uncovering facts about a program's performance is not enough to draw evaluative conclusions. Evidence must be understood to determine the practical significance of what has been learned. Interpretations draw on the information and perspectives of stakeholders and can be strengthened by their active participation.
- *Judgments* are statements made about the merit, worth, or significance of the program. Judgments are formed by comparing the findings and interpretations against one or more selected standards. Because multiple standards can be applied

to a given program, stakeholders might reach different or even conflicting judgments. This can trigger the need to clarify values and reestablish the bases on which the program should be judged.

- *Recommendations* are the actions proposed for consideration as a result of the evaluation. Recommendations for continuing, expanding, redesigning, or terminating a program are not solely based on a program's effectiveness (Scriven, 1998). They also take into consideration the context, particularly the organizational context, in which programmatic decisions will be made.

Tips for justifying conclusions include the following:

TIP 1 Summarizing findings using appropriate methods of analysis and synthesis.

TIP 2 Interpreting the significance of results for deciding what the findings mean.

TIP 3 Making judgments based on clearly stated values that classify a result as positive or negative and high or low.

TIP 4 Comparing results in a variety of ways such as with program objectives, a comparison group, national norms, past performance, or needs.

TIP 5 Proposing alternative explanations for findings and why they should or should not be discounted.

TIP 6 Making recommendations that are consistent with the conclusions.

TIP 7 Limiting conclusions to the situations, time frames, people, contexts, and purposes for which the findings are applicable (Joint Committee on Standards for Educational Evaluation, 1994).

Step 6—Ensure Use and Share Lessons Learned. It takes deliberate action to ensure stakeholders use the evaluation findings. Without a concerted effort, this may not happen. Consequently, preparation for this begins with

stakeholders as soon as possible and continues throughout the evaluation process. The five elements critical to ensuring evaluation finding are used include design, preparation, feedback, follow-up, and dissemination.

- *Design* refers to the way the evaluation questions, methods, and processes are structured. The design should enable the evaluation results to be used as intended. The process of creating the design should include stakeholders to add to the relevance, credibility, and overall utility of the evaluation.
- *Preparation* refers to the steps taken to get stakeholders ready to translate the evaluation finding into action. Preparing stakeholders to use the evaluation findings in steps gives them time to investigate the implications of the results and time to identify options for improving the program.
- *Feedback* is the back and forth commentary that goes on among everyone involved in the evaluation. The giving and receiving of feedback creates an atmosphere of trust among stakeholders, keeps the evaluation on track, and keeps everyone informed of its progress.
- *Follow-up* refers to the support users need during and after they receive the evaluation findings. Follow-up reminds users of the intended uses of the evaluation findings and prevents lessons learned from being lost or ignored. It increases understanding of what was found and the actions consistent with those findings. Follow-up also carries with it the responsibility for preventing misuse of evaluation results by stakeholders who might be tempted to take them out of context or use them for purposes other than those agreed upon. Active follow-up might prevent these and other forms of misuse by ensuring that evidence is not misinterpreted and not applied to questions other than those that were the focus of the evaluation.

- *Dissemination* is the process of sharing or communicating the procedures, results, and lessons learned from the evaluation to the appropriate audiences in a timely, accurate, and consistent fashion. The goal for dissemination is full disclosure and impartial reporting of the evaluation results and lessons learned. Although documentation of the evaluation is needed, a formal evaluation report may not always be the best way to share this information with all relevant audiences. Rather, evaluation reports should be tailored for the audience, include the focus of the evaluation, and list its strengths and weaknesses.

Following are tips to ensure findings are used and lessons learned are shared:

TIP 1 Design the evaluation so the results are compatible with users' intended uses.

TIP 2 Prepare stakeholders to use the results by practicing throughout the project how different conclusions would affect the program.

TIP 3 Provide regular feedback to stakeholders about interim findings, provisional interpretations, and decisions to be made that might affect the use of the findings.

Schedule follow-up meetings with intended users to facilitate the adaptation of evaluation conclusions into actions or decisions.

TIP 4 Use strategies tailored to meet stakeholders' needs for disseminating the procedures used and lessons learned from the evaluation.

Framework Standards

The standards recommended in the Framework are criteria for judging the quality of the evaluation activities and determining whether the activities are well designed and working as best as they can. The standards are grouped by the aspects of evaluation they address: utility, feasibility, propriety, and accuracy.

Utility Standards. The utility (usefulness) standards ensure that evaluations will serve the information needs of the intended users. They include

A. **Stakeholder identification.** Anyone involved in or affected by the evaluation should be identified so that their needs can be addressed.

B. **Evaluator credibility.** Those responsible for conducting the evaluation should be trustworthy and competent in performing the evaluation so that findings have maximum credibility and acceptance.

C. **Information scope and selection.** Information collected should address relevant questions about the program so that it is responsive to the needs and interests of stakeholders.

D. **Values identification.** The perspectives, procedures, and rationale used to interpret findings should be carefully described so that the bases for value judgments are clear.

E. **Report clarity.** Evaluation reports should clearly describe the program, including its context, purposes, procedures, and findings so that essential information is provided and easily understood.

F. **Report timeliness and dissemination.** Substantial interim findings and reports should be disseminated to intended users so that they can be used in a timely fashion.

G. **Evaluation impact.** Evaluations should be planned, conducted, and reported in ways that encourage follow-through by stakeholders so that the likelihood of its use increases.

Feasibility Standards. The feasibility standards ensure evaluations will be realistic, prudent, diplomatic, and frugal. They include

A. **Practical procedures.** Evaluation procedures should be practical while needed information is being obtained so that disruption is kept to a minimum.

B. **Political viability.** During planning and conducting the evaluation, consideration should be given to the various positions of interest groups so that their cooperation can be obtained and possible attempts to curtail the evaluation or bias or misapply the results can be averted or counteracted.

C. **Cost-effectiveness.** The evaluation should be efficient and produce valuable information so that expended resources can be justified.

Propriety Standards. The propriety standards ensure that an evaluation will be conducted legally, ethically, and with regard for the welfare of those involved in the evaluation, as well as those affected by its results. They include

A. **Service orientation.** The evaluation should be designed to assist organizations so that the needs of the target population are effectively addressed and served.

B. **Formal agreements.** All obligations of principal parties involved in an evaluation should be agreed upon in writing so that each must adhere to the conditions of the agreement or renegotiate it.

C. **Rights of human subjects.** The evaluation should be designed and conducted in a manner so that the rights and welfare of human subjects are respected and protected.

D. **Human interactions.** Those conducting an evaluation should interact respectfully with other persons associated with the evaluation so that participants are not threatened or harmed.

E. **Complete and fair assessment.** The examination and recording of the strengths and weaknesses of the program should be complete and fair so that the strengths can be enhanced and the weaknesses addressed.

F. **Disclosure of findings.** The principal parties to an evaluation should ensure that the full evaluation findings with pertinent limitations are made accessible so that those affected by the evaluation and any others with expressed legal rights to receive them.

G. **Conflict of interest.** Conflicts of interest should be addressed openly and honestly so that the evaluation processes and results are not compromised.

H. **Fiscal responsibility.** The distribution and spending of resources should reflect sound accountability procedures and be prudent and ethically responsible so that expenses are accountable and appropriate.

Accuracy Standards. The accuracy standards ensure that an evaluation will convey sufficient information about the determining features of the merit of the program. They include

A. **Program documentation.** Program documentation should be clear and accurate.

B. **Context analysis.** The program context should be examined in enough detail so that probable contextual influences on the program can be identified.

C. **Described purposes and procedures.** The purposes and procedures of the evaluation should be monitored and described in enough detail so that they can be identified and assessed.

D. **Defensible information sources.** The information sources used for an evaluation should be described in enough detail so that the adequacy of the information can be assessed.

E. **Valid information.** Data collection procedures should be developed and implemented so that they ensure valid interpretation for the intended use.

F. **Reliable information.** Information-gathering procedures should be developed and implemented so that they ensure sufficiently reliable information for the intended use.

G. **Systematic information.** Information collected, processed, and reported in an evaluation should be systematically reviewed so that errors can be corrected.

H. Analysis of qualitative information. The analysis of qualitative information should be done appropriately and systematically so that evaluation questions are answered effectively.

I. Justified conclusions. Conclusions should be explicitly justified so that stakeholders can assess them.

J. Impartial reporting. Reporting procedures should guard against distortion caused by the personal feelings and biases of anyone involved so that evaluation findings are reflected fairly.

K. Meta-evaluation. The evaluation should be evaluated formatively and summatively against these and other pertinent standards to guide its conduct appropriately so that on completion stakeholders can closely examine its strengths and weaknesses.

Using the standards to work through the steps of the Framework requires knowing which standards are relevant to what step. See **Table 7-6** for the Framework steps and their relevant standards.

Table 7-6 Framework steps and relevant standards

Step 1—Engage stakeholders

Standard	Standard group	Standard group item
Stakeholder identification	Utility	A
Evaluator credibility	Utility	B
Formal agreements	Propriety	C
Rights of human subjects	Propriety	D
Conflict of interest	Propriety	G
Meta-evaluation	Accuracy	L

Step 2—Describe program

Standard	Standard group	Standard group item
Complete and fair assessment	Propriety	C
Program documentation	Accuracy	A
Context analysis	Accuracy	B
Meta-evaluation	Accuracy	L

Step 3—Focus evaluation design

Standard	Standard group	Standard group item
Evaluation impact	Utility	G
Practical procedures	Feasibility	A

(continues)

Table 7-6 Framework steps and relevant standards *(continued)*

Political viability	Feasibility	B
Cost-effectiveness	Feasibility	C
Service orientation	Propriety	A
Complete and fair assessment	Propriety	E
Fiscal responsibility	Propriety	H
Describe purpose and procedures	Accuracy	C
Meta-evaluation	Accuracy	L

Step 4—Gather credible evidence

Standard	Standard group	Standard group item
Information scope and selection	Utility	C
Defensible information sources	Accuracy	D
Valid information	Accuracy	E
Reliable information	Accuracy	F
Systematic information	Accuracy	G
Meta-evaluation	Accuracy	L

Step 5—Justify conclusions

Standard	Standard group	Standard group item
Values identification	Utility	D
Analysis of quantitative information	Accuracy	H
Analysis of qualitative information	Accuracy	I
Justified conclusions	Accuracy	J
Meta-evaluation	Accuracy	L

Step 6—Ensure use and sharing of lessons learned

Standard	Standard group	Standard group item
Evaluator credibility	Utility	B

(continues)

Table 7-6 Framework steps and relevant standards   (continued)

Report clarity	Utility	E
Report timeliness	Utility	F
Evaluation impact	Utility	G
Disclosure of findings	Propriety	F
Impartial reporting	Accuracy	K
Meta-evaluation	Accuracy	L

Centers for Disease Control and Prevention. (2017b). *Evaluation standards.* Atlanta, GA: U.S. Department of Health and Human Services, Program Performance and Evaluation Office. Retrieved July 24, 2019, from https://www.cdc.gov/eval/standards/index.htm

Writing an Evaluation Plan and Timeline

The *evaluation plan* is part of the program plan and is developed during the planning stage of the planning process. To ensure it's a useful document:

1. develop it collaboratively with the stakeholders,
2. keep it flexible so it can be adjusted if there are program or priority changes,
3. cover multiple years of the program, if the program is ongoing,
4. address the entire program rather than focusing on one funding source or objective/activity (CDC, 2011).

The seven sections of the evaluation plan summarized next are based on the CDC Framework for Evaluation in Public Health (CDC, 2013).

Section 1—Title Page. The title page contains the name of the program, dates it covers, and the basic focus of the evaluation.

Section 2—Intended Use and Users. This section describes the purpose of the evaluation and its intended uses. This is particularly important as everyone involved in the evaluation should be on the same page with why the evaluation is being done and what the results will be used for. This section also identifies the primary users of the results. These are the people interested in, involved in, or affected by the program. From this group of users, establish an evaluation stakeholder working group of between 8 and 10 people who can serve as consultants throughout the evaluation (CDC, 2008). The description of intended uses and users in this section is also contained in Step 3 of the Framework—Focus Evaluation Design.

Section 3—Program Description. Including the program description in the evaluation plan clarifies its purpose, stage of development, activities, capacity for improving health, and its implementation context. It ensures everyone connected with the program, staff, and stakeholders are on the same page. It's a critical component of the plan because it sets the stage for identifying the evaluation questions, focusing the evaluation design, and connecting program planning with evaluation (CDC, 2011). The content of the program description in the evaluation plan is the same as that in Step 2 of the Framework—Describe Program, discussed previously.

Section 4—Evaluation Focus. This section of the evaluation plan focuses the evaluation design to reflect the stage of the program, its purpose, uses, and questions to be answered. It contains an explanation of how evaluation questions will be developed and selected. For example, one way is to have stakeholders submit questions based on the purpose of the evaluation and questions they'd like answered. These are then prioritized by an evaluation committee based on how consistent they are with the logic model, program description, and stage of development. Transparency in how evaluation questions are selected is critical for stakeholders to accept the evaluation results and possibly even for continued support of the program (CDC, 2011). This information is in Step 3 of the Framework—Focus Evaluation Design

In developing and selecting the evaluation questions, budget and resources need to be considered. Since the best evaluation design may not be feasible because of resource and budget limitations, it's recommended that a minimum of 10 percent of the overall program budget be allocated for evaluation activities (CDC, 2014).

It's helpful in this section to also determine the indicators for the evaluation questions. Indicators are what provide the information needed to answer the evaluation questions. These are the things that are read, seen or heard that "indicate" or show what has changed and by how much (Ontario Centre of Excellence for Child and Youth Mental Health, n.d.). For example, if the evaluation question is "Did the program decrease the incidence of driving while texting?"—an indicator might be the percent of change in the number of summonses given for driving while texting.

Section 5—Methods/Design. This section of the evaluation plan explains how the method or design for answering the evaluation questions will be selected. The information in this section is in Step 3 of the Framework—Focus Evaluation Design.

Section 6—Analysis and Interpretation: Planning for Conclusions. This section of the evaluation plan explains how data will be analyzed and includes a description of the process for interpreting the results. Also contained in this section is a description of who will receive the results. The content for this section is in Step 5 of the Framework—Justify Conclusions.

Planning for analysis and interpretation is directly tied to an evaluation timeline (see following) and available resources. It takes time and expertise to prepare data for analysis and to conduct the analysis, regardless of the type of data collected. Once data are analyzed, the results are interpreted in light of the program goals, context, and needs of the stakeholders.

It's critically important for the evaluation plan to include time for stakeholders to review conclusions drawn from the data. Planning for this increases the transparency of the processes used to arrive at conclusions and provides justification for them.

Section 7—Using, Disseminating, and Sharing Lessons Learned. This last section of the evaluation plan contains a clear description of how the evaluation findings or results will be used, who the intended users of the findings are, and how the findings will be shared with them. Consequently, the methods for dissemination are tailored to the users in terms of timing, style, tone, message source, method, and format. To enable this to happen, the plan for disseminating the findings should:

- focus on the needs of the specific user and include the types and levels of information needed in the form and language the user prefers.
- contain a variety of dissemination methods, including written information, electronic media, and person-to-person contact.
- share information that users have identified as important and information that users may not know to request, but are likely to need.

- establish clear avenues for users to make their needs and priorities known.
- use existing resources, relationships, and networks to share the information to the greatest extent possible while building new resources as needed by users.
- include effective quality control mechanisms to ensure that information included is accurate, relevant and representative.
- establish linkages to resources users may need to implement the information in the findings (National Center for the Dissemination of Disability Research, 2001).

An *evaluation timeline* is a table or chart used in conjunction with the plan to keep the evaluation on track. It contains the following information:

- the key evaluation questions.
- the indicators.
- the data collection method.
- the data collection instrument.
- who will collect the data.
- when the data will be collected.
- how the data will be analyzed and by whom (Smart, 2017).

See **Table 7-7** for an example.

Writing an Evaluation Report

Section 7 of the evaluation plan discussed earlier describes how the evaluation findings will be disseminated to those who need and will use the information. One way to do this is through an evaluation report, a written document that includes the *what, how,* and *why it matters* of the program (CDC, 2013).

What is the program's purpose, description, anticipated effects, and the way its activities are linked to the outcomes.

How is the program's implementation and whether it's being carried out with fidelity.

Why it matters is the program's rationale and its potential impact on public health (CDC, 2013).

The evaluation report format outlined below is based on the CDC Framework for Program Evaluation in Public Health. It's one way of organizing the report. Use it as a guide and adapt it as needed (CDC, 2013).

The basic elements of a final evaluation report include the following:

Title page: This first page or cover of the report includes the program title, dates, and the basic focus of the evaluation.

Executive summary: This is a brief summary that includes the program description, evaluation questions, evaluation design, key findings, and next steps.

Intended use and users: This section describes the purposes and intended uses of the evaluation findings, identifies the intended users of the findings, and the people who conducted the evaluation.

Program description: This section usually includes the logic model, a description of the program's stage of development, and a narrative description or the program's "story." It promotes an understanding of the program, explains the basis for the evaluation questions, and describes how they were prioritized.

Evaluation focus: This section explains how the evaluation questions were identified and prioritized based on the logic model, program description, stage of development, program and stakeholder priorities, intended uses of the evaluation, and feasibility.

Data sources and methods: Addressed in this section are the

Table 7-7 Sample evaluation timeline

Evaluation Question	Indicators	Data collection method	Data collection instrument	Sample	When will data be collected?	Who will collect data?	Who will analyze data?	How will data be analyzed?
Did the program reduce student vaccination barriers?	Percent of students reporting change in perception of vaccine efficacy Percent of students reporting elimination of injection—vaccine administration barrier with option of nasal spray vaccine administration	Survey	Questionnaire	Stratified random sample of residential undergraduate students by academic year	2 weeks after end of program	Program staff	Math faculty and graduate student	Quantitative analysis

Data from: Australian Institute for Family Studies, Child. (2017). How to develop a program evaluation plan. Retrieved March 6, 2020, from https://aifs.gov.au/cfca/expert-panel-project/program-planning-evaluation-guide/evaluate-your-program-or-service/how-develop-evaluation-plan evaluation indicators and performance measures, data sources, and the rationale for selecting the data collection methods used.

Results, conclusions, and interpretation: This section contains a description of the data analysis processes used, an interpretation of the results, and the actions or recommendations for next steps.

Use, dissemination, and sharing plan: In this last section, the plans for using the evaluation findings are discussed, including how they will be disseminated and shared.

Tools for clarity: To help clarify the information in the report the following are often included: a table of contents; lists of tables, charts, and figures; references; an acronym list; and appendices.

Chapter Summary

Evaluation occurs throughout the planning process starting with formative evaluation (needs assessment) during the assessment stage to determine needs and process evaluation during the planning and implementation stages to determine appropriateness of procedures, and concludes with summative (outcome and impact) evaluation in the final stage to determine program efficacy, strengths, and weaknesses. (See **Figure 7-3**.)

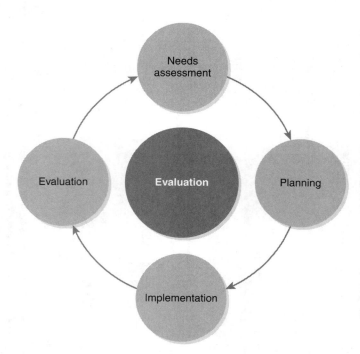

Figure 7-3 Evaluation in the planning process

Planning In Practice Chapter Activity

The 2015–2020 dietary guidelines for Americans recommend a daily intake of two cups of fruit and two and a half cups of vegetables (U.S. Department of Health and Human Services, 2015). However, only 1 in 10 Americans meets these recommendations (CDC, 2017b).

1. In small groups, brainstorm reasons why people might not eat the recommended daily amounts of fruit and vegetables.
2. Come to a consensus on the most likely cause of the problem of insufficient daily fruit and vegetable intake.
3. Formulate a possible solution to the problem based on the cause identified in the previous step.
4. Read the article below, and answer the questions that follow.

Article: *Washington state's fruit and vegetable prescription program: Improving affordability of healthy foods for low-income patients* (Marchinkevege, Auvinen, & Nambuthiri. 2019)

Link to article: https://www.ncbi.nlm.nih.gov/pmc/articles/PMC6716422/

Article Questions

1. What health problem did the program address?
2. What was the goal of the program?
3. Who were the "partners" in this program?
4. Who was the intended audience?
5. How did the program address the health problem?
6. Who designed the program, and what was it based on?
7. How did partners participate in the planning and implementation of the program?
8. How was the program tailored for contextual fit?
9. What constituted fidelity "dose" in this program?
10. Why was the process evaluation conducted?
11. How was the process evaluation conducted?
12. How were the process evaluation data analyzed?
13. What did the process evaluation reveal?
14. Why was the outcome evaluation conducted?
15. How were outcome evaluation participants selected?
16. What questions was the outcome evaluation designed to answer?
17. How were outcome evaluation data collected?
18. How were the outcome data analyzed?
19. What were the results of the outcome evaluation in relation to the evaluation questions?
20. Based on the evaluation results, was the program a success?
21. How was this approach to solving the problem of insufficient fruit and vegetable consumption similar to or different from the solution your small group formulated?

References

Baker, A., & Bruner, B. (2012). Appendix 10b—How big should the sample size be? *Integrating evaluative capacity into organizational practice: A guide for nonprofit and philanthropic organizations and their stake-holders.* Retrieved July 11, 2019, from http://evaluativethinking.org/evalthink.html

Banerjee, A.V., Duflo, E., Glennerster, R., & Kothari, D. (2010). Improving immunization coverage in rural

India: Clustered randomized controlled evaluation of immunization campaigns with and without incentives. *British Medical Journal, 340*(c2220). doi: https://doi.org/10.1136/bmj.c2220

Basch, C. E., Silepcevich, E. M., Gold, R. S., Duncan, D. F., & Kolbe, L. J. (1985). Avoiding type III errors in health education program evaluation: A case study. *Health Education Quarterly 12*(4), 315–31. doi: 10.1177/109019818501200311

Bertrand, J. (2006). Fundamentals of program evaluation. Johns Hopkins Bloomberg School of Public Health. Retrieved June 25, 2019, from http://ocw.jhsph.edu/courses/fundamentalsprogramevaluation/PDFs/Lecture7.pdf

Biron, C., Gatrell, C., & Cooper, C. L. (2010). Autopsy of a failure: Evaluating process and contextual issues in an organizational-level work stress intervention. *International Journal of Stress Management, 17*(2), 135–158. doi: 10.1037/a0018772

Boor, M., & Wood, F. (2006). *Keywords in qualitative methods: A vocabulary of research concepts.* Thousand Oaks, CA: Sage Publications. Retrieved June 17, 2019, from http://methods.sagepub.com/book/keywords-in-qualitative-methods/n69.xml

Bowie, L., & Bronte-Tinkew, J. (2008). Research to results: Briefs. Process evaluation. Retrieved March 3, 2020, from https://www.childtrends.org/publications/process-evaluations-a-guide-for-out-of-school-time-practitioners

Brinker, T. J., Stamm-Balderjahn, S., Seeger, W., Klingelhofer, D., & Groneberg, D. A. (2015). Education against tobacco (EAT): A quasi-experimental prospective evaluation of a multinational medical-student delivered smoking prevention program for secondary schools in Germany. *British Medical Journal, 5*(9), 1–7. https://doi.org/10.1136/bmjopen-2015-008093

Capwell, E. M., Butterfloss, F., & Francisco, V. T. (2000). Why evaluate? *Health Promotion Practice, 1*(1), 15–20. doi: 10.1177/152483990000100103

Center for Community Health and Development (CCHD). (2018a). Chapter 36, Section 1: A framework for program evaluation: A gateway to tools. Lawrence, KS: University of Kansas. Retrieved May 30, 2019, from the Community Tool Box: https://ctb.ku.edu/en/table-of-contents/evaluate/evaluation/framework-for-evaluation/main

Center for Community Health and Development. (CCHD). (2018b). Chapter 37, Section 4: Selecting an appropriate design for the evaluation. Lawrence, KS: University of Kansas. Retrieved July 15, 2019, from the Community Tool Box: https://ctb.ku.edu/en/table-of-contents/evaluate/evaluate-community-interventions/experimental-design/main

Centers for Disease Control and Prevention (CDC). (1999). Framework for program evaluation in public health. *Morbidity and Mortality Weekly Report (MMWR), 48*(RR-11):1–42. Retrieved July 18, 2019, from https://www.cdc.gov/mmwr/preview/mmwrhtml/rr4811a1.htm

Centers for Disease Control and Prevention (CDC). (2008). Introduction to process evaluation in tobacco use prevention and control. Retrieved May 26, 2019, from https://www.cdc.gov/tobacco/stateandcommunity/tobacco_control_programs/surveillance_evaluation/process_evaluation/index.htm

Centers for Disease Control and Prevention (CDC). (2011). *Developing an effective evaluation plan.* Retrieved July 5, 2019, from https://www.cdc.gov/tobacco/stateandcommunity/tobacco_control_programs/surveillance_evaluation/evaluation_plan/index.htm

Centers for Disease Control and Prevention (CDC). (2012a). *Introduction to program evaluation for public health programs: A self-study guide.* Atlanta, GA: U.S. Department of Health and Human Services, Centers for Disease Control and Prevention, Program Performance and Evaluation Office. Retrieved July 7, 2019, from https://www.cdc.gov/eval/guide/introduction/index.htm

Centers for Disease Control and Prevention. (CDC). (2012b). *Focus the evaluation design.* Retrieved June 10, 2019, from https://www.cdc.gov/eval/guide/step3/index.htm

Centers for Disease Control and Prevention (CDC). (2013). *Developing an effective evaluation report: Setting the course for effective program evaluation.* Retrieved July 26, 2019, from https://www.cdc.gov/eval/materials/developing-an-effective-evaluation-report_tag508.pdf

Centers for Disease Control and Prevention (CDC). (2014). *Best practices for comprehensive tobacco control programs—2014.* Retrieved July 26, 2019, from https://www.cdc.gov/tobacco/stateandcommunity/best_practices/index.htm

Centers for Disease Control and Prevention (CDC). (2017a). *A framework for program evaluation.* Retrieved May 30, 2019, from https://www.cdc.gov/eval/framework/index.htm

Centers for Disease Control and Prevention (CDC). (2017b). *Only 1 in 10 adults get enough fruits or vegetables.* Retrieved May 13, 2020, from https://www.cdc.gov/media/releases/2017/p1116-fruit-vegetable-consumption.html

Centers for Disease Control and Prevention (CDC). (2019). *What is program evaluation?* Retrieved May 29, 2019, from https://www.cdc.gov/eval/index.htm

Deepak, M. G. (2010). Missed vaccination—Violation of ethics? *British Medical Journal, 340*(c2220). https://doi.org/10.1136/bmj.c2220

Education Development Center, Prevention Solutions. (2018). Selecting an appropriate evaluation design. Retrieved July 26, 2019, from https://preventionsolutions.edc.org/sites/default/files/attachments/Selecting-an-Appropriate-Evaluation-Design.pdf

Esbensen, F., Osgood, W., Peterson, D., Taylor, T. J., Carson, D., Freng, A., & Matsuda, K. (2013). Process and outcome evaluation of the G.R.E.A.T. program. Retrieved July 1, 2019, from https://www.ncjrs.gov/pdffiles1/nij /grants/244346.pdf

Fetterman, D. M., Kaftarian, S. J., & Wandersman, A. (Eds.). (1996). *Empowerment evaluation: Knowledge and tools for self-assessment and accountability.* Thousand Oaks, CA: Sage Publications. http://dx.doi.org/10.4135/978145 2243573

Gargani, J., & Miller, R. L. (2016). What is program evaluation? *American Journal of Public Health, 106*(6), e.13. https://dx.doi.org/10.2105%2FAJPH.2016.303159

Gertler, P. J., Martinez, S., Premand, P., Rawlings, L. B., & Vermeersch, C. M. J. (2011). *Impact evaluation in practice.* Washington, DC: The World Bank. Retrieved February 29, 2020, from https://www.worldbank.org /en/programs/sief-trust-fund/publication/impact -evaluation-in-practice

Health Assessment and Research for Communities (HARC). (2016). Internal vs external evaluation: Pros and cons. Retrieved March 3, 2020, from https://harc data.org/internal-vs-external-evaluation/

Hutchins, S. S., Rosenthal, J., Easton, P., Swint, E., Guerrero, H., & Hadler, S. (1999). Effectiveness and cost-effectiveness of linking the Special Supplemental Nutrition Program for Women, Infants and Children (WIC) with immunization activities. *Journal of Public Health Policy, 20*(4), 408–426. doi: 10.2307/3343128

International Rescue Committee. (2018). Developing research questions for impact evaluations. Retrieved July 2, 2019, from https://www.rescue.org/resource /developing-questions-impact-evaluations

Joint Committee on Standards for Educational Evaluation. (1994). *Program evaluation standards: How to assess evaluations of educational programs* (2nd ed.). Thousand Oaks, CA: Sage Publications

Kaufman, R. (1988). Needs assessment: A menu. *Educational Technology, 28*(7), 21–23. doi: https://www .jstor.org/stable/44426572

King, T. L., Gullestrup, J., Batterham, P. J., Kelly, B., Lockwood, C., Lingard, H., Harvey, S. B., ... Milner, A. (2018). Shifting beliefs about suicide: Pre-post evaluation of the effectiveness of a program for workers in the construction industry. *International Journal of Environmental Research and Public Health, 15*(10), EII2106. doi: 10.3390/ijerph15102106

Knowledge for Health, Johns Hopkins Center for Communication Programs. (2017). Measuring success toolkit: Types of evaluation design. Retrieved July 14, 2019, from https://www.k4health.org/toolkits/mea suring-success/types-evaluation-designs

Linnan, L., & Steckler, A. (2002). Process evaluation for public health interventions and research: An overview. In A. Steckler & L. Linnan (Eds.), *Process evaluation for public health interventions and research* (pp. 1–23). San Francisco, CA: Jossey-Bass.

Lipsey, M. W. (1993). Theory as method: Small theories of treatments. *New Directions for Program Evaluation, 57,* 5–38. https://doi.org/10.1002/ev.1637

Mann, V., Eble, A., Frost, C., Premkumar, R., & Boone, P. (2010). Retrospective comparative evaluation the lasting impact of a community-based primary health care programme on under 5 mortality in villages around Jamkhed, India. *Bulletin of the World Health Organization, 88*(10), 727–736. Retrieved from https://www.ncbi.nlm.nih.gov/pmc/articles/ PMC2947035/

Metz, A. J. R. (2007). Why conduct a program evaluation? *Child Trends, #2007-31.* Retrieved May 30, 2019, from https://eric.ed.gov/?id=ED499616

Moore, G., Audrey, S., Barker, M., Bond, L., Bonell, C., Hardeman, W., Moore, L., ... Baird, J. (2014). Process evaluation of complex interventions. U.K. Medical Research Council (MRC) Guidance. Retrieved June 18, 2019, from https://www.bmj.com/content/350 /bmj.h1258

Murray, C., Aylward, P., Cooke, R., Martin, M., & Sidford, S. (n.d.). The planning and evaluation wizard: What is evaluation? Flinders University. Retrieved June 2, 2019, from http://www.flinders.edu.au/medicine /sites/pew/developing-a-project-and-evaluation-plan /evaluation-zone/about-evaluation/what-is-evalua tion.cfm

National Center for Mental Health and Youth Violence Prevention. (2004). National center brief: Evaluation designs and approaches. Retrieved July 15, 2019, from http://www.promoteprevent.org/sites/www.promote prevent.org/files/resources/evaluation_designs_appro aches%20(2).pdf

National Center for the Dissemination of Disability Research. (2001). *Developing an effective dissemination plan.* Austin, TX: Southwest Educational Developmental Laboratory, 2001. Retrieved July 28, 2019, from https://eric.ed.gov/?id=ED451653

Ontario Centre of Excellence for Child and Youth Mental Health. (n.d.). Program evaluation toolkit. Retrieved March 22, 2020, from https://www.cymh.ca/Modules /ResourceHub/?input=evaluation

Organization for Economic Cooperation and Development (OECD). (2006). Outline of principles of impact evaluation. Retrieved July 2, 2019, from http://www .oecd.org/dac/evaluation/dcdndep/37671602.pdf

Rural Health Information Hub (RHIhub). (2019). Evaluation design. Retrieved June 10, 2019, from https:// www.ruralhealthinfo.org/toolkits/rural-toolkit/4 /evaluation-design

Salabarria-Pena, Y., Apt, B. S., & Walsh, C. M. (2007). Practical use of program evaluation among sexually transmitted disease (STD) programs. Department of Health and Human Services, National Center for HIV, STD, and TB Prevention, Division of STD Prevention. Retrieved June 27, 2019, from https://www.cdc.gov /std/program/pupestd.htm

Santelli, J. S., Kantor, L. M., Grilo, S. A., Speizer, I. S., Lindberg, L. D., Heitel, J., Schalet, A. T. ... Ott, M. A. (2017). Abstinence-only-until-marriage: An updated review of U.S. policies and programs and their impact. *Journal of Adolescent Health*, *61*, 273–280. Retrieved July 8, 2019, from https://www.jahonline.org/article/S1054-139X(17)30260-4/fulltext

Saunders, R. P., Evans. M. H., & Joshi, P. (2005). Developing a process evaluation plan for assessing health program implementation: A how to guide. *Health Promotion Practice*, *6*(2), 134–147. doi: 10.1177/1524839904273387

Schneider, M., Hall, W. J., Hernandez, A. E., Hindes, K., Montez, G., Pham, T., Rosen, L., ... Steckler, A. (2009). Rationale, design and methods for process evaluation in the HEALTHY study. *International Journal of Obesity*, *33*(suppl 4), s60–67. doi: 10.1038/2009.118

Scriven, M. (1998). Minimalist theory of evaluation: The least theory that practice requires. *American Journal of Evaluation* 19, 57–70. https://doi.org/10.1016/S1098-2140(99)80180-5

Sexuality Information and Education Council of the United States (SIECUS). (2018). A history of federal funding for abstinence only until marriage programs. Retrieved July 8, 2019, from https://siecus.org/resources/a-history-of-abstinence-only-federal-funding/

Shantikumar, S. (2018). Public health textbook: Biases and confounding. Retrieved July 10, 2019, from https://www.healthknowledge.org.uk/public-health-textbook/research-methods/1a-epidemiology/biases

Smart, J. (2017). *How to develop a program evaluation plan*. Australian Institute for Family studies, Child Family Community Australia. Retrieved March 6, 2020, from https://aifs.gov.au/cfca/expert-panel-project/program-planning-evaluation-guide/evaluate-your-program-or-service/how-develop-evaluation-plan

Smith, M. K. (2012). Biased sampling and extrapolation. Retrieved July 13, 2019, from https://web.ma.utexas.edu/users/mks/statmistakes/biasedsampling.html

Smith, M. L., & Ory, M. G. (2014). Measuring success: Evaluation article types for public health education and promotion section of *Frontiers in Public Health*. *Frontiers in Public Health*, *2*, 2–6. doi: 10.3389%2Ffpubh.2014.00111

Social Security Administration. (1996). Maternal and child health services block grant. Retrieved July 8, 2019, from https://www.ssa.gov/OP_Home/ssact/title05/0500.htm

Spiegelmen, D. (2016). Evaluating public health interventions: Examples, definitions and a personal note. *American Journal of Public Health*, *106*(1), 70–73. https://doi.org/10.2105/AJPH.2015.302923

Statistics How To. (2014). Confidence level. Retrieved July 12, 2019, from https://www.statisticshowto.datasciencecentral.com/confidence-level/

Substance Abuse and Mental Health Services Administration. (2012). National Registry of Evidence-based programs and practices [PDF]. Retrieved June 6, 2019 from http://www.eblcprograms.org/docs/pdfs/NREPP_Non-researchers_guide_to_eval.pdf

Suresh, K. P. (2011). An overview of randomization techniques: An unbiased assessment of outcome in clinical research. *Human Reproductive Sciences*, *4*(1), 8–11. doi: 10.4103/0974-1208.82352: 10.4103/0974-1208.82352

The Pell Institute. (2019). Evaluation toolkit. Retrieved June 28, 2019, from http://toolkit.pellinstitute.org/evaluation-101/evaluation-approaches-types/

Tobacco Technical Assistance Consortium, Emory University. (n.d.). Types of evaluation. Retrieved June 28, 2019, from http://tacenters.emory.edu/resources/products_tools/tobacco/power-of-proof/types_eval/outcome/index.html

United Nations Evaluation Group (UNEG). (2008). *Core competencies for evaluators of the UN system*. New York, NY: Author. Retrieved July 18, 2019, from http://www.uneval.org/documentdownload?doc_id=1408&file_id=1850

United Nations Evaluation Group (UNEG). (2013). Impact evaluation in UN agency systems: Guidance on selection, planning, and management. Retrieved July 2, 2019, from http://www.uneval.org/document/detail/1433

United Nations Evaluation Group (UNEG). (2016). *Norms and standards for evaluation*. Retrieved June 3, 2019, from http://unevaluation.org/document/foundation-documents

United Nations Office on Drugs and Crime (UNODC). (2017). *Evaluation handbook: Why evaluate?* Retrieved June 5, 2019, from http://www.unodc.org/documents/evaluation/Evaluation_Handbook_new/UNODC_Evaluation_Handbook.pdf

U.S. Department of Energy, Office of Energy Efficiency and Renewable Energy. (n.d.). Program evaluation: Why, what, and when to evaluate. Retrieved June 5, 2019, from https://www.energy.gov/eere/analysis/program-evaluation-why-what-and-when-evaluate

U.S. General Accounting Office (U.S. GAO). (1991). *Designing evaluations*. Washington, DC: U.S. General Accounting Office, publication no. GAO/PEMD-10.1.4. Retrieved July 23, 2019, from https://www.gao.gov/products/PEMD-10.1.4

U.S. General Accounting Office (U.S. GAO). (1992). *Evaluation synthesis*. Washington, DC: U.S. General Accounting Office, publication no. GAO/PEMD-10.1.2. Retrieved July 23, 2019, from https://www.gao.gov/products/PEMD-10.1.2

U.S. General Accounting Office (U.S. GAO). (1998). *Managing for results: Measuring program results that are under limited federal control*. Washington, DC: U.S. General Accounting Office publication no. GAO/GGD-99-16. Retrieved July 23, 2019, from https://www.gao.gov/products/GGD-99-16

Vaughan, R. (2004). Evaluation and public health. *American Journal of Public Health*, *94*(3), 360. Retrieved May 30, 2019, from https://www.ncbi.nlm.nih.gov/pmc/articles/PMC1448255/

Watkins, R., West Meiers, M., & Visser, Y. L. (2012). *A guide to assessing needs: Essential tools for collecting information, making decisions, and achieving development results*. Washington, DC: World Bank. Retrieved October 1, 2018, from https://openknowledge.worldbank.org/handle/10986/2231

White, H., & Sabarwal, S. (2014). Quasi-experimental design and methods. *Methodological Briefs No. 8: Impact Evaluation 8*, UNICEF Office of Research, Florence. Retrieved July 16, 2019, from https://www.unicef-irc.org/publications/753-quasi-experimental-design-and-methods-methodological-briefs-impact-evaluation-no.html

World Health Organization (WHO). (2013). *WHO evaluation practice handbook*. Retrieved June 5, 2019, from https://apps.who.int/iris/handle/10665/96311

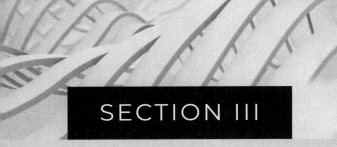

Planning Frameworks

CHAPTER 8

PRECEDE-PROCEED

STUDENT LEARNING OBJECTIVES

After reading this chapter, the student will be able to:

- Discuss the assumptions of the PRECEDE-PROCEED model.
- Explain the phases of the PRECEDE-PROCEED model.
- Identify the generic stages of program planning in the PRECEDE-PROCEED model.
- Plan a hypothetical program using the PRECEDE-PROCEED model.

Introduction

The acronym PRECEDE stands for: **P**redisposing, **R**einforcing, **E**nabling **C**onstructs in **E**ducational **D**iagnosis and **E**valuation. It's a systematic framework, a model, for establishing cause-and-effect relationships (Green & Kreuter, 1992) and a structure for assessing need and planning programs (Rural Health Information Hub [RHIhub], 2019).

The PROCEED acronym stands for **P**olicy, **R**egulatory, and **O**rganizational **C**onstructs in **E**ducational and **E**nvironmental **D**evelopment (Green & Kreuter, 1992). This portion of the model addresses the political, policy, and organizational barriers that hinder the use of resources, impede implementation and evaluation, and ultimately program outcomes (Green & Kreuter, 1992).

The original PRECEDE model was introduced in the early 1970s by Lawrence Green in response to demands at the time for health programs to demonstrate their cost-effectiveness and cost-benefits (Green, 1974). PRECEDE not only proved useful for this, but also as an organizing framework for planning and evaluating programs (Green, Levin, & Deeds, 1975). In the early 1990s, the model was expanded to include the PROCEED processes (Green & Kreuter, 1992).

Since its introduction, the model has been used, tested, and verified in over 960 published studies and thousands of unpublished programs in a range of public health settings spanning more than three decades (Green, 2016). It is one of the most commonly used planning frameworks in public health.

PRECEDE-PROCEED Assumptions

PRECEDE-PROCEED is predicated on the following basic assumptions about disease prevention, health promotion, and the community:

Assumption 1—Adoption of health promoting behaviors is almost always voluntary.

Health promotion program planning must involve the people whose behavior or actions are the focus of change (Center for Community Health and Development [CCHD], 2018).

Assumption 2—Health is a community issue (CCHD, 2018).

Health is influenced by community attitudes and shaped by its context and history (CCHD, 2018).

Assumption 3—Health must be considered within the larger context of quality of life (CCHD, 2018).

Health is one of many factors that make life better or worse for individuals and the community. It influences and is influenced by much more than what seems directly connected to it (CCHD, 2018).

Assumption 4—Health is more than physical well-being and the absence of disease, illness, or injury (CCHD, 2018).

Health reflects the combination of social, political, economic, ecological, and physical factors at play in individual lives and communities (CCHD, 2018).

PRECEDE-PROCEED Close-Up

The PRECEDE-PROCEED model has a total of eight phases, four subsumed under PRECEDE, which guide needs assessment and planning activities, and four under PROCEED, which guide implementation and evaluation activities. Although these eight phases present a strict process to follow, there is leeway for adapting the program design and methods to the specific issues, context, and needs (CCHD, 2018).

Table 8-1 PRECEDE-PROCEED phases

PRECEDE Phases	PROCEED Phases
Phase 1—Social assessment	Phase 5—Implementation
Phase 2—Epidemiological assessment	Phase 6—Process evaluation
Phase 3—Educational and ecological assessment	Phase 7—Impact evaluation
Phase 4—Administrative, organizational, and policy assessment	Phase 8—Outcome evaluation

It's important to note here that PRECEDE originally had five phases. In 1994 when the four phases of PROCEED were added, the whole model became nine phases. In 2005, Phases 2 and 3 of PRECEDE were collapsed into one (Green, 2016; Green & Kreuter, 2005), resulting in a reduction of the nine phases to the eight shown in **Table 8-1**. However, the literature continues to contain references to both the eight- and nine-phase versions of the model.

Additionally, in the original PRECEDE model, the term *diagnosis* was used to describe the focus of each phase. In 1999, the term was changed to *assessment*. Since then, both terms have been used interchangeably (Green, 2016; Green & Kreuter, 2005).

PRECEDE

Planning a program following the PRECEDE model begins with identifying what the community sees as its *social* problem, then identifying the outcome it wants from a program that addresses the problem and improves the quality of life. The model works to determine what must be done for these outcomes to happen (CCHD, 2018). The four phases of the PRECEDE portion of the model guide this process. They include social assessment, epidemiological assessment, educational and ecological assessment, and administrative, organizational, and policy assessment.

Phase 1—Social Assessment and Participatory Planning

In this first phase, the planning committee works with members of the community to identify the social problems and issues that are important to them, and what they want or need for their community (CCHD, 2018; Porter, 2016; RHIhub, 2019) relative to these. To ascertain this, a needs assessment is conducted to collect primary data from community members.

The results of the needs assessment will identify the problem the community members find most important and what they want and need to make the situation better. It may be the elimination of a problem, a solution to a long-standing issue, maintaining environmental progress made, or increasing the general quality of life in the community. (CCHD, 2018) This is the ultimate outcome the program aims to accomplish.

As an example, in response to the growing social problem of antibiotic-resistant bacteria from antibiotics overuse, especially in the treatment of mild respiratory infections in children, a team of researchers worked with parent and clinician advisory groups to develop a program to address the issue. Using PRECEDE-PROCEED as the framework to guide the process, they started by first determining the program outcome they wanted. They came to consensus on four possible areas of focus—antibiotic prescriptions, antibiotic consumption, experiences related to the care for respiratory infections, and the child's symptoms. Because the problem was the overuse of antibiotics, and because taking an antibiotic was contingent upon having a prescription, the agreed upon outcome of the program was a reduction in the number of prescriptions given to treat children with respiratory tract infections (Lucas, Ingram, Redmond, Cabral, Turnbull, & Hay, 2017).

Phase 2—Epidemiological Assessment

The epidemiological assessment focuses on identifying behavioral/lifestyle, environmental, and genetic factors that clearly influence the outcome the community identified it wanted in Phase 1. These are factors that both support accomplishing the outcome and the barriers that might hinder it (CCHD, 2018). Brainstorming with community members and other stakeholders to identify factors that would support or hinder the program's successful outcome is critical. Nominal group process can also be used to guide this type of discussion.

Once the possible influencing factors are known, they are prioritized (Porter, 2016). The aim here is to identify the most important factors, the greatest supports, and biggest barriers that can be addressed by a program (CCHD, 2018). Using the antibiotic overuse example again, if an influencing factor is lack of understanding by parents as to when antibiotics are and are not appropriate, can this be addressed by a program?

To identify the most important factors, each of them is discussed in terms of the following:

–   What would elimination of this barrier make possible that isn't possible already?
–   How does this factor create a barrier to the wanted or needed outcome?
–   Does this factor affect anything else besides the outcome wanted (CCHD, 2018)?

Most factors that can affect the outcome, either positively or negatively, fall under one of the following: behavior, lifestyle, environment (CCHD, 2018), or genetics (Green & Kreuter, 2005).

•   Behavioral factors

What are people doing that has to change for the needed/wanted outcome to happen? For example, if the outcome the community wants and needs is a safe park, what are people doing that has to change for a safe park to happen? What makes the existing park unsafe? If it's drug use and gangs, then those are the issues that need to be addressed for the outcome to happen.

- Lifestyle factors

Lifestyle factors reflect how people live their lives. How would lifestyle affect the needed/wanted program outcome?

Going back to the safe park example, how would lifestyle support or hinder the outcome of a safe park? People who had healthier lifestyles that included physical activity are more likely to be supportive than those with unhealthy lifestyles who are inactive. However, it might be that people with unhealthy lifestyles are inactive precisely because there is no safe place to walk and would support having a safe park.

- Environmental factors

Environmental factors that can affect the outcome of a program are more than those in the physical or natural environment such as water and air quality and open space. These are also factors in the social environment such as the influences of family, peers, culture, and attitudes; in the political environment such as laws governing individual behavior, for example, no smoking laws and seat belt laws. They also include factors in the economic environment such as housing, employment opportunities, and health care (CCHD, 2018). Going back to the safe park, what are the environmental factors that help or hinder accomplishing it? If there already is a park in the neighborhood, this would be a supporting factor for creating a safe park. But, a lack of open space to create a park would be a significant hindrance.

- Genetics

Genetics were added to the PRECEDE-PROCEED model as an outcome influencing factor in 2005 (Green, 2016). Although the contribution genetics makes to health, the quality of life, and ultimately the success of a program should be acknowledged, in practical terms, changes in genetics are obviously beyond the control of any program (Crosby & Noar, 2011).

Once the factors with potential to influence the desired outcome of the program are identified, one of them is chosen as the focus of the program. Specifically, what are people doing (behaviors or lifestyle) or what's going on in the environment that can lead to or prevent the changes needed (CCHD, 2018) to achieve the outcome?

To narrow down the factors, each is measured against the following criteria:

1. Is the potential factor important enough to have a real effect on the issue?
2. Can the potential factor be changed by a program with the available resources (CCHD, 2018)?

The process of narrowing down the factors and selecting the program focus is a group endeavor. The planning committee, which includes community members among other stakeholders, all have a voice in the decision. Using nominal group process to identify the focus will ensure that everyone's voice is heard.

Once the behavior, lifestyle, or environmental focus of the program is decided, measurable objectives for accomplishing the desired program outcome are developed (Porter, 2016). They are written following the SMART objective criteria discussed in Chapter 5, Planning.

Continuing with the previous example of a program to reduce the overuse of antibiotics, the epidemiological assessment found that the most significant behavioral factor associated with the problem was clinician prescribing decisions. Environmental factors contributing to the problem of antibiotics overuse were pressure from parents, schools, and childcare settings for antibiotics (Lucas et al., 2017). These became the focus of the program for which the objectives were developed.

Phase 3—Educational and Ecological Assessment

The educational and ecological assessments concentrate on identifying the predisposing, enabling, and reinforcing factors that drive the behavioral, lifestyle, and environmental factors identified in Phase 2 related to the problems identified in Phase 1. Consequently, these are the factors that must change before the desired outcome can be accomplished.

- Predisposing factors

Predisposing factors are the internal or intrapersonal influences that affect the likelihood of someone engaging in certain behaviors and avoiding others. They include knowledge, attitudes, beliefs, values, and self-efficacy. These factors are the ones often changed by educational programs (CCHD, 2018). For example, knowing how to cook affects the likelihood that someone will prepare meals at home rather than relying on fast food.

- Enabling factors

Enabling factors are the conditions that support a behavior, regardless of whether it's healthy or unhealthy. These include, for instance, availability of resources, access to services, laws or policies, and skills (CCHD, 2018). For example, a factor that enables the "unhealthy" behavior of avoiding routine dental checkups is not having dental insurance. Conversely, having dental insurance enables routine dental examinations.

- Reinforcing factors

Reinforcing factors are the attitudes of important people in our lives, and the community overall, that support or hinder adoption of healthy behaviors or environmental conditions (CCHD, 2018). These are the subjective norms in the Theory of Reasoned Action discussed in Chapter 2, Behavior Change Theories.

By answering the following two questions, the planning committee gains insight into the factors (predisposing, enabling, reinforcing) that need to be changed in order to accomplish the goals and objectives, the specific changes the program should aim to bring about (CCHD, 2018; Porter, 2016), who the intended audience should be, what the

program should look like to best accomplish the changes, the theory that should underlie it, and who should implement it (CCHD, 2018).

1. What must change in order to accomplish the outcome?
2. What will help bring about that change?

Going back to the antibiotic overuse example, the factors that *predisposed* clinicians to overprescribe included inflated estimation of parental pressure to prescribe and misinterpretation of parental concern for a request to prescribe. The factors that *enabled* clinicians to overprescribe antibiotics included clinical uncertainty of seriousness of the respiratory tract infection and the suspicion of a serious viral illness. (Note: Although antibiotics are not effective against viruses, the rationale for prescribing them to treat a viral infection was not given.) Last, the *reinforcing* factor for overprescribing was the desire of parents to have their children examined by a clinician when they were ill (Lucas et al., 2017), which again presents the issue of overestimation and misinterpretation of parental pressure to prescribe.

Phase 4—Administrative, Organizational, and Policy Assessment

The purpose of this phase is to identify the administrative, organizational, or policy factors that influence the kind of program that can be implemented (CCHD, 2018). For example, is there sufficient administrative support for the potential program? Does the potential program clash with the organizational culture? Are there agency policies in place that prohibit the type of program being planned?

Administrative and organizational factors include the following.

- Resources

In addition to money, resources include personnel, time, and space. This is the time in the planning process when the resources needs are compared to the resources available so any gaps between the two can be addressed (CCHD, 2018). For example, inadequate space was an issue for a teen pregnancy prevention program. One of the community agencies that agreed to implement the program usually met with their own clients at various sites through the community because they didn't have dedicated meeting space in their offices area. However, implementation of the pregnancy prevention program required the use of a consistent space with separate private rooms, which was not possible for the agency to obtain (Demby, Gregory, Broussard, Dickherber, Atkins, & Jenner, 2014).

- Organizational structure

How the implementing organization is structured can affect program implementation. Some organizations are hierarchical with everything working from the top down, while others are more democratic and collaborative, which gives everyone a voice, and some are a combination. The organizational structure and program design should be compatible and flexible enough to make adjustments when necessary (CCHD, 2018).

For example, it's the organizational structure of the Drug Abuse Resistance Education (D.A.R.E.) that enables it to rapidly disseminate new prevention strategies to the local level. Its structure is that of a top-down corporation with a president and directors at the national level, each responsible for national oversight of a key function such as communications, training, development and implementation, education, and marketing, among others. At a regional level, there are several directors each responsible for five to seven states who serve as their link to the national office. At the state level there is a D.A.R.E. organization, which is the link to the local programs (Merrill, Pinsky, Killeya-Jones, Sloboda, & Dilascio, 2006).

- Organizational procedures

These are the ways the organization functions, how it does things, how it carries out its work. For a program to be successful, procedures have to focus on the goals, rather than on the organization's convenience or traditional methods (CCHD, 2018). For instance, if the organization's usual program registration procedure includes showing identification, a driver's license or other government-issued identification, but the program's intended audience includes undocumented immigrants, this is a barrier to their participation and would need to be suspended.

- Organizational culture

An organization's culture is its system of beliefs, values, and behavioral norms (Schein, 2017) that affect, among other things, how staff interact with one another and their supervisors, how program participants are treated, and how the organization views its work and mission. The organizational culture affects the "fit" between the organization and the program (CCHD, 2018). If some aspect of the program doesn't mesh with the culture, it may hinder the success of the program.

Organizational culture proved to be a sticking point for the implementation of safety plans at two water utility companies in two developing countries. Water safety plans are a comprehensive approach for "source to tap" water risk assessment and management with the primary aim of protecting public health. They are needed to combat widespread illness and death caused by unsafe drinking water in developing nations (Summerill, Pollard, & Smith, 2010).

Although the organizational culture of both companies was different, the culture of each contributed to ineffective program implementation at both. In one company it was a lack of effective communication in a top-down organizational structure and a perceived lack of time and resources committed to implementing the plans. Communication was also an issue in the second company, as well. Only in this case, the structure was decentralized, which limited opportunities for interaction between different groups responsible for the different aspects of the company's functions. As this was a private company, profits competed with other outcomes, including water quality (Summerill et al., 2010).

- Policies and regulations

Policy and regulatory issues are the internal and external rules of an organization that can impact a program (CCHD, 2018).

Internal policies and regulations include the following:

- *Staff:* Are staff considered employees who take orders, colleagues who contribute to the workings of the organization, or collaborators who jointly own the organization? How staff are treated affects the amount of freedom they have to be creative and take initiative (CCHD, 2018).
- *Program participants:* Are program participants treated authoritatively as subordinates that the organization is doing something to or for, or respectfully as equal partners working together to initiate change (CCHD, 2018)?
- *Collaboration:* Do the organization's policies encourage collaboration with other organizations and agencies as much as possible, or discourage collaborative work (CCHD, 2018)?
- *Professional ethics:* Are staff expected to follow a professional code of ethics, either an internal organizational one, or a professional association's that covers confidentiality, inappropriate relationships, abuse of position, reporting (or nonreporting) of specific kinds of illegal behavior, and other professional expectations (CCHD, 2018)?

External policies and regulations include the following:

- *Funders' requirements:* Funders may have restrictions on the types of programs the organization can implement, even if it's something the funder isn't directly funding (CCHD, 20018a). For example, the

federal government forbids the use of federal funds to advocate for or promote gun control (Rostron, 2018). It prohibits the use of federal funds in programs (organizations or agencies) where abortion is a method of family planning (U.S. Department of Health and Human Services, 2019) and where it's referred, promoted, encouraged, or advocated. Organizations and agencies that engage in these prohibited activities must separate their abortion-related activities physically and financially if they want to receive federal funding. This means they must have separate facilities for abortion and non-abortion services, including separate exam and waiting rooms, entrances and exits, websites, and staff, and separate accounting, medical records, and workstations (Congressional Research Service, 2019).

- *Oversight agency regulations:* These are the regulations of state or federal agencies that an organization may be required to follow (CCHD, 2018). For example, the Health Resources and Services Administration (HRSA) has oversight for the federally funded Health Center Program. Community organizations designated as health centers under this program are required to provide comprehensive, culturally competent primary care services and supportive services such as health education, translation, and transportation to provide access to care. They are required to provide services regardless of the patient's ability to pay, operate under the direction of a patient-majority governing board, and develop systems of patient-centered care that responds to the unique needs of medically underserved areas and populations, and meet requirements for key management and clinical staff. HRSA provides oversight and support for compliance with these requirements and takes action for noncompliance (HRSA, n.d.).

- *Laws:* These are federal and state laws or local ordinances the organization must abide by (CCHD, 2018). For example, needle exchange laws differ state by state as do laws governing gun ownership, gambling, and driving age.
- *Unstated community policies:* There may be certain actions or programs that are just unacceptable to the community or other stakeholders (CCHD, 2018). For example, a program that promotes children walking or biking to school may be unacceptable in certain communities while the same program would be supported in another. This is where working closely with community members is invaluable.

At the end of the four phases of PRECEDE, a needs assessment will have been completed, the data from it analyzed, the problem identified, and what the community wants and needs from a program determined. A program plan will have been developed that includes goals and objectives, strategies, activities and actions, a timeline, and an evaluation plan. With this done, it's time to proceed to PROCEED.

PROCEED

PROCEED focuses on the implementation and evaluation processes of program planning. Although evaluations are conducted in this portion of the model, the preparatory work for them is done throughout the planning process. For example, evaluation is addressed in the PRECEDE phases through the collection of baseline data and developing measurable objectives necessary for the impact evaluation in Phase 7 and outcome evaluation in Phase 8.

Phase 5—Implementation

This is the action phase of the PRECEDE-PROCEED model when the program is implemented. The focus is on assessing what the program was intended to be, what it is, and where the gaps are between the two (Green, 2016). In this phase the concern is with implementing the program with fidelity, and addressing issues that arise related to contextual fit, characteristics of the community, organization, and/or program that might have an impact on its successful outcome. (See Chapter 6, Implementing, for a more detailed discussion.)

Phase 6—Process Evaluation

This phase of the model is the evaluation of "how" program implementation is being carried out, that is, the extent of implementation fidelity. In the context of PRECEDE-PROCEED, the process evaluation helps identify reasons why the gaps found in Phase 5 exist and the relationships between program components (Green, 2016). (See Chapter 7, Evaluating, for a more detailed discussion of process evaluation.)

Phase 7—Impact Evaluation

The impact evaluation determines the program's intended and unintended consequences and its positive and negative effects (Green, 2016). It confirms if the changes expected in the behavioral and environmental factors are happening (CCHD, 2018). (See Chapter 7, Evaluating, for a more detailed discussion of impact evaluation.)

Phase 8—Outcome Evaluation

The outcome evaluation enables a determination to be made of the extent to which the results the community needed and wanted were attained (Green, 2016). However, sometimes the outcome effects aren't apparent for years as with lifestyle changes to reduce the risk of heart disease or cancer (CCHD, 2018). (See Chapter 7, Evaluating,

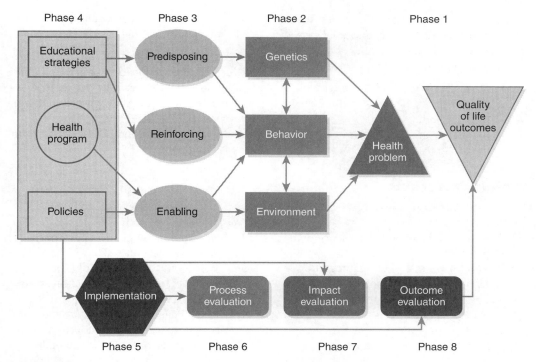

Phase 4   Phase 3   Phase 2   Phase 1

Phase 5   Phase 6   Phase 7   Phase 8

Figure 8-1 PRECEDE-PROCEED flowchart

Data from Green, L. (2016). The Precede-Proceed model of health program planning and evaluation. Retrieved March 29, 2020 from http://www.lgreen.net/precede.htm

for a more detailed discussion of outcome evaluation.)

Unlike other planning models that work toward identifying the desired end result, the PRECEDE-PROCEED model *begins* by identifying the desired end result and works backward to plan a program to accomplish it. Consequently, the flowchart in **Figure 8-1**, begins on the right with Phase 1 and moves to the left.

Chapter Summary

PRECEDE-PROCEED is a planning framework that starts with identifying the desired program outcome relative to the health problem and works backward to identify factors contributing to the health problem, which suggest possible solutions for the problem that lead to the desired outcome.

Planning in Practice Chapter Activity

Personal health behaviors are leading contributors to health status. Health-promoting behaviors are often mundane actions such as handwashing, eating fruits and vegetables, walking, and sleeping. When health-promoting behaviors are not practiced, the risk of disease increases. For example, when dental hygiene is lax, there is an increased risk of gum disease and dental cavities, but also of oral cancer, heart disease, and pneumonia.

1. In small groups, brainstorm reasons why some people brush and floss their teeth and others don't.
2. Assign one group member to record the group responses.
3. Read the article below, and answer the questions that follow.

Article: *Application of the PRECEDE-PROCEED planning model in designing an oral health strategy* (Binkey & Johnson, 2014)

Article link: https://www.ncbi.nlm.nih.gov/pmc/articles/PMC4199385/

(Note: Download the PDF to see the article page numbers.)

Article Questions

1. What health problem was the focus of this article?
2. Who was the intended audience of the program?
3. What was the goal of the program?
4. How and why was the PRECEDE-PROCEED model adapted?
5. What theory and constructs were used to guide program development?
6. How was the social assessment conducted in Phase 1, and what were the results?
7. What factors did the epidemiological assessment in Phase 2 reveal as contributing to the health problem?
8. What did the behavioral assessment in Phase 2 reveal as contributing to the health problem?
9. What factors did the environmental assessment in Phase 2 identify as contributing to the health problem?
10. What factors did the educational and ecological assessments in Phase 3 reveal as contributing to the health problem?
11. How did the authors use the information they gathered during the first three phases of the PRECEDE-PROCEED model?
12. How did the program align with results of the assessments in Phases 1–3?
13. What contextual factors did the authors identify as possible threats to the effectiveness of the program?
14. In the Phase 4 administrative and policy assessments, what factors were identified as necessary for an oral health program?
15. What did the pilot study conducted in Phase 5 assess?
16. What will implementation in Phase 6 entail?
17. For phases 7 and 8, how will evaluation participants be chosen?
18. How will possible contamination of program results be reduced?
19. When will attainment of outcomes (goal) be measured?
20. Think back to the responses your small-group brainstorming session generated about why people do or don't brush and floss. Were the factors identified in the assessments for this program among them? If not, why not?

References

Center for Community Health and Development [CCHD]. (2018). Chapter 2, Section 2: PRECEDE/PROCEED. Lawrence, KS: University of Kansas. Retrieved August 5, 2019, from the Community Tool Box: https://ctb.ku.edu/en/table-contents/overview/other-models -promoting-community-health-and-development /preceder-proceder/main

Congressional Research Review. (2019). Title X family planning program: 2019 final ruling. Retrieved August 21, 2019, from https://crsreports.congress.gov

/search/#/?terms To Search=title%20X%20final%20 rule &orderBy=Relevance

Crosby, R., & Noar, S. M. (2011). What is a planning model? An introduction to PRECEDE-PROCEED. *Journal of Public Health Dentistry, 71*, S7–S15. doi: 10.1111/j.1752-7325.2011.00235.x

Demby, H., Gregory, A., Broussard, M., Dickherber, J., Atkins, S., & Jenner, L. W. (2014). Implementation lessons: The importance of assessing organizational "fit" and external factors when implementing evidence-based teen pregnancy prevention programs. *Journal of Adolescent Health, 54*, S-37–44. http://dx.doi.org/10.1016/j.jadohealth .2013.12.022

Green, L.W., Levine, D.M., & Deeds, S. (1975). Clinical trials of health education for hypertensive patients: Design and baseline data. *Preventive Medicine, 4*(4), 417-425. https://doi.org/10.1016/0091-7435(75)90 030-4

Green, L. W. (1974). Toward cost-benefit evaluations of health education: Some concepts, methods and examples. *Health Education Monographs, 2*(1) suppl. 34–64.

Green, L. W. (2016). PRECEDE-PROCEED. Retrieved August 11, 2019, from http://lgreen.net/precede.htm

Green, L. W., & Kreuter, M. W. (1992). CDC's planned approach to community health as an application of PRECEDE and an inspiration for PROCEED. *Journal of Health Education, 23*(3), 140–147. https://doi.org/10 .1080/10556699.1992.10616277

Green, L. W., & Kreuter, M. W. (2005). *Health program planning: An educational and ecological approach* (4th ed.). New York: McGraw-Hill.

Health Resources and Services Administration [HRSA], (n.d.). Health center program requirements. Retrieved April 1, 2020, from https://bphc.hrsa.gov/program requirements

Lucas, P. J., Ingram, J., Redmond, N. M., Cabral, C., Turnbull, S. L., & Hay, A. D. (2017). Development of an intervention to reduce antibiotic use for childhood coughs in UK primary care using critical synthesis of multi-method research. *BMC, Medical Research Methodology, 17*(1), 175. https://dx.doi.org/10.1186%2Fs 12874-017-0455-9

Merrill, J. C., Pinsky, I., Killeya-Jones, L. A., Sloboda, Z., & Dilascio, T. (2006). Substance abuse prevention infrastructure: A survey based study of the organizational structure and function of the D.A.R.E. program. *Substance Abuse Treatment Prevention and Policy, 1*(25). https://doi.org/10.1186/1747-597X-1-25

Porter, C. M. (2016). Revisiting Precede–Proceed: A leading model for ecological and ethical health promotion. *Health Education Journal, 75*(6), 753–764. https://doi.org/10.1177%2F0017896915619645

Rostron, A. (2018). The Dickey Amendment on federal funding for research on gun violence: A legal dissection. *American Journal of Public Health, 108*(7), 865–867. https://dx.doi.org/10.2105%2FAJPH.2018 .304450

Rural Health Information Hub [RHIhub]. (2019). PRECEDE-PROCEED. Retrieved August 5, 2019, from https:// www.ruralhealthinfo.org/toolkits/health-promotion /2/program-models/precede-proceed

Schein, E. H. (2017). *Organizational culture and leadership* (5th ed.). Hoboken, NJ: Wiley.

Summerill, C., Pollard, S. J. T., & Smith, J. A. (2010). The role of organizational culture and leadership in water safety plan implementation for improved risk management. *Science of the Total Environment, 408*(20), 4319–4327. https://doi-org.ezproxy.wpunj.edu/10 .1016/j.scitotenv.2010.06.043

U.S. Department of Health and Human Services. (2019). Statues and regulations: Title X notice of final rule. Retrieved August 21, 2019, from https://www.hhs .gov/opa/title-x-family-planning/about-title-x-grants /statutes-and-regulations/index.html

CHAPTER 9

Mobilizing for Action Through Planning and Partnerships (MAPP)

STUDENT LEARNING OUTCOMES

After reading this chapter the student will be able to:

- Discuss the principles underlying MAPP.
- Identify the generic steps of program planning in the MAPP phases.
- Plan a hypothetical program using the MAPP process.

Introduction

In 1988, the Institute of Medicine (IOM) published *The Future of the Public's Health in the 21st Century,* a report that basically said the public health system in the United States was a mess. As expected, it became the impetus for the creation and implementation of a multitude of assessments, standards, and improvement processes (National Association of County and City Health Officers [NACCHO], 2013a).

One of the improvement processes was the Assessment Protocol for Excellence in Public Health (APEX-PH). Developed by the NACCHO with support from the Centers for Disease Control and Prevention (CDC), APEX-PH was a way for health departments to assess the health status of their communities and to establish a leadership role in the community. It was updated and revised regularly throughout the 1990s (NACCHO, 2013a).

In 1997, the IOM published another report, *Improving Health in the Community: A Role for Performance Monitoring,* which emphasized the importance of having the community actively involved in monitoring public health performance, and included a detailed accounting of what a plan for improving community health should entail. In response to this, public health practitioners asked for a community-driven process they could use to help them in this endeavor (NACCHO, 2013a).

After gathering substantial input from the field and reviewing the literature, NACCHO, again with support from the CDC, evolved APEX-PH into Mobilizing for Action Through

Planning and Partnerships, or MAPP. MAPP provided the structure and guidance for the planning process that practitioners wanted (NACCHO, 2013a).

MAPP is a planning framework that helps communities prioritize public health issues, identify resources for addressing them, and take action to improve conditions to support healthy living. The successful use of the MAPP framework depends on one (or more) community organizations taking a leadership role and serving as the MAPP facilitating organization, as well as participation of people who work, learn, live, and play in the community (NACCHO, 2013a, 2019).

MAPP Up-Close

While similar in some ways to other planning models, MAPP is unique in that it's a community-owned process that relies on wide representation and participation of local public health system entities. It uses both qualitative and quantitative data gleaned from four different assessments to inform the development, implementation, and evaluation of plans to improve the health of a community (NACCHO, 2013a).

MAPP is based on the following seven principles:

Principle 1—Work from a shared vision.
A healthy community is possible when stakeholders have a shared a vision of how they can work together to create one (Center for Community Health and Development [CCHD], 2018).

Principle 2—Encourage open dialogue.
When stakeholders can voice their opinions, discuss their differences, and come to compromise or common ground, it leads to resolution and problem solving. It also establishes trusting, collaborative relationships (CCHD, 2018).

Principle 3—Create partnerships. Permanent change in a community

requires collaboration of everyone working together to avoid duplication; provide services to those in need; share effective procedures, practices, and resources; and plan together (CCHD, 2018).

Principle 4—Use systems thinking.
Problems occur within systems. It's only when the system in which the problems are taking place is understood that the problems can be solved (CCHD, 2018).

Principle 5—Use data.
Only with data and a clear understanding of the needs and wants of community members can conclusions be drawn, strategies devised, and actions planned to address the problem conditions in the community (CCHD, 2018).

Principle 6—Think strategically.
It takes planning—setting goals, analyzing a situation, and setting a course of action—to control a situation and accomplish a desired outcome (CCHD, 2018).

Principle 7—Celebrate success.
When success is recognized and celebrated publicly, achievement is sustained (CCHD, 2018).

These seven principles are integrated into the six phases of the MAPP process—organizing, visioning, assessing, identifying issues, formulating goals and strategies, and taking action (planning, implementing, and evaluating). They are summarized in the following sections from the NACCHO (2013a) handbook, *Mobilizing for Action Through Planning and Partnerships*.

Phase 1—Organizing for Developing Partnerships

In preparation for MAPP, the facilitating organization establishes a MAPP Core Group consisting of two to three people. The Core Group is responsible for organizing the MAPP process, operational and logistical aspects, planning oversight, staffing, and working collaboratively with community members and public health partners (NACCHO, 2013a).

The Core Group begins organizing the MAPP process by completing the seven steps of Phase 1.

Step 1.1 Determine Need. The first task of the Core Group is to determine the need for conducting a MAPP process. This determination is based on the compelling nature of this small group's responses to the following questions:

– Why should the community complete a Mapp process?
– What critical issues will a MAPP process address?
– Who or what is the driving force behind conducting a MAPP process?
– What outcome is wanted from doing a MAPP process (NACCHO, 2013a)?

Step 1.2 Identify Participants. If the need for a MAPP process is established, the next step is for the Core Group to identify the people who will participate in the process.

• Define the "community."

The first action the Core Group takes to identify the MAPP participants is to define the geographic parameters of the "community" that is the focus of the MAPP process. Is the "community" a neighborhood, a town/city, a county, a portion of the state (northern, mid, southern, eastern, western)? For example, in one large city that undertook a MAPP process, the "community" was defined as a specific neighborhood, while another MAPP process defined "community" as an area that included one city and five counties. (NACCHO, 2013a).

• Identify existing partnerships.

Next, the Core Group lists the community partnerships the facilitating organization already has in place that might contribute to the MAPP process (NACCHO, 2013a).

• Identify potential partnerships.

With existing partnerships identified, potential partnerships are identified next. To facilitate this, the Ten Essential Public Health Services are used as the basis for a brainstorming session to determine who in the community is responsible for providing them. (See **Figure 9-1**.) This enables the Core Group to identify *potential* partner organizations.

The MAPP process also relies on input from people and organizations with knowledge about the social, economic, institutional, and other contextual factors that directly or indirectly affect the health of the people in the community. In some cases, these entities don't consider themselves part of the public health system and may or may not provide an essential public health service. But they are important to consider as potential partners, nonetheless. These might include:

– civil rights organizations.
– labor organizations.
– minority, religious, and immigrant population organizations.
– english as a foreign language groups.
– housing authorities.
– service providers for the homeless.
– community development and organizing organizations.
– women's rights organizations.
– gay, lesbian, bisexual, transgender organizations.
– child advocacy groups.
– developmental and physical disability rights organizations.
– mental health advocacy organizations (NACCHO, 2013a).

Other key potential partners are the community members themselves. Community members have unique insight into the issues that affect their ability to live healthy lives and the community resources available for initiatives

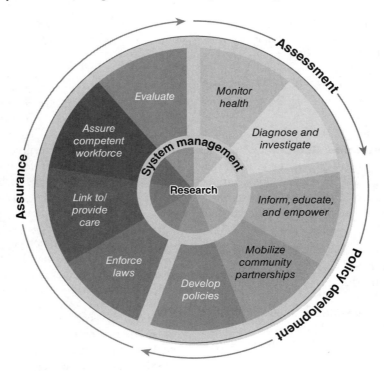

Figure 9-1 The 10 essential public health services

Centers for Disease Control and Prevention. (2018). The ten essential public health services. https://www.cdc.gov/publichealthgateway/publichealthservices/essentialhealthservices.html

to improve their health. They can provide valuable guidance on strategies that might or might not work and can be instrumental in program implementation. Community members include those individuals who live, work, learn, or play in the community as defined by the Core Group (NACCHO, 2013a).

• Invite potential partners.

Once the list of potential partners is completed, each is invited to participate in the MAPP process. An individual, tailored communication is created for each of them, whether it's a letter, email, or phone call. A blanket email is not used (NACCHO, 2013a).

Tailoring an invitation to each individual or organization takes time. Ideally, it should explain how their participation in the MAPP process aligns with their organization's mission, benefits the individual or the organization,

and contributes to the success of the MAPP process and a healthier community (NACCHO, 2013a).

Step 1.3 Plan the Process. It's important for the Core Group to include all partners in the MAPP process from the very beginning and to keep them involved throughout all the phases. This ensures community ownership of the process and supports collaboration (NACCHO, 2013a).

Planning the MAPP process begins with the Core Group completing the following:

• Convening a MAPP partner meeting

The purpose of this first MAPP partner meeting is to introduce the partners to each other, establish partner expectations, and obtain commitment for carrying out MAPP tasks (NACCHO, 2013a).

• Obtaining commitments

One way the Core Group can obtain commitments from MAPP partners is to provide them with a document that explains the six phases of the MAPP process and the associated roles and responsibilities, asking them to volunteer for tasks that are in line with their strengths, capabilities, and interests. The results of this exercise are shared with the group. A designated "recorder" keeps track of who volunteered for what on flip charts for each of the six phases/tasks. At the end of the sharing session, volunteers are asked to come forward for tasks left uncovered (NACCHO, 2013a).

• Recruiting Steering Committee members

In addition to the Core Group, a Steering Committee is needed. The Steering Committee is composed of 10–20 partners recruited by the Core Group to provide guidance and direct the MAPP process throughout. The Steering Committee is akin to a board of directors. It should be composed of representatives from the entire local public system as well as the community (NACCHO, 2013a).

Step 1.4 Identify Resources Needed.

The Core Group identifies the resources needed to complete the MAPP process and determines which are available and which need to be obtained. Determining resource needs for staff, data collection, meeting space, travel expenses, printing, consultants, and education and training early in the process allows the MAPP partners to plan how unavailable resources will be obtained (NACCHO, 2013a).

In terms of resources, the following are considered:

• Staff

Are there enough staff available at the different partner organizations to carry out the responsibilities of the MAPP process?

If there are, can enough time be allotted for them to participate in the MAPP process?

• Data collection

What data collection and analysis resources are available in terms of people, hardware, and software?

The resources needed for data collection depend on *how* data will be collected, by whom, and from whom. Resource needs for a telephone interview are very different than those needed for a mailed paper-and-pencil survey.

• Meeting space, meals/refreshments

Having meeting space available is not the same as having *appropriate* meeting space. How suitable is available space in terms of accessibility by public transportation, parking, safety, the condition of the physical space—heating, cooling, capacity, seating? Meeting space should be easily accessed, comfortable, and inviting for partners to encourage their attendance.

At minimum, refreshments (coffee, tea, water) should be provided at all meetings. If resources are available, providing a light meal is always appreciated by participants.

• Travel reimbursement

Reimbursing travel costs incurred by partners to attend meetings can be expensive. These costs include a per mile reimbursement in addition to tolls and parking fees. How partners' travel expenses will be handled needs verification. This is particularly important if MAPP partner meetings are planned outside of regular working hours. If these costs are covered for partners from community agencies, then they should be included as expenses for reimbursement for community members.

If the MAPP plan calls for hiring consultants, some include travel expenses in their overall fee; others separate these out. These expenses also need verification.

• Printing costs

The resources needed for printing depend on which reports and materials are likely to be distributed in hard copy, and to whom. Printing may be one resource that a partner organization can provide.

• Consultant fees

Consultants don't come cheap! Before hiring consultants, it's important to investigate if the needed expertise is available within a partner organization. If not, determine if the best use of available resources (funds) is a flat fee per project or an hourly fee, which for a statistical consultant is about $140/hour on average (Payscale.com, 2019) and may or may not include travel and other expenses.

• Educational and training materials

If educational and training materials are going to be produced "in house" by one of the partner organizations, the organization may cover the cost.

Once the resources needs are identified, the information is used to develop a budget. (See **Table 9-1**.) It's also the basis for brainstorming possible funding sources.

Step 1.5 Assess Readiness. In this step, the Core Group conducts a readiness assessment to determine if the elements needed to proceed with the MAPP process are in place. To complete this assessment, the Core Group comes to consensus about the following:

Organizational leadership supportive of MAPP process

Support for MAPP process that outweighs opposition to it

Availability of needed resources

The MAPP process and outcomes

How to proceed

The planning scope

The planning time frame

Staff and technical support

Involvement of a majority of public health partners (NACCHO, 2013a)

Step 1.6 Determine MAPP Process Management. How the MAPP process is managed is critical to its success. The Core Group delineates its roles and responsibilities for carrying out the tasks involved, and those of the Steering Committee, subcommittees, and community members (NACCHO, 2013a). **Table 9-2** presents these by phase for each group.

Step 1.7 Conduct Process Evaluation. Process evaluations are conducted by the Core Group on a regular basis with the frequency at its discretion (monthly, quarterly, etc.). In addition, the Core Group chooses the data collection methods used and selects the participants from whom data are collected.

For example, the Core Group might conduct a process evaluation of Phase 1 at the end of a quarterly Steering Committee meeting by asking those present to complete an anonymous paper-and-pencil questionnaire or by emailing them the questionnaire, providing a link to an online questionnaire, or by conducting a group discussion to elicit answers to the following questions:

– Does the planning process encourage active participation by our public health partners?
– Does the planning process make good use of participants' time?
– Does the planning process encourage and build commitment from our public health partners? If not, what can we do to improve this?
– Was the atmosphere set among participants one of openness and sustained commitment?
– Are all the appropriate people involved in the process?
– Will the planning process structure result in a realistic plan?
– Were the participants/public health partners clearly informed about the activities associated with the MAPP process, their responsibilities, how long the process will take and the anticipated end results (NACCHO, 2013a)?

Table 9-1 Sample budget worksheet

Resource needed	Estimated cost	Potential funding source	Potential in-kind	Alternative to resource
PERSONNEL				
Half-time MAPP coordinator	$35,000 annually	Grant		Rotate coordinator role among MAPP partner agencies
CONSULTANTS				
Statistician	$5,000 contract	Grant	University partner	Community volunteer
SUPPLIES				
Flip charts	$120 (10 @ $20 each)	Chamber of Commerce	School district	Hold meetings in locations with whiteboards.
TRAVEL				
MEETINGS				
PRINTING and POSTAGE				
MISC				

Modified from National Association of City and County Health Officials (NACCHO). (2013). Mobilizing action through planning and partnerships (MAPP): A user's handbook. NACCHO.

Table 9-2 MAPP roles and responsibilities

	Core Group	Steering Committee	Subcommittee	Community
Phase 1 Organizing	Initiate MAPP process. Organize and plan MAPP process. Identify available and needed resources. Conduct readiness assessment. Recruit Steering Committee members. Propose subcommittee membership.	Begin meeting. Suggest recruitment of additional committee members. Approve MAPP process plan. Identify resources to meet needs. Make recommendations for subcommittee members, and approve final subcommittee membership.		Assist with recruiting community members for Steering Committee. Ensure broad community awareness of MAPP process.
Phase 2 Visioning	Plan visioning sessions. Secure visioning session facilitator(s). Work with them to prepare for visioning session(s). Summarize visioning session results. Draft vision statement values.	Oversee and participate in the Visioning phase. Develop a plan for getting broad community participation. Identify community members to participate in visioning session(s).		Ensure community receives announcements and updates through multiple communication avenues. Promote Visioning session(s) to encourage community participation.
Phase 3 Assessing	Community Health Status Assessment (CHSA)			
	Support activities of Steering Committee and CHSA subcommittee. Assist with data collection and analysis. Assist Community Health Profile development, presentation, and distribution of assessment results. Ensure CSHA, Steering Committee, and subcommittee activities are connected.	Oversee CHSA subcommittee activities. Identify data sources for CHSA subcommittee. Select locally appropriate indicators. Provide input into Community Health Profile development.	Oversee Community Health Status Assessment (CHSA). Secure community members to participate in planning and conducting CHSA. Collect and analyze CSHA data. Develop Community Health Profile using CSHA results. Distribute assessment results to community.	Disseminate Community Health Profile throughout the community. Involve community members in the CHSA subcommittee.

(continues)

Table 9-2 MAPP roles and responsibilities

Community Themes and Strengths Assessment (CTSA)

Support Steering Committee and CTSA subcommittee activities. Ensure CTSA, Steering Committee, and subcommittee activities are connected. ■ Participate in activities as needed	Oversee subcommittee activities. Provide recommendations for gaining broad community participation in assessment. ■ Participate in activities as needed	Form subcommittee with expertise in community engagement, knowledge of community, and in data collection and analysis, oversee the CTSA. Engage community members to participate in CTSA planning and implementation and to provide feedback in CTSA. ■ Prepare for CTSA activities, and ensure effective implementation. ■ Oversee implementation of activities. ■ Compile results	*Broad community participation is essential.* ■ Promote broad community participation in all assessment activities. ■ Ensure the community receives announcements and updates through a broad spectrum of community mechanisms (media, word of mouth, etc.). ■ Ensure participation of community members representing the diversity of the community, including those disproportionately affected by poor health outcomes or community conditions.

Local Public Health System Assessment (LPHSA)

Support Steering Committee and subcommittee activities. ■ Ensure connectivity between methods and promotion of all MAPP assessments	Oversee subcommittee activities. ■ Assist in ensuring broad LPHSA participation in LPHSA. ■ Participate in Essential Services Orientation session. ■ Respond to performance measures instrument. ■ Discuss results, and identify challenges and opportunities.	Convene a subcommittee, if preferred, to oversee LPHSA. ■ Engage community members to participate in LPHSA planning and implementation. ■ Prepare for LPHSA activities and ensure effective implementation. ■ Ensure facilitation and recording of all LPHSA sessions.	Engage community members in the LPHSA subcommittee; additional community participants can be recruited if desired.

(continues)

Table 9-2 MAPP roles and responsibilities

Forces of Change Assessment (FoCA)				
	Prepare for and plan brainstorming session(s). ■ Identify and secure session facilitator(s), and engage with them in preparing for visioning session(s). ■ Summarize and compile the assessment results. ■ Ensure connectivity between methods and promotion of all MAPP assessments.	Entire committee should participate in brainstorming session(s) to identify influential forces. ■ Identify opportunities and threats for each force.	None recommended; however, some Steering Committees may want to designate a FoC subcommittee to conduct the responsibilities identified for the Core Group	None recommended; however, some Steering Committees may want to designate a FoC subcommittee to conduct the responsibilities identified for the Core Group
Phase 4 Identifying	Compile and summarize results from four MAPP Assessments. ■ Plan process to identify strategic issues. ■ Provide staff support at meeting(s) in which strategic issues are identified. ■ Summarize the results of the meeting(s).	Approve general process for identifying strategic issues. ■ Participate (entire committee) in meeting(s) at which strategic issues are identified and analyzed.	Charge small groups with specific tasks related to identifying strategic issues, if preferred.	Engage community through the Steering Committee.
Phase 5	Prepare information to assist in developing strategies and goals. ■ Plan process to formulate goals and strategies, including identifying and supporting subcommittee(s) if needed. ■ Plan and staff the meeting(s) where goals and strategies are formulated. ■ Summarize the meeting(s) results. ■ Draft the planning report to guide next steps.	Participate (entire committee) in meeting(s) at which strategies and goals are selected and confirmed. ■ Oversee development of the planning report, and adopt the plan. ■ Ensure community member review and buy-in of strategic issues.	May be formed to discuss each strategic issue in-depth and identify the goals, strategies, and barriers.	Obtain community input into feasible and effective strategies. ■ Obtain broad community buy-in of strategies and goals in some manner.

(continues)

Table 9-2 MAPP roles and responsibilities

(continued)

Phase 6	Provide support to ensure process sustains itself and action occurs. ■ Recruit additional participants for plan implementation and evaluation as needed. ■ Support subcommittees and Steering Committee as needed.	Oversee action planning, implementation, and evaluation across all strategies. ■ Oversee recruitment of additional participants to assist in plan implementation and evaluation as needed. ■ Secure and/or assist in ensuring resources needed for implementation and evaluation are available.	Form subcommittee(s) or small groups to oversee implementation and evaluation. ■ Form small groups to oversee action plans for each strategy and report back to Steering Committee as requested.	Ensure community is aware of action and progress. ■ Engage community members in implementation to increase likelihood of success.

Reproduced from National Association of County & City Health Officials (US). (2013). Mobilizing Action through Planning and Partnerships (MAPP): A users handbook. NACCHO. Retrieved from http://eweb.naccho.org/eweb/DynamicPage.aspx?WebCode=proddetailadd&ivd_qty=1&ivd_prc_prd_key=8cb05f83-90\4e-471b-b588-8c51e9628c8b&Action=Add&site=naccho&ObjectKeyFrom=1A834/91A-9853-4C87-86A4-F7D95601C2E2&DoNotSave=yes&ParentObject=CentralizedOrderEntry&ParentDataObject=Invoice%20Detail

The aim of the process evaluation for Phase 1 is to find out the following:

- If there are community members or public health partners missing from the MAPP process, and if so, who.
- If there are aspects of the process in need of improvement.
- If there is anything about the process that needs clarification (NACCHO, 2013a).

In summary, Phase 1 answers the following questions:
1. Who is included in the MAPP process?
2. How ready is the community to conduct a MAPP process?
3. What resources are needed to implement a MAPP process?
4. How will the community work through the phases of a MAPP process (NACCHO, 2013a)?

Phase 2—Visioning

The focus of the seven steps of Phase 2 is developing community values and vision statements. This is done through visioning. Visioning is a process that entails MAPP partners, including community members, coming to consensus about what they value most in the community and the image they share of what they want their community to become. It serves as an inspiration for working together to make the vision a reality (Municipal Research and Services Center [MRSC], 2018; NACCHO, 2013a).

Community values are the core principles or standards honored by community members. They shape the character and development of the community and guide its goals, objectives, activities, projects, budgets, and services (City of Livingston, n.d.). They are the characteristics and attributes the community cherishes and wants (City and County of Denver, 2019) and reflect how people will behave with each other (Arnold, 2012).

The following are examples of community values:

- Affordable housing.
- Environmental stewardship.
- Diverse employment opportunities.
- Transportation choices.
- Community engagement.
- Outdoor lifestyle (City and County of Denver, 2019).

A vision statement conveys a community's hopes for the future. Ideally, it is understood and shared by community members, diverse, from a local perspective, inspiring and uplifting, and easily communicated (CCHD, 2018b).

Following are examples of community vision statements:

Our vision of Lakewood is a thriving, urban, South Puget Sound city possessing the core values of family, community, education and economic prosperity. We will advance these values by recognizing our past, taking action in the present and pursing a dynamic future. (City Council of Lakewood, Washington, 2015, p. 2)

Santa Cruz County is a healthy, safe and more affordable community that is culturally diverse, economically inclusive and environmentally vibrant. (Santa Cruz County, 2019, para. 1)

Denver is a healthy and prosperous community that thrives on civic engagement and collaboration to enhance the quality of our natural, social, and built environments for current and future generations and serves as a model for others to do the same. (City and County of Denver, 2019, para. 4)

The seven steps of Phase 2 summarized here aim to answer the following questions:

- Where does the community see itself in 3 to 5 years?
- What values will support the community as it goes through the MAPP process (NACCHO, 2013a)?

Step 2.1 Review Existing Community Vision and Values Statements. An often-used phrase in public health is *"Don't reinvent the wheel."* Before creating vision and values statements, existing ones are reviewed to determine if, with adaptation, any are applicable. The Core Group and Steering Committee can brainstorm these and decide if any represent the views of community members and public health partners. If none do, then new ones are crafted (NACCHO, 2013a).

Step 2.2 Design the Values and Visioning Process. The process of designing values and vision statements begins with planning how MAPP partners and community members will share their values and vision. Common ways communities obtain this information is through discussions or brainstorming sessions, community surveys, interviews, or some combination of these. The Steering Committee provides input into which of these methods would work best in the community, keeping in mind that the aim is to have the greatest community participation possible (NACCHO, 2013a).

If the Steering Committee decides to conduct a group brainstorming session, it's helpful to have a facilitator. Ideally, this person should have experience managing these types of sessions in a neutral and fair manner (NACCHO, 2013a).

Step 2.3 Conduct the Values and Visioning Session. In planning the values and visioning session, the following need to be decided (NACCHO, 2013a):

- Where and when will the session take place?

Because the aim is to have maximum community participation, it's important to take into consideration the day of the week that's most likely to draw people to the meeting. Generally, Mondays and Fridays are not good meetings days, which leaves a day midweek as the better option and Tuesday as the best choice (Staley, 2016).

Although attending a meeting during regular daytime working hours is generally not an issue for public health partners, it could be for community members. Consequently, it might be best to hold the session in the evening to encourage community member attendance. Public health practitioners typically have flexible hours to accommodate attending meetings and other events held outside the regular workday.

Where the event is held can impact attendance. The location should be easy to get to, be familiar to the participants, have sufficient parking and/or be accessible by mass transit, and be considered safe by the community. The size of the room should be appropriate for the number of people expected—not too big or too small, but just right, have good acoustics so everyone can be heard, and have a good layout so everyone can be seen. The space should be in good repair, clean, with no off-putting odors, have comfortable seating, and be easily accessible in the building.

- Who will participate in the session?

All MAPP partners and community members who made a commitment to participate in the MAPP process are invited. However, agencies and community members who were not able to commit to participating in the MAPP process are also invited because they may be interested in contributing to developing the vision and values statements.

- Who will facilitate the session?

It's beneficial to have an experienced facilitator manage the session. An experienced facilitator is one that:

- guides participants through the brainstorming process and draws out their opinions and ideas without offering his/her own.
- makes participants feel comfortable voicing their opinions and ideas.
- prevents disruptions from people trying to dominate the conversation, going on unrelated tangents, having side conversations, and attacking other's ideas (CCHD, 2019a).

- Who will record the session?

A brainstorming session produces a plethora of ideas, opinions, suggestions, decisions, and actions, all of which are recorded in the meeting minutes. Meeting minutes are the official record keeping documents that provide a summary of the discussions, decisions, and next steps agreed upon during the meeting. Given their importance, it's critical that the person designated to take the minutes is:

- a good listener and pays attention.
- assertive enough to speak up and ask for clarification during the meeting.
- organized and prepared.
- knowledgeable about the topic of the meeting.
- a good writer (uses correct spelling, grammar, and punctuation).
- a critical thinker and can sort through information (Bennet, 2017).

The minutes are distributed to all the meeting participants. They are used by the Core Group and Steering Committee in formulating the vision and values statements.

- What materials are needed for the session?

The mix and array of materials needed for a brainstorming session vary depending on the number of participants, room size, session format—small-group discussion or one big discussion, and availability of technology. At the least, a flip chart and an easel, poster-size paper to hang on a wall, or a whiteboard and markers are needed to record suggestions and ideas. In addition, registration materials including name tags, sign-in sheets, and agendas are also necessary.

- What questions will guide the session?

The session is driven by questions that provoke thoughts and ideas from participants about their vision for the community and the values they want sustained. The questions are developed before the meeting by the Steering Committee and used to prompt discussion at the meeting.

Examples of questions to elicit community values include:

- What values do you think the community has in common (Foundation for Intentional Community [FIC], 2019)?
- What is the one thing you think everyone in the community should believe (FIC, 2019)?
- What three core values and beliefs do you think drive our community (Olsen, 2019)?

Examples of questions to elicit ideas about a community vision include:

- What characteristics would make ours a healthy community for those who live, work, play, and learn here (NACCHO, 2013a)?
- If anything is possible, what is your dream for our community (CCHD, 2019b)?
- What kind of community would you like to create (CCHD, 2019b)?
- In 10 years, what would our community look like if it was the best it could be (Food and Agricultural Organization of the United Nations [FAO], 2019)?

At the values and visioning session, participants are greeted, asked to sign in at the registration table, where they receive a name tag, and are directed to the refreshments. The meeting should start on time with a member of the Core Group or Steering Committee welcoming everyone, introducing the Core Group and Steering Committee members, and explaining the purpose of the session and its importance to the MAPP process. Next, participants should be asked to introduce themselves to everyone in the room. To further build support among them, an ice breaker exercise is often done at this point (NACCHO, 2013a).

Once introductions are complete, the process of gathering information from the participants begins. One way of doing this is to:

- provide participants with the list of questions developed by the Steering Committee to prompt their values.
- allot no more than 15 minutes for participants to write down their responses.
- ask each participant to share the value that is most significant to them.
- record their responses on a flip chart or whiteboard at the front of the room.
- facilitate a group discussion of the ideas shared by the participants.
- organize the ideas into themes, and come to consensus about the concepts that will be in the values statements (NACCHO, 2013a).

This process is repeated to develop the visioning statement. However, if there are time constraints, a second meeting is scheduled (NACCHO, 2013a).

The most successful values and visioning sessions have the following five characteristics in common:

1. They promote a shared understanding of the whole community and aim to engage the entire community and key stakeholders.
2. They seek to identify a community's core values.
3. They explore emerging trends driving the community's future.
4. They produce a statement describing the community's preferred future.
5. They promote a strategic plan and serve as a roadmap to move the community closer to its vision (Ames, 2010).

Step 2.4 Formulate the Vision and Values Statements. Following the values and visioning session, a small group (subcommittee) of Steering Committee members compile the session results and begin drafting the values and vision statements (NACCHO, 2013a). Because the values are reflected in the vision, it's best to begin by drafting the values statement first.

Guidelines for developing value statements include:

- avoiding overly general words and phrases (Ashe-Edmunds, 2017).
- avoiding vague wording (Mulholland, 2018).
- keeping the list of values to a maximum of seven, preferably three (Ashe-Edmunds, 2017; Mulholland, 2018).

Each value statement contains the following three elements:

1. The value
2. A definition of the value
3. Key behavioral attributes of the value (Arnold, 2012)

Following is an example of a well-written value statement that meets these criteria:

> **Equity:** *Access for all.*
> *We provide accessible, affordable experiences and spaces for all Philadelphians. (City of Philadelphia, 2018, para. 1)*

Equity—is the value

Access for all—is the definition of the value

We provide…—is the behavioral attribute of the value.

Guidelines for developing a vision statement include:

- keeping it short, no more than two sentences.
- keeping it clear, avoid ambiguous words.
- keeping it simple, avoid jargon or buzz words the average person wouldn't understand.
- keeping it future focused.
- keeping it ambitious, but achievable.
- keeping it aligned with the community values (Wright, 2019).

The following vision statement meets these criteria:

Cambridge is a forward-thinking, welcoming, and diverse city. We enjoy a high quality of life and thrive in a sustainable, inclusive, and connected community. (City of Cambridge, 2019, p. 26)

A good example of all the guidelines are seen below in the vision and community values statements of Portland, Oregon (City of Portland, 2010, para. 8).

Vision

The Office of Community and Civic Life (of Portland) works toward a future where the community is a full and equal decision-making partner in all aspects of the City of Portland.

Community Values
Inclusion—No one gets left out

– *We are committed to equal participation and the continuous development of organized and meaningful inter-cultural relationships.*
– *Our neighborhood system strives to fully engage residents of Portland from all cultural, social and economic walks of life.*
– *We aspire to understand and honor the diversity of ways in which our communities communicate and participate, and ensure that our processes and opportunities reflect that understanding.*

Shared Power and Governance

– *We continuously strive to level the playing field for those that want to participate.*
– *We seek the most effective ways to include and respond to the community and eliminate attitudes and behaviors that exclude or isolate community voices.*
– *We work for equal access, equal opportunity, and equity in our work, in ways that are culturally-diverse, culturally-specific, and multicultural.*

– *We incorporate the flexibility to adjust whenever necessary in order to eliminate barriers to genuine collaboration with community.*
– *There is always room for those who want to participate.*

Relationships—the cornerstone of our work

– *The foundation of our work is a belief in effective, equitable and collaborative relationships with government and community partners.*
– *We seek to maintain the highest community trust through accountability and transparency in our processes and decisions.*
– *We value our community relationships and show it by being flexible and listening— ensuring timely, accurate and helpful responses to those who work with us or seek our services.*
– *We approach our work with humility and the understanding that we learn together. We embrace and encourage youth input and involvement.*

Social Sustainability—people are our most important resource

– *We use an equity lens to make decisions collaboratively with community partners.*
– *We strive to provide more choices for people who may have fewer choices.*
– *We recognize that involving and connecting people with government and with each other results in the most sustainable efforts for the City.*

Drafting the values and vision statements is not a quick process. It takes patience and wordsmithing to reach agreement on statements that reflects the thoughts and ideas of the community. When the final draft statements are ready, the subcommittee shares them with the full Steering Committee and Core Group, visioning session participants, MAPP partners, and community members for comment. They are revised if needed and final statements developed (NACCHO, 2013a).

Step 2.5 Keep Vision and Values Statements Alive. Once the values and vision statements are finalized, it's important to keep them alive or top-of-mind by everyone involved in the MAPP process. The Steering Committee, Core Group, MAPP partners, and community members use the following questions to guide a brainstorming session on how to ensure this happens:

- What can keep the community aware of the vision and value statements on a continuous basis?
- What are some ways to incorporate the vision and value statements in communications with the community?
- When and where is it appropriate and useful to read the statements aloud?
- What are some possible locations for displaying the value and vision statements (NACCHO, 2013a)?

Step 2.6 Celebrate Success. During this step, the completion of Phase 2 is celebrated, and the contribution MAPP partners made to its success are recognized (NACCHO, 2013a). It's important to keep costs and resource availability in mind when planning this event.

Step 2.7 Conduct Process Evaluation. The process evaluation for Phase 2 is done to ascertain if the values and visioning session was collaborative, and if it resulted in shared values and vision statements. To determine this, session participants are surveyed for their responses to the following questions:

Was the process collaborative? If not, why not?

What would increase collaboration in future phases?

Did the process lead to a shared vision and value statements? If not, why not?

Are there any aspects of the process that need improvement (NACCHO, 2013a)?

In summary, Phase 2 answers the following questions:

1. Where does the community see itself in 3 to 5 years?
2. What values will support the community as it goes through the MAPP process (NACCHO, 2013a)?

Phase 3—Assessing

This phase of the MAPP process focuses on collecting needs assessment data. While it's akin to the generic needs assessment stage discussed in Chapter 4, it differs in that there are four distinct assessments each conducted by a separate subcommittee. The four assessments are:

- The Community Health Status Assessment, which provides data on health conditions in the community.
- The Community Themes and Strength Assessment, which identifies community assets and issues of importance to community members.
- The Local Public Health System Assessment, which measures how well local public health partners work together to deliver the 10 essential public health services.
- The Forces of Change Assessment, which identifies forces affecting the community and their associated threats and opportunities (NACCHO, 2013a).

These assessments are done in any order that works best for a given community. For example, communities with an abundance of secondary quantitative data might consider starting with the Community Health Status Assessment because it's quick and easy to complete. Communities conducting a visioning session might also collect data for the Community Themes and Strengths Assessment at the session. Asking participants to think about community themes and strengths is a good brainstorming prompt for eliciting their thoughts about a long-term vision for the community as well as a way of collect the assessment data (NACCHO, 2013a).

Since the four assessments focus on different aspects of the community, the steps for completing each one are presented separately in the following sections.

Community Health Status Assessment (CHSA)

The purpose of the CHSA is to assess the health status, quality of life, and risk factors of the people in the community, which requires quantitative data. Because it's likely that the public health MAPP partners already have this information, the Steering Committee explores what's available, from whom, and finds out the willingness of those with the data, to share it (NACCHO, 2013a).

After the existing data are reviewed, the Steering Committee identifies information gaps, using the following questions as a guide:

- Does the existing data reflect all segments of the community and public health system?
- Which segments of the community are not reflected in the existing data (NACCHO, 2013a)?

This assessment entails completing the following eight steps:

CSHA Step 1—Create CSHA Subcommittee. The Steering Committee is responsible for creating a CHSA subcommittee whose sole function is to conduct the CHSA, including accessing and analyzing data and creating a data management system. Public health partners with the expertise needed to complete these tasks include statisticians or epidemiologists at a local hospital or university (NACCHO, 2013a).

CHSA Step 2—Create Health Inequity Indicator List. In this step, the CHSA subcommittee creates a list of health inequity

indicators or signs. Health *inequities* are health differences between population groups that are avoidable, unnecessary, unjust (Boston Public Health Commission [BPHC], 2018), and reducible through appropriate government actions (World Health Organization [WHO], 2017). They are rooted in unfair social conditions in which people are born, grow, live, and age that increase susceptibility to poor health (BPHC, n.d.; WHO, 2017).

Disparities or *inequalities* on the other hand, are differences in health status or health determinants between different population groups. Inequalities, for instance, may result from conditions that are *unavoidable* such as biological variations (genetics, age, gender) (WHO, 2019). Because inequalities and inequities are not the same, the terms are not interchangeable.

As an example, girls generally weigh less at birth than boys. This is a health *inequality*. It's rooted in genetics and therefore, unavoidable. However, that babies born to black women are more likely to die before their first birthdays than babies born to white women is a health *inequity* because the difference in mortality rates has been linked to the stress of racism experienced by black women, which is unfair, avoidable, and based in social injustice (BPHC, n.d.).

In developing the list of health inequity indicators, the CHSA subcommittee should:

1. Keep in mind that health inequities are rooted in imbalances in the distribution of power and resources relative to gender, race, class, sexual orientation, and other aspects of identity, which result in unequal social, economic, and environmental conditions (National Academies of Sciences, Engineering and Medicine, 2017).
2. Reference the vision statement and interests of the public health MAPP partner organizations.
3. Determine which of the following data categories related to the social determinants

of health are most important, and then discuss specific indicators in the chosen categories:

Social and community context, for example, civic participation, incarceration, discrimination, social cohesion (*Healthy People*, 2020).

Neighborhood and built environment, for example, access to healthy food, crime and violence, housing quality, environmental conditions (*Healthy People*, 2020).

Health and health care, for example, health behaviors, quality of life, maternal and child health, social and mental health, chronic and infectious disease, injury and death, access to health resources and care (*Healthy People*, 2020; NACCHO, 2013a).

Education, for example, high school graduation, language and literacy, early childhood education (*Healthy People*, 2020).

Economic stability, for example, employment, income, poverty, housing instability, food security (*Healthy People*, 2020; NACCHO, 2013a).

Common social determinant indicators include:

- Household income
- Percent of people and households living in poverty
- Percent of renters in a neighborhood
- Percent of car ownership
- Neighborhood allocation of city or county budget
- Unemployment rate
- Neighborhood home foreclosure rate
- Value of owner-occupied housing (NACCHO, 2013a)

CHSA Step 3—Collect Indicator Data. Much, if not all, of the data needed by the CHSA subcommittee is likely available from secondary sources. Consequently, CHSA subcommittee members should confer with representatives from the local health department, state health department, hospitals, community health centers, schools, law enforcement, and other public health and community organizations that collect health data to find out what they have, and what they are willing to share (NACCHO, 2013a).

Online sources of secondary health data include:

U.S. Census Bureau—www.census.gov/acs/www/

County Health Rankings—www.countyhealthrankings.org

Health Information Warehouse—http://healthindicators.gov

Healthy People 2020—www.healthypeople.gov (NACCHO, 2013a)

National Center for Health Statistics—https://www.cdc.gov/nchs/index.htm

National Institutes of Health: Health Data Resources—https://www.nihlibrary.nih.gov/resources/subject-guides/health-data-resources

State centers for health statistics databases

Primary data is only collected if it's absolutely necessary (NACCHO, 2013a). It's costly in terms of time and money, neither of which is likely to be in abundance.

Indicators that identify segments of the community affected by health inequities and disparities provide the most important data for the CHSA and include the following:

- Income
- Race/ethnicity
- Immigration status
- Gender/sexual identity
- Education
- Age
- Employment status
- Homeownership and housing status (NACCHO, 2013a)

CHSA Step 4—Organize and Analyze Data. At a minimum, data analysis should include socioeconomic status, mortality rates, gender, age, race, ethnicity, geographic area, and other population subgroups in the community, if there are any. It's helpful if trends over time are shown, and if results are compared with similar communities or state averages and national targets such as those in the *Healthy People* objectives (NACCHO, 2013a).

A good statistical method to identify differences in health status among different community groups is cross-tabulation. For example, prevalence rates of diabetes can be cross-tabulated by race or age, heart disease can be cross-tabulated by employment status or gender to reveal any differences in disease occurrence by these social or economic indicators (NACCHO, 2013a).

Analyzing data to produce meaningful results takes someone with statistical analysis expertise. If no one on the CHSA subcommittee or otherwise involved in the MAPP process can competently enter the data, analyze it, and interpret the results, a consultant should be brought in to complete this task.

CHSA Step 5—Compile and Disseminate Results. The results of the data analysis are compiled into a report that should present the results in chart form along with a written interpretation. The report is shared with the Steering Committee, Core Group, MAPP partners, and community members. The report format, whether it's a hard copy, online/electronic, or slide presentation (NACCHO, 2013a), depends on which is the most efficient and effective way of sharing it with the different groups. For example, community members attending a meeting might get a hard copy report with public health partners getting an emailed electronic copy.

CHSA Step 6—Create Monitoring Systems. Since the CHSA data are a snapshot in time and continuously changing, a sustainable, easily updated system to track changes in the community's health status over time is needed. Although the MAPP process is not repeated every year, the next time it is, having a system in place that tracked changes in the health status data will support the process (NACCHO, 2013a).

To create a sustainable system to monitor health status indicators, a clear understanding of roles, leadership, coordination, and communication are needed. While one public health partner organization can take the lead, other partners should contribute to monitoring the data, also (NACCHO, 2013a).

The CHSA subcommittee is responsible for creating this tracking system. To accomplish this, decisions about the following are needed:

- Frequency of data collection
- Quality of data collected
- Inclusion of peer, state, or national data for comparison
- Modification or addition of indicators
- Complexity of the data system
- Maintenance of the data system
- Communication mechanisms to support use of the data system use (NACCHO, 2013a)

CHSA Step 7—Create Challenges and Opportunity Lists. In this step, the CHSA subcommittee uses the assessment results to create a summary list of 10–15 health status issues that present a challenge or opportunity. The following questions are useful in sorting these issues out from the CHSA results.

- Does the health issue affect a large number of people?
- Are there serious consequences if the issue is not addressed?
- Is there evidence of wide inequity between groups or increasing trends?
- Is the issue amendable to proven interventions?
- Does the issue have potential for improvement over the long term?
- If the issue is addressed, is there potential for a breakthrough in improving community health?

– Has this issue persisted in the community and been unsolvable?

– Is it possible to monitor this issue (NACCHO, 2013a)?

CHSA Step 8—Share Results. The final step of the CHSA is sharing the results with the Steering Committee, Core Group, MAPP partners, and community members.

Community Themes and Strengths Assessment (CTSA)

The purpose of the CTSA is to identify community thoughts, experiences, opinions, and concerns. To accomplish this, qualitative data about quality of life issues are needed. Because this type of data is often collected by public health partners, the Steering Committee identifies what data are available, from whom, and the willingness of those with the data to share it. The design of the CTSA is influenced by how useful the existing data was in informing past improvements. (NACCHO, 2013a).

CTSA Step 1—Create Subcommittee. The first step in conducting this assessment is for the Steering Committee to create a CTSA subcommittee. Members of the CTSA subcommittee should have an interest and/or expertise in collecting quality of life data, and skills to identify ways of encouraging the community at large and specific population group to participate in the CTSA (NACCHO, 2013a).

CTSA Step 2—Choose Data Collection Methods. The CTSA involves collecting data through:

1. Open discussions to hear the concerns, opinions, and comments of the community.
2. Surveys to identify quality of life perceptions.
3. Asset mapping to determine the resource capacity of the community members, organizations and institutions (NACCHO, 2013a). *Asset mapping* is the systematic

process used to catalogue the services, skills, and benefits available in a community (Rural Health Information Hub [RHIhub], 2019). The map provides a visual representation of the assets or resources in the community that can improve the quality of community life (CCHD, 2019c).

Assets are untapped potential in the community that when accessed can improve conditions in the community (University of Memphis [UofM], 2019). They include the people, associations, institutions, built and natural environment, and businesses that already exist. For example:

People—with special talents, skills, and abilities, older adults, youth, parents, artists, or entrepreneurs (RHIhub, 2019; UofM, 2019)

Associations—civic groups, environmental groups, education groups (PTA), block group, charitable organizations, animal protection/care groups (RHIhub, 2019)

Institutions—educational institutions (schools, colleges, universities), hospitals, museums, social service agencies, libraries, nonprofits (RHIhub, 2019)

Physical structures/space—parks, playgrounds, campsites, ponds/lakes, bike paths, community centers, roads, recreation facilities (UofM, 2019; RHIhub, 2019)

Businesses—chamber of commerce, banks, credit unions, merchants, business associations (RHIhub, 2019)

Knowing what the community's assets are is essential to the development of a "doable" program. In preparation for identifying and eventually mapping them, the CTSA subcommittee answers the following questions:

– How is the community defined?

For the CTSA, the definition of "community" is the same as what was established by the Core Group in Phase 1.

– Who will identify the assets?

The work of identifying community assets could be done by a small group of community members, representatives from MAPP public health partner organizations, a community organization or agency (CCHD, 2019c), or a combination of them.

Regardless of who else is involved in identifying assets, community members must be involved so they can share their insight. The adage *"Beauty is in the eye of the beholder"* holds true in this situation. While someone from outside the community may see an abandoned building as an eyesore, someone living in the community may see it as a "potential" community center. However, as tempting as it might be for the CTSA subcommittee to ask a community member to take on this task, unless the geographic boundaries of the "community" are limited, it's too much work for one person.

– What is the time frame for completing the CTSA?

The more time allotted for identifying a community's assets, the more assets that can be identified (CCHD, 2019c). The amount of time needed to complete a thorough appraisal of assets depends on the number of people available to complete the task and the size of the community in terms of population, services, organizations, institutions, and space. A rural community with a sparse population, few services, and few businesses will take less time than a densely populated urban community with many services, institutions, and businesses.

– What resources are available for the CTSA?

Asset mapping is a labor-intensive undertaking. It requires available resources in terms of personnel, time, funding, equipment, and technical expertise.

With these questions answered, the CTSA subcommittee decides which asset identification approach will work best, group or individual (CCHD, 2019c).

Group asset identification

A group asset approach entails compiling a list of all the associations, institutions, and organizations in the community. In addition to the general knowledge of the CTSA subcommittee members and knowledge of the community groups, other resources for identifying assets include community websites, local or county chambers of commerce, community or town directories, community calendars, friends, neighbors, colleagues. When the list of assets is complete, it's organized in some logical way—alphabetically, geographically, or functionally (education, health care, social service) and ready to be used to create the map (CCHD, 2019c).

Individual asset identification

Identifying assets of individuals is more challenging than identifying those of groups. Not only are there many more individuals in a community than there are groups, but it's impossible to know what someone's assets are without asking them, which is time consuming (CCHD, 2019c).

If individual asset identification is the approach the CTSA subcommittee chooses to use, decisions are needed about the following:

1. Geographic area

Individual asset identification is usually conducted in a small area. For example, a neighborhood (CCHD, 2019c), census tract, or school district instead of a whole community or county. The resources available for the CTSA in terms of personnel, time, and money are important determining factors here (CCHD, 2019c).

2. Number of people

How many people in the geographic area are the staff going to collect data from—all adults living or working in the area, a percentage of the adult population, as many as the staff can identify in a specific time frame? Again, this decision relates back to CTSA resource availability (CCHD, 2019c).

3. Type of information

Before the collection of information can begin, clarification is needed from the CTSA subcommittee about the type of general information it wants—skills, interests, or both, and what specific information it wants about that information. For example, if the CTSA subcommittee wants information about skills, what skills does it want to know about—office skills, parenting skills, or tutoring skills, construction skills? The same goes for interests. What interests does the subcommittee consider assets important enough to find out about (CCHD, 2019c)?

The CTSA subcommittee can narrow down the focus of the information it wants by answering the following questions:

- Why is the information needed?
- What will the subcommittee do with the information (CCHD, 2019c)?

4. Data collection

The CTSA subcommittee is responsible for drafting the questions that will be used to elicit the information they want from community members. These questions are submitted to the Steering Committee, Core Group, and MAPP process community member for review and feedback. The feedback is used to revise the questions, if necessary (NACCHO, 2013a).

When the questions are completed, the CTSA subcommittee next decides which data collection methods would work best given the geographic area. For example, if a survey is best, what type of survey—one that's mailed, emailed, completed on the phone, door to door, or during individual or group interviews (CCHD, 2019c)?

Because it's important to gather data from individuals or groups that represent the community's diversity, most communities use mixed methods of data collection (NACCHO, 2013a). **Table 9-3** presents a sampling of these methods. A more detailed discussion of them is in Chapter 4, Assessing Need.

CTSA Step 3—Gather Data. In preparation for data collection, the CTSA subcommittee addresses the following:

Who will data be collected from?

What data will be collected?

When will data collection begin and end?

Where will data collection take place, in which geographic area?

How will data be collected, through which methods (NACCHO, 2013a)?

CTSA Step 4—Review Data and Summarize Results. At the end of the data collection period, the CTSA subcommittee reviews the results, identifies assets, and summarizes the data into a short one- to two-page report (NACCHO, 2013a). The data are then used to create an asset map.

Two common ways of creating an asset map are by either using a large existing street map of the community or producing a computer-generated map (Google My Maps is a popular method, and it's free) (University of California Agriculture and Natural Resources [UCANR] n.d.). Armed with a "map" of the community, CTSA subcommittee members work together to plot or mark the map with the identified assets. When plotting assets on a paper map, pins, markers or tabs are used to identify the asset location. When plotting assets on a computer program (such as Google My Map), icons are used (UCANR, n.d.).

Not only should the map contain the name and location of the asset, but also why it's an asset. For example, if a community center is identified as an asset, it's important to note on the map who it's an asset to, who in the community uses it, who might also use it, what activities it's used for, and what might it be used for? Is the asset usable as is, or is it a potential asset (UCANR, n.d.)? (See **Figure 9-2**.) If individual assets are identified rather than group assets, it's not practical or even possible to plot them on a geographic map (UCANR, n.d.).

Table 9-3 Community themes and strengths assessment (CTSA) data collection methods

Method	Advantage	Disadvantage
Town hall meeting Large open meeting (up to 100 people) for community members to share their concerns, voice their opinions, and offer their comments.	Publicizes the MAPP process and CTSA. Can be repeated multiple times.	Can be difficult to get broad community involvement. Meeting can be dominated by one vocal group or individual.
Focus group Small group (8–10) of invited community members who respond to predetermined questions.	Small group allows participants to build upon each other's comments. Specific discussion questions guide session minimizing "going off topic."	Group can be dominated by one vocal participant. Small-group environment may hamper honesty. Limited number of participants may not reflect community-at-large.
Windshield or walking survey A driving or walking tour around the community taking note of the environment.	Can be done with a few people. Can identify assets (i.e., parks and playgrounds) and issues (littered lots and abandoned houses).	Assets and issues depend on the viewer's perception.
Photovoice A walking tour of up to 10 people taking pictures of whatever strikes them that is compiled into a book with a narrative of each picture provided by the photographer.	Attracts younger participants. Presentation of results are engaging. Some assets and issues are better conveyed in pictures rather than words.	Assets and issues worthy of being photographed depend on the viewer's perception. Requires a camera and ability to process photos.
Interviews One-to-one interviews can be done with key community leaders or members of a specific group.	Can gather in-depth information. Builds awareness of the CTSA and the MAPP process Is interactive.	Time consuming. Input limited to a small number of people.
Surveys Can be done through written questionnaires, by phone or in-person or electronically.	Can reach a large number of people in a short amount of time. Can generate specific data and/or open-ended responses.	May be difficult to reach some community groups. Does not provide in-depth feedback. Issues addressed limited to questions on the survey. Not interactive.

Data from National Association of County & City Health Officials (US). (2013). Mobilizing Action through Planning and Partnerships (MAPP): A user's handbook. NACCHO.

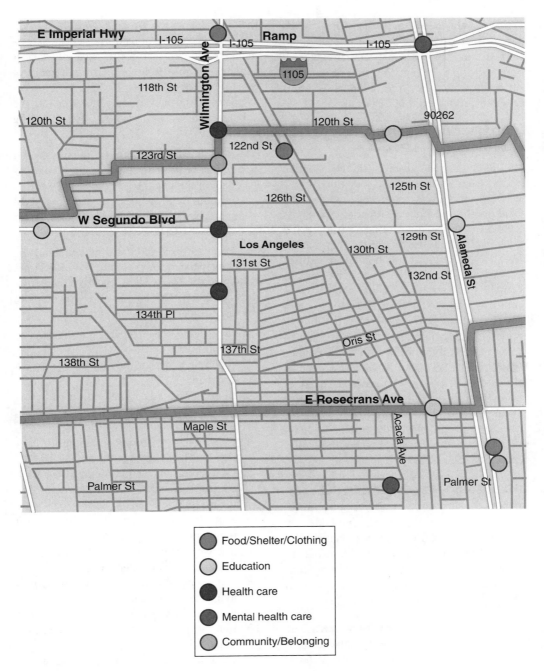

Figure 9-2 Asset map

Data from Healthy-Children-Healthy City Asset Mapping Project at http://www.healthycity.org/

CTSA Step 5—Share Results with Community. The CTSA results (written summary and the asset map) are shared with those who participated in the assessment, community members, the Steering Committee, Core Group, and MAPP partners.

Local Public Health System Assessment—LPHSA

The LPHSA gauges how well the local public health system delivers the 10 essential public health services as measured against the National Public Health Performance Standards [NPHPS or the Standards] using the NPHPS Local Assessment Instrument (CDC, 2018b; NACCHO, 2013b). The Standards are optimal performance expectations of what should occur in the community rather than what is minimally expected (NACCHO, 2013a), not only of the local public health system, but all entities in the community that contribute to the provision of public health services (See **Figure 9-3**.) Consequently, the LPHSA is useful in identifying service areas in need of improvement, strengthening local and state partnerships, and ensuring that the public health system can effectively provide the day-to-day essential services and respond to emergencies (NACCHO, 2013b).

LPHSA Step 1—Create LPHSA Subcommittee. In forming the LPHSA subcommittee, the Steering Committee should identify members who are from diverse segments of the local public health system and knowledgeable about the organizations providing essential public health services and the recipients of the health services (NACCHO, 2013a).

LPHSA Step 2—Plan Assessment. The LPHSA is conducted at a meeting that takes 4 to 5 months to plan. Planning begins with the LPHSA subcommittee reviewing the NPHPS Local Assessment Instrument and the accompanying Local Implementation Guide and the Facilitator Guide (NACCHO, 2013c). This familiarizes the subcommittee members with

the implementation process, timeline (NACCHO, 2013a), questions on the Local Assessment Instrument, and the type of data it generates. **Table 9-4** provides a summary of this information.

Reviewing these documents prepares the subcommittee members for brainstorming sessions to:

identify the community members and public health partners to invite to participate in the LPHSA.

reframe or revise questions on the Local Instrument if they want more focused data (NACCHO, 2013a).

Detailed discussion and guidance on the decisions needed for planning the LPHSA are contained in NACCHO's Local Implementation Guide (NACCHO, 2013c). The steps in the LPHSA planning process include:

1. Identifying a lead organization, group, or committee.
2. Selecting a method for conducting the assessment.
3. Identifying the best method for gathering information about how essential services are fulfilled.
4. Developing a plan and timeline for conducting the assessment.
5. Developing an orientation for MAPP public health partners who will participate in the assessment.
6. Securing support of public health leads at the highest levels possible.
7. Securing facilitators to guide participants through the assessment process.
8. Identifying potential public health partners to invite to participate in the assessment.
9. Finalizing assessment date and location.
10. Inviting potential public health partners to participate.
11. Conducting a participant orientation.
12. Conducting a facilitator training.
13. Preparing assessment meeting materials.
14. Coordinating meeting site logistics (equipment, name tags, refreshments, parking, signage, etc.) (NACCHO, 2013c).

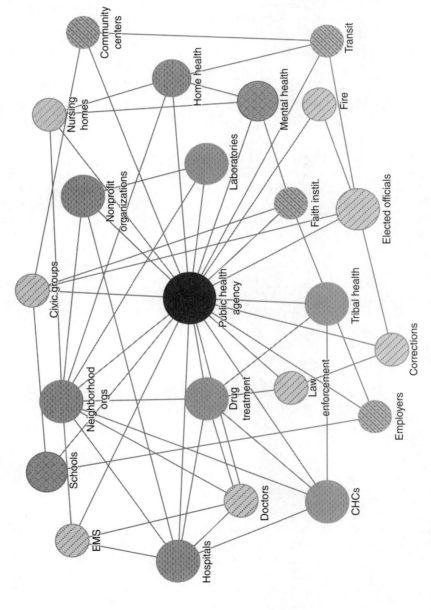

Figure 9-3 The local public health system

Table 9-4 Local assessment instrument and essential public health services

Essential Service	Responsibility Essential Service encompasses	Local Assessment Instrument and Essential Service assessment
1—Monitor health status to identify and solve community health problems.	Assessing community health status. Identifying health threats. Determining service needs. Attending to needs of high-risk groups. Identifying health-related community assets. Interpreting and sharing data. Collaborating to manage information systems.	What is going on in the community? Do we know how healthy the community is?
2—Diagnose and investigate health problems and hazards in the community.	Accessing public health laboratory able to do rapid screening and high-volume testing. Establishing infectious disease/epidemiology program. Creating ability to do disease outbreak investigations.	How ready is the local public health system to respond to health problems or hazards? How quickly does the public health system find out about problems? How effective is the public health system's response to problems?
3—Inform, educate, and empower people about health issues.	Creating community development interventions. Establishing social marketing and public media communication. Providing health information resources for the community. Working jointly with health education programs throughout the community.	How well is the community kept informed about health issues?
4—Mobilize community partnerships and actions to identify and solve problems.	Facilitating partnerships not typically considered health related. Undertaking health improvement screening, rehabilitation, and support projects. Building a coalition to improve community health.	How well does the public health system engage people in local health issues?
5—Develop policies and plans that support individual and community health efforts.	Ensuring leadership development. Ensuring community and state-level planning for health improvement. Developing and tracking health objectives for continuous quality improvement. Establishing evaluations with medical/healthcare system to define policies for prevention and treatment services.	What local government and private-sector policies promote health in the community? How well is the public health system setting healthy local policies?

(continues)

Table 9-4 Local assessment instrument and essential public health services   *(continued)*

Essential Service	Responsibility Essential Service encompasses	Local Assessment Instrument and Essential Service assessment
6—Enforce laws and regulations that protect health and ensure safety.	Enforcing sanitary codes. Protecting drinking water. Enforcing air quality standards. Initiating activities for animal control. Follow-up on hazards, injuries, and diseases identified in occupational and community settings. Monitoring medical service quality of laboratories, home health care providers, and nursing homes. Reviewing applications for new drugs, biologics, and medical devices.	Is the enforcement of health regulations technically competent, fair, and effective?
7—Link people to needed personal health services, and ensure the provision of health care when otherwise unavailable.	Ensuring an effective entry for people into a coordinated system of care. Providing culturally and linguistically appropriate materials and staff to ensure special populations are linked to services. Ensuring management of care is ongoing. Ensuring transportation services. Organizing health education/promotion/ disease prevention interventions for vulnerable populations.	Are people in the community receiving the health services they need?
8—Ensure competent public and personal healthcare workforce.	Educating, training, and assessing personnel to meet needs for health services. Establishing processes for professional licensing. Adopting programs for continuing improvement and lifelong learning. Establishing partnerships with professional programs to ensure student community learning experiences. Providing continuing education in leadership and management for those in executive positions.	Are the public health staff competent? Are the healthcare staff competent? How can the public health system ensure staff stay current?

(continues)

Table 9-4 Local assessment instrument and essential public health services *(continued)*

Essential Service	Responsibility Essential Service encompasses	Local Assessment Instrument and Essential Service assessment
9—Evaluate effectiveness, accessibility, and quality of personal and population-based health services,	Assessing the effectiveness of programs by monitoring and evaluating implementation, outcomes, and effect. Providing information needed for allocating resources and revising programs.	Is the public health system meeting the needs of the population it serves? Is the public health system doing the right things? Is the public health system doing things right?
10—Research for new insights and innovative solutions to health problems.	Establishing a continuum of innovation, from field-based efforts to more academic efforts that encourage new directions in scientific research. Linking with institutions of higher education and research. Creating capacity to conduct epidemiologic and economic analyses and health services research.	Is the public health system discovering and using new ways to meet its responsibilities?

Data and developed from National Association of City and County Health Officials [NACCHO]. Version 3.0 Local Assessment Instrument. Retrieved September 18, 2019 from https://www.naccho.org/programs/public-health-infrastructure/performance-improvement/community-health-assessment/local-assessment-and-governance-tools

LPHSA Step 3—Conduct the Assessment. The LPSHA meeting leader should follow the guidance offered in the NACCHO Local Assessment Facilitator Guide [Facilitator Guide] (NACCHO, 2013d). In summary, the Facilitator Guide recommends the following meeting format:

Participant welcome and LPHSA subcommittee introductions

Assessment process overview

Essential Services and National Public Health Performance Standards review

NPHP Standards discussion

Performance measure scoring

Consensus building

Results discussion

LPHSA Step 4—Review Results, Identify Opportunities and Challenges. In this step, the LPHSA subcommittee sorts the

performance results of each Essential Public Health Service into one of the following categories:

Category 1—Successful service performance, maintain efforts.

Category 2—Successful service performance, reduce resources.

Category 3—Challenging service performance, needs increased activity.

Category 4—Challenging service performance, needs more coordination (NACCHO, 2013a).

Detailed guidance for this step is provided in NACCHO's Local Assessment Implementation Guide (NACCHO, 2013c).

LPHSA Step 5—Share Results. The LPHSA results are shared with the MAPP partners and the community at large. This is done at meetings, via the community's website, in the local newspaper, through social media, or by any other means that information such as this is conveyed in the community. It's important to encourage community feedback and to provide a mechanism through which feedback can be submitted (NACCHO, 2013a).

Forces of Change Assessment—FoC

The Forces of Change (FoC) assessment is done to identify the phenomena that can affect the community and the local public health system, now or in the future. Forces are separated into the following three categories:

1. *Trends*, which are patterns of change that occur over time. For example, population growth or decline, special education needs, immunization rates.
2. *Events*, which are unusual or important occurrences that may happen only one time. For example, opening of a new community center, a dam break, or a chemical spill.
3. *Factors*, which are distinct aspects of the community. For example, close proximity to the ocean, an isolated mountainous location, a large ethnic population (NACCHO, 2013a).

FoC Step 1—Create FoC Subcommittee.
In creating the FoC subcommittee, the Steering Committee identifies individuals who are knowledgeable about the trends, events, and factors in the community, the opportunities they offer, and the threats they pose. Individuals who might be appropriate include long-term community residents, elected public officials, business leaders, and agency or organization directors (NACCHO, 2013a).

FoC Step 2—Complete Assessment.
To complete the FoC assessment, the subcommittee members engage in a brainstorming session to identify the forces at play in the community and their related opportunities and threats.

In preparation, subcommittee members should know:

- the definition of "forces of change" as the trends, factors, and events that presently impact the community or may impact it in the future.
- the forces in the community related to its social, political, economic, environmental, technological, scientific, legal, and ethical conditions.
- how to identify a force of change as being something that has happened in the community recently that affected or may affect the public health system or the community; a trend occurring now that will affect the community or the public health system in the future; a characteristic of community or state that poses or may pose an opportunity or threat; something that is happening or may happen that is posing or may pose a barrier to achieving the community's shared vision (NACCHO, 2013a).

During the brainstorming session, the FoC subcommittee members identify forces in the community and their related opportunities and threats by answering the following questions:

- What patterns or trends in decisions, policies, investments, rules, and laws affect the health of the community?
- Who is benefiting from these decisions, policies, investments, rules, and laws?
- Who is harmed by these decisions, policies, investments, rules, and laws?
- What institutions or people can create, enforce, implement, and change these decisions, policies, investments, rules, and laws?
- Who or what supports or opposes actions that contribute to health inequity?
- What opportunities are available to influence decisions, policies, investments, rules, and laws to benefit all groups?
- What present and future forces reinforce health inequity? How can the community reduce or prevent them?
- What present and future forces reinforce health equity? How can the community take advantage of these forces?

Table 9-5 Sample forces of change (FoC) assessment

Force	Trend	Factor	Event	Opportunity created	Threat posed
Weak economy	x			Increased partnerships and collaboration Increased entrepreneurship	Increased unemployment and underemployment Increased uninsured and underinsured Increased home foreclosures and housing issues
Built environment		x		Providing walking, running and biking trails Creating safe public space	Less open space for public recreation areas Limited affordable housing options
Contaminated water supply			x	Enacting stronger environmental protection laws	Lasting damage to wildlife and plants Increased risk of cancer and neurological problems

Data from Delaware Department of Health and Social Services, Division of Public Health (2012). The first Delaware state health improvement plan: Forces of change assessment. Retrieved September 23, 2019 from https://dhss.delaware.gov/dhss/search.html?s#stq=MAPP%202012

The forces identified from these questions are then compiled into one list. Each force on the list is designated a trend, event, or factor, along with the opportunities it creates or the threats it poses to the community or the public health system (NACCHO, 2013). **Table 9-5** is an example of what this might look like.

FoC Step 3—Summarize Findings. The FoC subcommittee summarizes key findings from the assessment into a two- to three-page report.

FoC Step 4—Share Results. The FoC Assessment report is shared with the subcommittee members who participated in the assessment brainstorming session, the Steering Committee, Core Group, and the MAPP partners and community members. This is accomplished in any number of ways, including electronically on the community's website or emailed, through social media, in hard copy at meetings, or through more traditional means in a local newspaper (NACCHO, 2013a).

In summary, the assessment in Phase 3 answers the following questions:

1. What is the health status of the community?
2. What is important to the community?
3. What is the community's perception of quality of life?
4. What assets are available to improve community health?
5. What are the local public health system's activities, competencies, and capacities?
6. What does the local public health system do to provide the 10 essential public health services?
7. What is happening or might happen that affects the community's health or the public health system?
8. What threats or opportunities do these happenings produce (NACCHO, 2013a)?

Phase 4—Identifying Strategic Issues

Phase 4 focuses on using the data generated from the four assessments completed in the previous phase to identify the strategic issues for the community and the public health system. Strategic issues are the policy choices or critical challenges that are standing in the way of the community achieving its vision (NACCHO, 2013a).

Step 4.1 Determine Method for Completing Phase. To begin Phase 4, the Core Group summarizes the data from the four assessments. The Core Group and Steering Committee then meet to decide on a process for identifying the strategic issues in the assessment results.

The following questions guide this determination:

– What will ensure the public health partners and community members understand the assessment results?
– What process will enable the local public health system partners and community members to identify the strategic issues from the assessment data summaries?
– What process will enable the prioritization of the strategic issues?
– What will ensure everyone is aware of the strategic issues (NACCHO, 2013a)?

Step 4.2 Present Summarized Assessment Data. At a meeting of the Steering Committee, MAPP partners, and community members to identify the strategic issues, the Core Group presents the summarized assessment data and a list of the challenges and opportunities the results pose (NACCHO, 2013a). The data presented differ for each assessment as follows:

- Community Health Status Assessment—the health conditions that exist in the community.
- Community Themes and Strengths Assessment—reasons why the health conditions (identified in the CHSA) exist, assets available for use in the community, what's important to the community, and what the quality of life is like in the community.
- Local Public Health System Assessment—weaknesses in the public health system that need improvement, strengths in the public health system that are available for use, capability/capacity opportunities that exist.
- Forces of Change Assessment—forces affecting actions taken, what is happening or might happen that will affect the local public health system or the community (NACCHO, 2013a).

Step 4.3 Brainstorm Themes and Potential Strategic Issues and Supporting Data. Using the assessment summaries, participants at the strategic issues meeting brainstorm to identify themes common to at least three assessments. Providing participants with a format to follow helps in this undertaking (NACCHO, 2013a). An example of a format is presented in **Table 9-6**.

Table 9-6 Sample strategic issue theme and supporting data

Theme	Supporting Data			
Community design	CHSA	CTSA	LPHSA	FoC
	Chronic disease rates		Workforce development needs	Economic development changes

Data from National Association of County & City Health Officials (US). (2013). Mobilizing action through Planning and Partnerships (MAPP): A user's handbook. NACCHO.

At the end of the brainstorming time period, meeting participants share their results with each other (NACCHO, 2013a). One way to facilitate this is to record verbal responses on flip charts or whiteboards.

Step 4.4 Prioritize Strategic Issues.
Even though all the issues raised by the meeting participants will have importance, there are some that will have *strategic* importance. These are the issues that have significant consequences for the community and public health systems (NACCHO, 2013a).

To determine which issues are "strategic," each issue is assessed against the following nine criteria. The more "yes" answers an issue generates, the more strategic it is. After the strategic issues have been identified, they are prioritized (NACCHO, 2013a).

1. Is the issue related to the community vision?
2. Does the issue or will the issue affect the entire community?
3. Does the issue affect the community now or will it affect it in the future?
4. Will the issue necessitate a change in how things function?
5. Is the solution to this issue obscure?
6. Is leadership support needed to address this issue?
7. Does this issue result in long-term consequences, if it's not addressed?
8. Is more than one organization needed to address the issue?
9. Is this issue creating tension in the community (NACCHO, 2013a)?

Although there is no one best way to prioritize the strategic issues, one possible technique for the Steering Committee to use is nominal group process (NACCHO, 2013a). Briefly, this process entails the following:

– Reviewing the strategic issues.
– Clarifying any misconceptions or misunderstanding.
– Having each committee member rank each of the strategic issues with the highest priority issue receiving the highest ranking. For example, if there are 3 strategic issues, the one with the highest priority is ranked "3," the lowest priority is ranked "1."

When the committee members complete their ranking of each strategic issue, the rankings from each member for each issue are totaled. The issue with the highest total ranking score is the highest priority. (See **Table 9-7**.)

Table 9-7 Nominal group process strategic issue prioritization
Ranking scale: 1 = lowest priority, 3 = highest priority.

	Unemployment	Low childhood immunization rates	Aging population
Participant 1	2	3	1
Participant 2	3	1	2
Participant 3	1	2	3
Participant 4	1	3	2
Total ranking	7	9	8

Data from National Association of County & City Health Officials (US). (2013). Mobilizing action through Planning and Partnerships (MAPP): A user's handbook. NACCHO.

Step 4.5 Disseminate Priority Strategic Issue Results. The priority strategic issues are shared with the MAPP partners and the community at large (NACCHO, 2013a). It's always beneficial to ask MAPP community members for guidance on how to best disseminate the results to the community-at-large because this varies from community to community.

Step 4.6 Conduct Process Evaluation. Upon completion of Phase 4, the Core Group conducts a process evaluation by asking those who attended the strategic issues meeting the following questions:

- Were the data from the four MAPP assessments effectively analyzed and synthesized?
- Was an effective process used to identify the policy choices or challenges that need attention in order for the community to achieve its vision?
- Was there assurance that partners collectively identified with and felt ownership of the strategic issues?
- Were partners assured that strategic issues were not biased by any one individual or agency's agenda?
- Was there assurance that the strategic issues resonate with the community (NACCHO, 2013a)?

> In summary, Phase 4 answers the following questions:
> 1. What issues are critical to the local public health system's success?
> 2. What critical challenges or fundamental policy choices need attention before the community can achieve its vision?

Phase 5—Formulating Goals and Strategies

This phase of the MAPP process is akin to the planning stage in the generic planning process discussed in Chapter 5. The focus is on developing goals and strategies to address the prioritized strategic issues identified in Phase 4.

Step 5.1 Determine the Process for Developing the Goals and Strategies. The Core Group is responsible for making the following decisions related to developing goals and strategies:

- What format will work best for developing the goals and strategies—for example, a series of short, weekly meetings or a day-long retreat (NACCHO, 2013a)?
- Who will participate in the process (NACCHO, 2013a)—a subcommittee, all MAPP partners, only the Steering Committee and Core Group?
- Who will guide/facilitate the process (NACCHO, 2013a)—someone from "outside" or a MAPP partner?
- What method will work best for coming to consensus on the goals and strategies (NACCHO, 2013a)—nominal group process, open discussion, small groups?

With these issues decided, the Core Group sets a date, time, and location for a goals and strategies meeting, invites participants, secures a facilitator, develops a meeting agenda, and develops and prepares meeting materials.

Step 5.2 Develop Goals to Address Priority Strategic Issues. The first task at the goals and strategies meeting is to develop the goals for each of the priority strategic issues. One way this is done is for participants to brainstorm each of the issues, either individually or in small groups, using the following questions as a guide:

- What, if anything, is currently under way to address the issue?
- What resources, if any, are currently available to address the issue?
- Who in the community is likely to support working on this issue, and to what extent?

– What are the potential community, legal, technical, or financial barriers to addressing this issue?
– What are some possible goals for addressing this issue (NACCHO, 2013a)?

Following the brainstorming exercise, each participant or group of participants develops a potential goal related to the strategic issue (NACCHO, 2013a).

Step 5.3 Generate Strategies. After the potential goals are developed, strategies to reach the goals are generated. Individually, in small groups or in an open discussion, one strategy is developed for each potential goal. To move the process of strategy development along, the following are determined:

– What past action/strategy related to the strategic issue, has worked?
– What past action/strategy related to the strategic issue has not worked?
– What strengths exist in the community related to the strategic issue and the goal?
– What opportunities exist in the community related to the strategic issue and the goal?
– What threats exist in the community related to the strategic issue and goal that need mitigating?
– What new insights from the assessments might support a strategy to achieve the goal (NACCHO, 2013a)?

The answers to these questions are used to develop strategies to achieve each potential goal.

Step 5.4 Brainstorm Potential Barriers to Strategy Implementation. In the process of developing strategies, consideration is given to potential barriers to their implementation. Addressing barriers while the strategies are still in the developmental stage increases the likelihood that if implemented, they'll produce the desired results (NACCHO, 2013a). Barriers might include inadequate resources, lack of community support, antiquated technology, or legal/policy issues (NACCHO, 2019).

Step 5.5 Detail Strategy Implementation. . This step focuses on drafting details for the implementation of each potential strategy, including:

– specific actions needed to implement the strategy.
– organizations and individuals whose involvement and support are needed.
– resources needed and their potential sources.
– proposed implementation timeline (NACCHO, 2019, 2013a).

Step 5.6 Select and Adopt Strategies. Because all the potential strategies are not suitable for implementation, the Steering Committee uses the PEARL test to choose which are suitable by considering each one against the following five criteria:

Propriety: Is the strategy consistent with public health principles and essential services?

Economics: Is the strategy financially possible and makes economic sense to implement?

Acceptability: Is the strategy something the stakeholders and community will accept?

Resources: Is the strategy supported by MAPP partners with staff, expertise, and/or space needed for implementation?

Legality: Is the strategy legal to implement (NACCHO, 2013a)?

Strategies that don't meet all the criteria are either revised or eliminated (NACCHO, 2013a).

Step 5.7 Conduct Process Evaluation. Phase 5 of the MAPP process focuses on identifying the priority strategic issues and developing the goals and strategies for addressing them. To determine if this is accomplished, the Core group conducts a process evaluation to answer the following questions:

- Was an effective process used to formulate the goals and strategies?
- Was there assurance that the goals and strategies reflect what the community wants to achieve?
- Were the goals and strategies formulated so they enable the development of practical work plans (NACCHO, 2013a)?

As discussed in previous phases, there are a variety of ways to conduct the process evaluation, including: an open discussion at the end of a Steering Committee meeting, by completing a paper-and-pencil, online or emailed evaluation form.

In summary, Phase 5 answers the following questions:

1. What are the long-term goals related to the priority strategic issues?
2. What can the community do to reach these goals (NACCHO, 2013a)?

Phase 6—Taking Action (Planning, Implementing, and Evaluating)

Phase 6 addresses the generic planning stages of planning, implementation, and evaluation. It's during this phase that the goals and strategies developed in Phase 5 are used to create an overall plan. The overall plan is composed of multiple separate work plans for implementing the strategies and achieving the goals (NACCHO, 2013a).

The work plans are usually implemented by Action Teams. Action Teams are composed of community members and representatives of various community organizations and agencies that have been involved in the MAPP process all along as well as those new to it. Successful implementation of the work plans depends on these diverse entities working together. Consequently, transparency, effective communication, trust, and leadership are critical (NACCHO, 2013a).

Step 6.1—Organize for Planning, Implementation, and Evaluation. This first step of Phase 6 focuses on setting up the structure for the remaining steps. It involves the Steering Committee creating the Action Teams and tasking them with developing measurable objectives and activities to meet a goal (NACCHO, 2013a).

The process of forming Action Teams entails:

- Identifying the Action Teams needed

A separate Action Team is needed for each goal, strategic issue, or strategy (NACCHO, 2013a), with the Steering Committee deciding which of these the teams will address. Consequently, the number of teams needed and their tasks depends on the goals, strategies, or strategic issues identified previously.

- Inviting people to participate on each team

Depending on the focus of the Action Team (goal, strategic issue, or strategy) individuals and organizations with expertise or interest in it are invited to participate on the team.

- Creating a process for facilitating accountability

Having the Action Teams report their progress to the Steering Committee is essential to the Committee's oversight responsibilities for the Action Phase (NACCHO, 2013a). The process might entail a periodic written report, an oral presentation at a regular meeting of the Steering Committee, or submission of minutes from team meetings.

Step 6.2—Develop SMART Objectives. Each Action Team develops SMART objectives for the goal, strategic issue, or strategy their team is assigned (NACCHO, 2013a). In addition to meeting the SMART criteria, objectives also contain a quantitative baseline and indication of its desired result—increase, decrease, or stability (maintenance) (NACCHO, 2013a).(How to write SMART objectives is discussed in Chapter 5, Planning.)

Step 6.3—Establish Accountability. Achieving the goals and realizing the community's vision takes collaboration by MAPP partners and community members from the very beginning of the MAPP process. When this exists, there is a greater likelihood of commitment to and accountability for implementing plans (NACCHO, 2013a).

In addition, as the Action Phase unfolds, the Steering Committee is in regular contact with the Action Teams. This gives team members an opportunity to share challenges they're having and work with the Steering Committee to identify remedies (NACCHO, 2013a).

Step 6.4—Develop Implementation/ Action Work Plans. With the objectives written, the Action Teams develop plans for implementing the activities associated with them. The implementation/action plans include the following:

- The strategic issue, goal, or strategy that is the focus of the implementation plan.
- The objective associated with the strategic issue, goal, or strategy.
- The start and end dates for implementing actions to accomplish the objective.
- The steps for implementing the actions.
- The individual, group or organization responsible for completing the steps.
- Potential collaborators or partners who should participate in the implementation.
- The evaluation criteria to determine if the actions implemented were successful in meeting the objective.
- Special resource needs (Institute of Cultural Affairs, 2019; NACCHO, 2013a).

Step 6.5—Review Plans for Coordination Opportunities. The Steering Committee reviews the completed implementation/ action plans submitted by the Action Teams, makes suggestions for revisions, and identifies opportunities for coordinating actions/activities across them. Steering Committee feedback to the Action Teams is used to revise the plans (NACCHO, 2013a).

Step 6.6—Take Action—Implement The Plans. Using the plans as their guide, the Action Teams begin implementing the activities they developed. As implementation progresses, data are collected to monitor progress toward meeting the objectives and ultimately achieving the community goals and realizing its vision (NACCHO, 2013a). (This step is equivalent to the implementation stage of the generic planning process discussed in Chapter 6, Implementing.)

Step 6.7—Conduct Process and Outcome Evaluations. The process evaluation for this phase provides answers to the following questions:

- Was the assessment data used effectively to inform planning in this phase?
- Were objectives identified for or related to each goal and strategy?
- Was the division of labor and organization structure used effectively?
- Was system partner ownership of activities ensured?
- Was energy and progress sustained throughout the phase?
- Were evaluation results used effectively to improve activities?
- What worked well in this MAPP process?
- What changes are recommended for the next MAPP process (NACCHO, 2013a)?

In addition to process evaluations, outcome evaluations are done at least once every 12 months to determine the extent of progress the community is making toward meeting its goals and objectives and, ultimately, realizing its vision (NACCHO, 2013a). A more detailed discussion of evaluation is in Chapter 7, Evaluating.

In summary, Phase 6 answers the following questions:

1. What will happen to ensure the vision is realized?
2. Who (individual or organization) will make it happen?
3. How will it happen?

4. What will indicate improvements occurred?
5. How can continual improvement occur (NACCHO, 2013a)?

The MAPP process is a roadmap for planning. (See **Figure 9-4**.) Its foundation is the partnerships between the local public health system and the people it serves in the community where they live, work, and play. Its success lies in the collaborative effort of the partners working toward a healthier community.

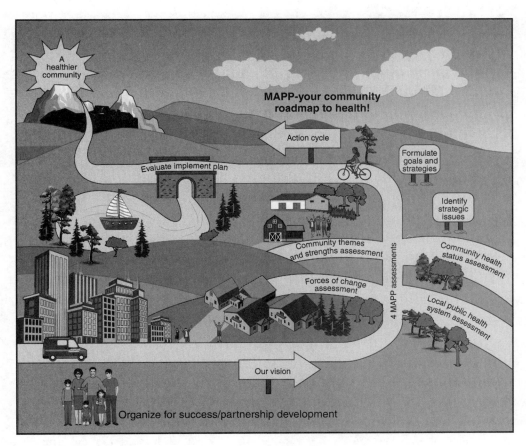

Figure 9-4 MAPP roadmap

Chapter Summary

MAPP is a health planning model grounded in collaboration among the community's public health entities committed to identifying the health issues of greatest importance to the community, the health status of the community, the strengths and weaknesses of the public health system, and factors that may change them all, and developing programs to improve them all.

Planning in Practice Chapter Activity

If you were asked to identify the greatest health-related issue in your community, what would it be? (Record your answer.)

1. In a small group, share your responses.
2. Choose one of the issues from among the many identified by the group, and brainstorm which of the MAPP assessments would enable verification that the issue is, in fact, a problem in the community.
3. Brainstorm ways the problem might be addressed.

4. Next, read the following report and answer the questions below.

Report: *Multnomah County Community Assessment Mobilizing for Action through Planning and Partnerships (MAPP) to Identify Health-Related Priorities Summary Report* (Sorvari & Mowlds, 2011)

Link to report PDF: https://multco.us/file/16662/download

(Note: Click on "Summary report" to download report PDF

Article Questions

1. Who were the partners that comprised the MAPP advisory group?
2. Who comprised the "staff" of the MAPP process?
3. How often did the Advisory Group (AG) meet during the course of the MAPP process?
4. Why was the Community Themes and Strengths Assessment (CTSA) conducted?
5. What was the first step taken in conducting the CTSA?
6. What was done with the results from the first step of the CTSA?
7. What were the top three results from the first step of the CTSA?
8. What did the AG do with the findings from the first step of the CTSA, and what did it recommend as a result, for whom?
9. What role did the AG play in implementing its recommendations?

10. What barriers limited completion of the AG's recommendations?
11. What was the purpose of the community health focus groups conducted as the second step of the CTSA assessment?
12. Who developed the CTSA focus group questions?
13. How were focus group participants recruited?
14. What were the focus group participants asked to do prior to the start of the group discussion?
15. How many focus groups were conducted and by whom?
16. What was learned from the focus groups? (Summarize the findings.)
17. What was the purpose of conducting a community health survey as part of the CTSA?
18. What were the demographics of the priority populations sought as

participants for the survey, where were they recruited, and by whom?

19. What were the results of the survey? (Summarize.)

20. How did the results of the primary data collected from the CTSA focus groups and survey mesh with the themes on the preliminary health issues inventory created with secondary data during the first step of the CTSA?

21. Which themes were supported by primary data from both the focus groups and survey?

22. Which health status indicators did the county health department regularly review?

23. How were the results of the health status indicator reviews shared?

24. What factors were used to assess the health status indicators?

25. What criteria did a health status indicator have to meet in order to be included in the Community Health Status Assessment?

References

Ames, S. (2010). The new Oregon model: Envision—plan-achieve. *Journal of Future Studies, 15*(2), 163–166. Retrieved September 9, 2019, from https://jfsdigital.org/articles-and-essays/2010-2/vol-15-no-2-december/symposium-guest-editor-jan-lee-martin/the-new-oregon-model-envision-plan-achieve/

Arnold, K. (2012). Definition and benefits of a values statement. Retrieved September 6, 2019, from http://www.extraordinaryteam.com/definition-and-benefits-of-a-values-statement/

Ashe-Edmunds, S. (2017). How to write a values statement. Retrieved September 6, 2019, from https://bizfluent.com/how-8707684-write-values-statement.html

Bennet, R. (2017). Skills required to be a good minute taker. Retrieved October 3, 2019, from https://www.practicallyperfectpa.com/2017/skills-required-to-be-a-good-minute-taker/08/24

Boston Public Health Commission. (2018). The guide to advance racial justice and health equity. Retrieved January 20, 2021 from https://bphc.org/whatwedo/racialjusticeandhealthequity/Documents/BPHC%20The%20Guide%20To%20Advance%20Racial%20Justice%20and%20Health%20Equity.pdf

Center for Community Health and Development [CCHD]. (2018). Chapter 2, Section 13: MAPP: Mobilizing for action through planning and partnerships, Lawrence, KS: University of Kanas. Retrieved August 27, 2019, from https://ctb.ku.edu/en/table-of-contents/overview/models-for-community-health-and-development/mapp/main

Center for Community Health and Development [CCHD]. (2019a). Chapter 16, Section 2: Developing facilitation skills, Lawrence, KS: University of Kanas. Retrieved September 5, 2019, from https://ctb.ku.edu/en/table-of-contents/leadership/group-facilitation/facilitation-skills/main

Center for Community Health and Development [CCHD]. (2019b). Chapter 8, Section 2: Proclaiming your dream: Developing mission and vision statements, Lawrence, KS: University of Kanas. Retrieved September 5, 2019, from https://ctb.ku.edu/en/table-of-contents/structure/strategic-planning/vision-mission-statements/main

Center for Community Health and Development [CCHD]. (2019c). Chapter 3, Section 8: Identifying community assets and resources, Lawrence, KS: University of Kanas. Retrieved September 15, 2019, from https://ctb.ku.edu/en/table-of-contents/assessment/assessing-community-needs-and-resources/identify-community-assets/main

Centers for Disease Control and Prevention [CDC]. (2018a). The ten essential public health services. Retrieved August 27, 2019, from https://www.cdc.gov/publichealthgateway/publichealthservices/essentialhealthservices.html

Centers for Disease Control and Prevention [CDC]. (2018b). National public health performance standards. Retrieved September 17, 2019, from https://www.cdc.gov/publichealthgateway/nphps/index.html

City of Cambridge. (2019). Envision Cambridge. Retrieved September 9, 2019, from https://www.cambridgema.gov/CDD

City of Philadelphia. (2018). Vision, mission and values. Retrieved September 9, 2019, from https://www.phila.gov/departments/philadelphia-parks-recreation/about/vision-mission-and-values/

City of Portland. (2010). Mission, goals and values. Retrieved September 9, 2019, from https://www.portlandoregon.gov/civic/29128

City and County of Denver. (2019). Denver's sustainability vision. Retrieved September 3, 2019, from https://www.denvergov.org/content/denvergov/en/office-of-sustainability/about-us/denver-s-sustainability-vision.html

City Council of Lakewood, Washington. (2015). Resolution No. 2015-30: A resolution of the city council of Lakewood, Washington, adopting a community vision statement for the city. Retrieved September 3, 2019, from https://cityoflakewood.us/city-council/city-council-goals/

Food and Agriculture Organization of the United Nations [FAO]. (2019). FAO capacity development: Visioning exercise. Retrieved September 5, 2019, from http://www.fao.org/capacity-development/resources/practical-tools/multi-stakeholder-processes/visioning/en/

Foundation for Intentional Community [FIC]. (2019). Setting community goals and values in a visions statement. Retrieved September 5, 2019, from https://www.ic.org/wiki/setting-community-goals-and-values-in-a-vision-statement/

Healthy People 2020 [Internet]. Washington, DC: U.S. Department of Health and Human Services, Office of Disease Prevention and Health Promotion. Retrieved April 16, 2020, from https://www.healthypeople.gov/

Institute of Cultural Affairs. (2019). Technology of participation. Retrieved October 1, 2019, from https://www.ica-usa.org/apps/search?q=technology+of+participation

Mulholland, B. (2018). Value statement: Defining the heart of your company. Retrieved September 6, 2019, from https://www.process.st/value-statement/

Municipal Research and Services Center [MRSC]. (2018). Creating a community vision. Retrieved September 2, 2019, from http://mrsc.org/getdoc/c11bbf9d-34e8-4b57-94d0-e27bc38bfec9/Creating-a-Community-Vision.aspx

National Academies of Sciences, Engineering and Medicine. (2017) *Communities in action: Pathways to health equity.* https://doi.org/10.17226/24624. Retrieved April 16, 2020, from https://www.nap.edu/download/24624

National Association of County and City Health Officials [NACCHO]. (2013a). Mobilizing action through planning and partnerships (MAPP): A users handbook. Retrieved August 23, 2019, from http://eweb.naccho.org/eweb/DynamicPage.aspx?WebCode=proddetailadd&rivd_qty=1&rivd_prc_prd_key=8cb05f83-904e-471b-b588-8c51e9628c8b&Action=Add&site=naccho&ObjectKeyFrom=1A83491A-9853-4C87-86A4-F7D95601C2E2&DoNotSave=yes&ParentObject=CentralizedOrderEntry&ParentDataObject=Invoice%20Detail

National Association of County and City Health Officials [NACCHO]. (2013b). National public health performance standards: Local assessment instrument [PDF]. Retrieved September 19, 2019, from https://www.naccho.org/programs/public-health-infrastructure/performance-improvement/community-health-assessment/local-assessment-and-governance-tools

National Association of County and City Health Officials [NACCHO]. (2013c). National public health performance standards: Local implementation guide [PDF]. Retrieved September 19, 2019, from https://www.naccho.org/programs/public-health-infrastructure/performance-improvement/community-health-assessment/local-assessment-and-governance-tools

National Association of County and City Health Officials [NACCHO]. (2013d). National public health performance standards: Local assessment facilitator guide [PDF]. Retrieved September 19, 2019, from https://www.naccho.org/programs/public-health-infrastructure/performance-improvement/community-health-assessment/local-assessment-and-governance-tools

National Association of County and City Health Officials [NACCHO]. (2019). Mobilizing for action through planning and partnerships. Retrieved August 23, 2019, from https://www.naccho.org/programs/public-health-infrastructure/performance-improvement/community-health-assessment/mapp

Olsen, E. (2019). Core values. Retrieved September 5, 2019, from https://onstrategyhq.com/resources/core-values/

Rural Health Information Hub [RHIhub]. (2019) Identify assets/resources available. Retrieved September 15, 2019, from https://www.ruralhealthinfo.org/toolkits/rural-toolkit/1/asset-identification

Santa Cruz County. (2019). Vision Santa Cruz County. Retrieved September 3, 2019, from http://www.santacruzcounty.us/VisionSantaCruz.aspx

Staley, O. (2016). The best day and time to hold a meeting. Retrieved October 7, 2019, from https://qz.com/work/653033/heres-the-best-day-and-time-to-hold-a-meeting/

University of California, Agriculture and Natural Resources [UCANR]. (n.d.). Community mapping toolkit. Retrieved September 17, 2019, from https://ucanr.edu/?search=1&q=asset+mapping+toolkit

University of Memphis [UofM], (2019). Module 4—Asset based community engagement. Retrieved September 15, 2019, from https://www.memphis.edu/ess/module4/page4.php

World Health Organization [WHO]. (2017). 10 facts on health inequities and their causes. Retrieved September 11, 2019, from https://www.who.int/features/factfiles/health_inequities/en/

Wright, T. (2019). How to write a good vision statement. Retrieved September 6, 2019, from https://www.executestrategy.net/blog/write-good-vision-statement

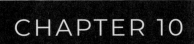

CHAPTER 10

Mobilize, Assess, Plan, Implement, Track (MAP-IT)

STUDENT LEARNING OUTCOMES

As a result of reading this chapter, the student will be able to:

- Explain the tasks in the six steps of the MAP-IT framework.
- Identify the generic steps of program in the MAP-IT framework.
- Plan a hypothetical program using the MAP-IT framework.

Introduction

Mobilize, Assess, Plan, Implement, Track (MAP-IT) was developed by the Centers for Disease Control and Prevention as a framework for planning and implementing public health programs to meet the *Healthy People 2020* objectives (U.S. Department of Health and Human Services [USDHHS], n.d.). Although it was created for this specific purpose, the steps of the framework are applicable in the planning and implementation of health programs in general.

MAP-IT Up-Close

Using the MAP-IT framework entails involving all stakeholders in the community in the planning process; assessing needs and assets based on the realities of the community; developing a plan with timelines, objectives, action steps, and task assignments for meeting the objectives; and integrating evaluation activities throughout the process to allow for adjustments along the way (Center for Community Health and Development [CCHD], 2019a). These undertakings are subsumed under the following five steps of the MAP-IT framework:

> **M**obilizing partners
>
> **A**ssessing community needs
>
> **P**lanning programs
>
> **I**mplementing programs
>
> **T**racking progress (USDHHS, n.d.)

Step 1—Mobilize Partners

Recognizing that improving the health of a community is a group effort, the first step of the MAP-IT framework entails forming a coalition. A coalition is a group composed of individuals and representatives from different organizations and agencies with a common interest that come together to work toward a common goal (CCHD, 2019b).

However, sometimes forming a coalition is easier said than done with the following issues often needing resolution:

- Sharing/turf issues

    Organizations are often hesitant to share their work, populations, and especially their resources. To resolve turf issues, they may need convincing that working together is a benefit and allows them to better address their core missions (CCHD, 2019b).

- Historical issues

    Some potential coalition members may have had difficult past experiences working with each other, which may cause them to decline the invitation to participate in the coalition (CCHD, 2019b). To address past issues, having different representatives from the participating agencies if possible or avoiding assigning people with difficult histories to the same tasks or committees may resolve the problem.

- Control issues

    Oftentimes people who see themselves as having authority (politicians, business leaders, or those with advance degrees) take charge of solving the problem without involving those affected by the problem. These people, while well-meaning, have an off-putting know-it-all attitude, which does not bode well for the functioning of a coalition. To address this, creating and sustaining a participatory, inclusionary atmosphere with equal voice for all participants is needed to curtail dominance by a few (CCHD, 2019b).

- Funding/resource issues

    Securing the resources necessary to run the coalition is a common problem. Care is needed to avoid funding from a source that will push the coalition in a direction that conflicts with its focus or requires action too quickly to effectively address the problem the coalition is working toward solving (CCHD, 2019b).

- Leadership issues

    A coalition, regardless of its reason for being, is a collaborative endeavor that needs collaborative leadership (CCHD, 2019b). Collaborative leadership is a process for sharing responsibility in addressing a problem and coming to a resolution where everyone has an equal voice and works together. While there is a designated person tasked with leading the coalition, this person's role in a collaborative leadership environment is to guide and coordinate the process to allow the group to decide on the actions it will take to accomplish its goals (CCHD, 2019c).

- Cost issues

    The actual or perceived costs of working with a coalition may outweigh the benefits for some potential coalition members. The challenge in this situation is to find ways to decrease the cost and increase the benefit of participation in the coalition (CCHD, 2019b).

    Establishing the coalition starts with identifying potential coalition members. They should include broad representation of agencies and organizations in the community as well as community members (USDHHS, n.d.). For example:

    Governmental health agencies such as the local or county health department or health clinics

    Nonprofit agencies such as those that advocate for children, older adults, pregnant women, or those affected by specific diseases or disorders

    Healthcare organizations such as hospitals/medical centers

Higher education institutions such as universities and colleges

Community leaders from religious institutions, school districts, businesses, and government

Those affected by the issue, and those who can affect the issue (CCHD, 2019b)

Once the list of potential coalition members is created, but before they are invited, the following questions need answers:

— How many members should the coalition have?
— What type of skills should members have?
— How many hours per month should members expect to commit to coalition activities and for how long?
— Which population groups should the coalition represent?
— When, where, and how often will the coalition meet?
— Who will lead the coalition and by what process should their selection take place?
— Who are the coalition's strongest supporters (CCHD, 2019b)?

The next step is to set a date, place, and time for an initial coalition meeting and invite the potential members. Invitation is made in person, by phone, email, and/or hard copy letter. Regardless of the invitation method, the following is conveyed:

• Description of the coalition's tentative purpose
• Date, place, and time of the initial meeting
• Instructions for responding and a respond by date
• Name, phone number, and email address of a contact person for more information

Immediately after receiving notice of potential members' intention to attend the meeting, a confirmatory email containing the purpose, date, time, location of the meeting and the contact person's information is sent. It's wise to send a reminder email with the same information 3–4 days before the scheduled meeting.

The purpose of the initial coalition meeting is to bring the members together, define their roles, assign responsibilities, and identify the coalition's mission and vision (CCHD, 2019a). This session is akin to Step 2.3 of the MAPP process discussed in Chapter 9.

In addition to establishing the coalition, the initial meeting should also aim to engage the members. The greatest threat to a coalition's continuance is disengaged members. Engaging members in the work of the coalition begins at the beginning, which is why having members participate in the visioning process is so important, as is assigning them meaningful tasks to complete.

For example, members can:

• Provide opportunities for community input at their meetings or events.
• Create and present education and training programs that support the coalition's mission and vision.
• Hold fundraising events to support the financial needs of the coalition.
• Sponsor policy initiatives that further the coalition's mission and vision.
• Provide technical assistance for program planning and evaluation (USDHHS, n.d.).

In summary, Step 1 answers the following questions:

What is the coalition's vision and mission?
Who should the coalition represent?
Who are potential coalition members?
What is the reason for bringing potential members together (USDHHS, n.d.)?

Step 2—Assess

The aim of this step is to assess the community's needs and identify its assets. Data collected from these assessments is used by the coalition to identify what the community's actual needs are versus what some coalition members may *think* they are (CCHD, 2019a) and what the community would *like* to do versus what it *can* do (USDHSS, n.d.), given the resources available. Different methods of collecting needs assessment data are discussed in Chapter 4, Assessing Needs.

When data collection is completed, coalition members work together to prioritize the needs taking into consideration feasibility, effectiveness, and measurability (CCHD, 2019a). Having coalition members work together to set priorities is another way of keeping them engaged and sustaining the coalition.

Setting priorities is done by consensus, with coalition members agreeing on the issues needing immediate attention and those that can wait until a later date (CCHD, 2019a). (See Chapter 9, MAPP Step 4.4, for a detailed explanation of how this is done.)

Once coalition members agree on the priorities, the focus shifts to the assets/resources available to address them. Community assets are more than financial and include the professional expertise at organizations, agencies, and academic institutions in the community; infrastructure such as parks, office space, bus routes, housing; technology such as computers, access to databases, websites; data such as census information, morbidity and mortality rates, demographics (CCHD, 2019a). (See Chapter 9, MAPP Step CTSA 3.2, for a detailed description of how to assess community assets.)

Step 3—Plan

This step of MAP-IT entails developing a program plan to address the priority issues, which include the following:

- Measurable goals and objectives with a target of change from the baseline. (See **Figure 10-1**.)
- Realistic, doable strategies for reaching the goals and objectives, preferably evidence-based.
- Actions/tasks for implementing the strategies.
- Assignments for task completion.
- Resources needed to implement the strategies.
- Means of evaluating strategy effectiveness.
- A realistic timeline for completion (CCHD, 2019a).

Having coalition members participate in developing the program plan is another way to keep them engaged. For instance, some members could research the literature for examples of evidence-based programs that address the priority health issues, or participate in a strategy brainstorming session (USDHHS, n.d.), or assess assets within their own organization.

For each strategy developed and included in the program plan, indicators for monitoring its implementation process, performance, and outcomes are also developed. This MAP-IT step is aligned with the generic planning stage discussed in Chapter 5, Planning.

Step 2 answers the following questions:
Who is affected by what (public health issue) and how?
What resources are available?
What resources are needed (USDHHS, n.d.)?

Step 3 answers the following questions:
What are the goals?
What will the coalition do in order to reach the goals?
Which coalition members will do what?
How will the coalition know when it reaches its goals?

Objective: Reduce the annual number of newly diagnosed cases of diabetes by 10 percent from the present 10 per 1,000 population ages 18–65 to 9 new cases per 1,000 population ages 18–65.

Figure 10-1 Target of change from baseline

Data from U.S. Department of Health and Human Services [DHHS]. (n.d.). *MAP-IT: A guide to using Healthy People 2020 in your community.* Atlanta, GA: U.S. Department of Health and Human Services, Office of Disease Prevention and Health Promotion.

Step 4—Implement

With the detailed program plan developed and agreed to by the coalition members, it's ready for implementation. Implementation requires coordination to make sure things get done how and when they are supposed to. Having a point person helps (CCHD, 2019a; USDHHS, n.d.). To avoid conflict and stay true to the collaborative nature of the coalition, the members should agree on who will serve in this capacity.

Coalition members should implement those aspects of the program plan assigned to them in the established time frame. To ensure this is happening, the indicators for monitoring the implementation process, performance, and outcomes developed during the previous planning step are used (CCHD, 2019a). For a detailed discussion of implementation, see Chapter 6, Implementing.

Step 4 answers the following questions:
Is the coalition following its program plan?
Is there anything it can do better?

Step 5—Track

This final step in the MAP-IT process focuses on tracking outcomes. This is done through ongoing data collection, analysis, and reporting (CCHD, 2019a; USDHHS, n.d.).

Tracking and evaluation are key to the long-term success of the coalition's endeavors. Given the importance of evaluation, having expert assistance in the collection, analysis, and interpretation of the data is vital. If coalition members don't have staff with this expertise, then assistance should be sought from a university, state center for health statistics, or a consultant (CCHD, 2019a; USDHHS, n.d.).

Of particular concern in this step are the following:

- Data quality: The quality of the data is negatively impacted when the structure of the questions used to generate the data and the processes used for collection are not standardized (CCHD, 2019a).
- Data limitations: Efforts are needed to avoid overreliance on self-reported data. Data generated from self-reports, typically questionnaires, are often unreliable. This happens when questions ask for sensitive or personal information such as incidents of abuse, violence, or drug and alcohol use, which results in people underestimating or underreporting occurrences. It also happens from faulty recall of events. The longer the recall period (how many alcoholic drinks did you have in the past month vs. how many did you have in the past 24 hours), characteristics of the health issue (chronic or acute), and participant characteristics (age, literacy level) all can lead to less-than-accurate reporting (Althubaiti, 2016).
- Data validity and reliability: Revisions of survey questionnaires or development of new data collection systems can affect reliability and validity. This is a situation where the expertise of a statistician is needed (CCHD, 2019a).
- Data availability: In order to ensure that data needed to track progress is available, its collection is done on a regular basis and in concert with the evaluation schedule in the work plan (CCHD, 2019a).

It's important to keep the community abreast of the coalition's efforts and progress. Press releases, postings on the community and coalition members' websites, and on social media done regularly, are some ways of doing this.

Step 5 answers the following questions:
Where were evaluations done?
Was the work plan followed?
What changed?
Were the goals reached (USDHHS, n.d.)?

Chapter Summary

MAP-IT is a five-step planning framework that entails the creation of a community coalition to undertake assessing community needs, planning programs to address those needs, implementing the planned programs, and tracking (evaluating) their effectiveness.

Planning in Practice Chapter Activity

Imagine you're newly employed at a county health department in a different state far from where you call "home." After a recent meeting, your supervisor congratulates you on being assigned to develop programs to address the health needs of the county's Bangladeshi American community. You're anxious about this assignment because you don't know anything about the people, their community, health issues, culture, and so on.

1. Why would MAP-IT be a good planning framework for you to use?
2. In mobilizing the community, who would you invite to participate on a coalition to planning a program?
3. What needs assessment method would you suggest the coalition use to learn about the health needs of the community, and why?
4. Assume the results of the needs assessment indicate that the greatest

health issues facing the Bangladeshi American community in the county are cardiovascular diseases, in particular, hypertension, stroke, and heart attack, and the health behaviors increasing their risk seem to be diet related. What is one action that could be implemented as part of a program to address this issue?

Read the article below and answer the questions that follow.

Article: *MAP-IT in action: Developing a plan to improve the food systems frequented by Bangladeshi Americans living in Hamtramck, Michigan* (Caboral-Stevens, Gee, Kachaturoff, & Wu, 2019)

Article link: http://www.ijsrp.org/research-paper-0919.php?rp=P939100

(Click on Download to access article PDF)

Article Questions

1. What organization led to the development of this program?
2. What secondary data support the authors' contention that South Asians are an important focus for public health?
3. Why were Bangladeshi Americans identified as the priority population for this program?
4. Once the authors identified the priority population, they began building a coalition as the first step of the MAP-IT framework. Who comprised the membership of the coalition?
5. Which of the coalition members was identified as the partner most needed to move the program forward, and why?
6. What is the focus of the assessment step of the MAP-IT framework in this program?
7. What will the needs assessment include?
8. Which of the assessment activities listed above will result in the creation of a map, and what will it be used for?
9. What are the overall goals of the program?
10. What are the aims of the strategic plans?

11. What actions will implementation of the strategic plans entail to meet the aims of the program?
12. In addition to actions for implementing the strategic plans, what other actions were part of the implementation plan?
13. How will program progress be tracked (evaluated?)
14. How do the activities undertaken in the assessing, planning, and implementing components of the MAP-IT framework for this program compare to those of the hypothetical program you developed for the Bangladeshi American community?

References

Althubaiti, A. (2016). Information bias in health research: Definition, pitfalls and adjustments. *Journal of Multidisciplinary Healthcare, 9,* 211–217. doi: 10.2147/JMDH.S104807 Retrieved October 17, 2019, from https://www.ncbi.nlm.nih.gov/pmc/articles/PMC 4862344/

Center for Community Health and Development [CCHD]. (2019a). Chapter 2, Section 14: MAP-IT: A model for implementing *Healthy People 2020.* Lawrence, KS: University of Kanas. Retrieved October 9, 2019, from https://ctb.ku.edu/en/table-of-contents/overview /models-for-community-health-and-development /map-it/main

Center for Community Health and Development [CCHD]. (2019b). Chapter 5, Section 15: Coalition building I: Starting a coalition. Lawrence, KS: University of Kanas. Retrieved October 9, 2019, from https://ctb.ku.edu /en/table-of-contents/assessment/promotion-strategies /start-a-coaltion/main

Center for Community Health and Development [CCHD]. (2019c). Chapter 13, Section 11: Collaborative leadership. Lawrence, KS: University of Kanas. Retrieved October 9, 2019, from https://ctb.ku.edu/en/table-of -contents/leadership/leadership-ideas/collabora-tive-leadership/main

U.S. Department of Health and Human Services [DHHS]. (n.d.). *MAP-IT: A guide to using Healthy People 2020 in your community.* Retrieved October 15, 2019, from https://www.healthypeople.gov/2020/tools-and -resources/Program-Planning

CHAPTER 11

Intervention Mapping (IM)

STUDENT LEARNING OUTCOMES

After reading this chapter the student will be able to:

- Explain the core processes of IM.
- Discuss the tasks associated with the six steps of the IM process.
- Use IM to develop a hypothetical program.

Introduction

Intervention Mapping (IM) was developed in the late 1990s to improve the process of designing and developing programs (Bartholomew, Parcel, & Kok, 1998). It's based on a social ecological approach that recognizes behavior as a function of people and the physical, social, and organizational environments in which they live. It emphasizes participation of all stakeholders in the planning process to ensure relevance, acceptability, contextual appropriateness, and implementability (Kok, Peters, & Ruiter, 2017). As its name implies, the process of IM entails producing "maps" or matrices that guide the development, implementation, and evaluation of behavior change programs (Bartholomew et al., 1998; Kok et al., 2017).

IM Up-Close

The IM framework consists of six core processes and six planning steps. The core processes increase the planning committee's understanding of the health problem and guide decision making throughout the six-step planning process (Bartholomew Eldredge et al., 2016).

Core Processes

When program planners don't have a thorough or complete understanding of the problem they are trying to address, don't use theory to understand the behavior driving the problem, and/or don't use or have observational or research data, they often don't develop effective programs. To minimize or eliminate these issues, the following six core processes are used: posing questions, brainstorming, reviewing literature, reviewing theories, assessing research needs, and developing a list of answers (Bartholomew Eldridge et al., 2016).

- Posing questions

    The first core process, posing questions, ensures that the people involved in planning the program thoroughly understand the problem that needs solving and have insight into its background and underlying causes (Bartholomew Eldridge et al., 2016; Buunk & Van Vugt, 2013). Having members of the planning committee address the following questions can bring this about:

- What is the problem?
- Why is it a problem?
- Who is affected by the problem?
- What are the consequences if the problem is not resolved?
- What behaviors increase risk or cause the problem?
- What determinants increase the risky behaviors?
- Is the problem solvable?
- What would change the risky behaviors (Bartholomew Eldridge et al., 2016; Buunk & Van Vugt, 2013)?

- Brainstorming

The second core process, brainstorming, is used to answer the questions posed. Brainstorming entails planning committee members sharing their unedited answers to the questions with the rest of the group. Their answers are recorded as "conditionally" valid responses (Bartholomew Eldridge et al., 2016).

- Reviewing literature

A literature review is done to gather evidence that supports or rejects the conditionally valid responses. While a literature review is usually a time-consuming, formal, systematic process and a project in itself, for this purpose, a simple review using the following questions as a guideline suffice:

- What question needs answering?
- What evidence will answer the question?
- What is the search strategy for finding the evidence?
- What criteria does the evidence have to meet for inclusion?
- What criteria would exclude the evidence?

- What evidence from the search meets the criteria for inclusion?
- What metric will determine the strength of the evidence?
- How will the planning group document answers to the questions?
- How will the planning group summarize the finding and draw conclusions based on the evidence (Bartholomew Eldridge et al., 2016)?

The planning committee uses the results of the literature review to revise the list of conditionally valid responses. Responses that are supported by evidence in the literature remain on the list of possible causes, risk behaviors, determinants, and consequences of the health problem. Those that are not supported by evidence are removed (Bartholomew Eldridge et al., 2016).

- Reviewing theories

Theory review entails another literature review, but this time with a focus on identifying theories that might explain the underlying cause of the problem and provide a basis for a program. This review can be conducted by issue, concept, or theory (Bartholomew Eldridge et al., 2016).

Conducting a literature review using an issue approach entails using the health issue, for example, childhood obesity, as the search term. The results are then examined for theories used to address the issue of childhood obesity (Bartholomew et al., 1998).

The concept approach entails matching ideas about the behavioral causes of the problem that were generated during the brainstorming session to theoretical constructs (Bartholomew et al., 1998; Buunk & Van Vugt, 2013). Conducting the literature search this way will turn up the theories (Bartholomew Eldridge et al., 2016). For example, if during a brainstorming session on childhood obesity, one possible cause suggested was parents' perceived inability to cook healthy foods, this is an issue of parental self-efficacy. Using self-efficacy as the search term will results in references to Social Cognitive Theory, Health Belief Model, and Self-Efficacy Theory.

The third way to review the literature for possible theories is to start by considering the more frequently used theories and their applicability to the problem and the question responses (Bartholomew et al., 1998; Buunk & Van Vugt, 2013). Then, use the most applicable theories as the search terms for the literature review.

- Assessing research needs

The previous core processes provide information from the literature that fits with, suggests changes to, or adds to the conditional responses and explanations of the problem's causes. Sometimes, however, this information raises more questions and the need for further research. This core process, then, focuses on using qualitative or quantitative methods to obtain missing data and fill in the gaps (Bartholomew Eldridge et al., 2016; Bartholomew et al., 1998).

- Developing a working list of answers

This final core process entails using results from the literature and theory reviews and any assessments or research that was conducted to develop a list of possible determinants of the problem and methods for addressing it (Bartholomew Eldridge et al., 2016; Buunk & Van Vugt, 2013). The aim is to have determinants that are credible, supported with evidence, and methods that can change the behaviors and/or environmental conditions causing the problem (Bartholomew et al., 1998).

IM Framework Steps

The core processes are integrated into the six program planning steps of the IM framework. Each step is completed in order as the preceding step serves as the foundation for the next step (Fernandez et al., 2019).

The six planning steps are as follows:

Step 1—Create Logic Model of the Problem

The first step of the IM framework includes forming a planning committee, conducting a needs assessment, creating a logical model of the problem, and developing program goals. It consists of the following four tasks (Bartholomew Eldridge et al., 2016):

Task 1.1—Forming a Planning Committee. Ideally, the planning committee should consist of residents of the community, representatives from the population affected by the problem, and representatives from community agencies or organization with an interest in the problem and the potential to implement a program. Having these stakeholders on the planning committee ensures that issues important to the community are addressed, that questions asked in the needs assessment are relevant to the problem, and that local factors influencing context and behaviors are taken into consideration (Tufel-Shone, Siyuja, Watahomigie, & Irwin, 2006). For a more detailed discussion of forming a planning committee see Chapter 3, Preparing for Planning, and Chapter 9, MAPP, Step 1.2.

Task 1.2—Conducting a Needs and Asset Assessment, and Creating a Logic Model. Conducting a needs assessment is the first undertaking of the planning committee. To complete this, the IM framework uses the core processes and an adaptation of the four steps of the PRECEDE model to create a logic model of the health problem (Bartholomew Eldridge et al., 2016). (For more information on PRECEDE-PROCEED, see Chapter 8. For more information on conducting a needs assessment, see Assessing Needs, Chapter 4.)

The needs assessment begins with an analysis of the health problem and/or the population at risk to identify the behavioral and environmental causes of the problem and its determinants (Bartholomew Eldridge et al., 2016; Kok et al., 2017). In addition, the environmental

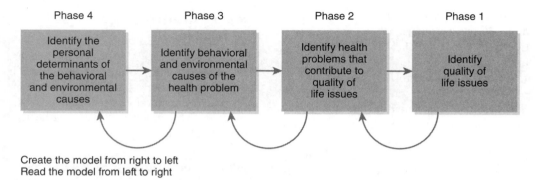

Create the model from right to left
Read the model from left to right

Figure 11-1 Logic model of the problem

Data from Bartholomew Eldredge, L.K., Markham, C.M., Ruiter, R.A.C., Fernandez, M.E., Kok, G., & Parcel, G.S. (2016). *Planning health promotion programs: An intervention mapping approach* (4th ed). San Francisco: Jossey-Bass.

context of the population is analyzed from four ecological model perspectives: interpersonal, organizational, community, and societal to identify factors contributing to the health problem (Bartholomew Eldridge et al., 2016). (For more information about the Ecological Model, see Chapter 2, Health Behavior Theories.)

Using a mixed methods approach to conduct the needs assessment produces the qualitative and quantitative data needed to answer the following questions:

- What is the health problem of concern?
- Who has the problem or is the population at risk?
- How prevalent is the problem?
- What is the incidence of the problem?
- How is the problem distributed throughout the population?
- What are the demographic characteristics of the population at risk?
- What are the characteristics of the community (resources, strengths) in which the problem exists or where the population at risk lives?
- Which segments of the community are most affected by the health problem?
- Where/how can a program reach those most affected or at greatest risk of the problem (Bartholomew Eldridge et al., 2016)?

The needs assessment data are used to complete the first four adapted phases of PRECEDE to create a logic model of the causes of the problem. (See **Figure 11-1**.) The model is created from right to left, starting with the quality-of-life issues identified by the needs assessment, moving left toward identifying the personal determinants of the issues. It is read from left to right reflecting how the factors collectively contribute to or cause the health problem and quality of life issues (Bartholomew Eldridge et al., 2016). (For more detailed discussion of logic models, see Chapter 5, Planning.)

Task 1.3—Describing the Program Context. The context or population within which the problem exists is an important factor in the development, planning, and implementation of a program. For this reason, an asset assessment is completed in addition to the needs assessment. (For a detailed discussion of asset mapping, see Chapter 9, MAPP.)

The asset map in the IM framework reflects assets from the social, information, policy/practice, and physical environments.

- Social environment assets

Assets in the social environment include the abilities and skills of individuals, social cohesion and identity, personal income, and existing organizations/groups such as local businesses, faith-based groups, and coalitions (Bartholomew Eldridge et al., 2016) that would support implementation of the program.

- Information environment assets

Assets in the information environment might include the communication channels in the community such as the local newspaper, radio station, television channel, or website (Bartholomew Eldridge et al., 2016) that would support informing the community about the program.

- Policy or practice environment assets

Assets in the policy or practice environment include local, state, or national policies; town ordinances; school policies; or family practices (Bartholomew Eldridge et al., 2016) that would support development and implementation of the program.

- Physical environment assets

Assets in the physical environment include those in both the built environment such as office buildings and schools, and in the natural environment such as parks and unused land that would support the planning committee in choosing a setting for the program (Bartholomew Eldridge et al., 2016).

Task 1.4—Developing Program Goals.
The final task in Step 1 is determining the priority health problems from all the health problems identified in the needs assessment. The priority health problems are the ones that the program will address and the ones for which goals are needed. These are arrived at by assessing each health problem using the following factors to identify the problems that are more important, relevant, and changeable (Bartholomew Eldridge et al., 2016). (For a detailed explanation of the priority setting process, see Chapter 9, MAPP.)

o The difficulty of changing the problem
o The consequences of ignoring the problem
o The cost of solving the problem
o The community's values relative to the problem
o Competing priorities at the local, state, and national levels

o Political and public expectations
o Available assets

Once the planning committee has determined the priority health problems, the intended audience, and the factors (behavioral, environmental, and personal) contributing to the problems, work begins on developing program goals. In IM, program goals are defined as "changes in health, quality of life, behavioral or environmental factors" (Bartholomew Eldridge et al., 2016, p. 227). (For a detailed discussion of developing program goals, see Chapter 5, Planning.)

Step 2—Developing Program Objectives, Outcomes, and a Logic Model of Change

The second step of IM focuses on developing the objectives and outcomes for the program goals set in the previous step and creating a logic model of change. Completing the following five tasks accomplishes this.

Task 2.1—State Expected Outcomes for Health Behavior and Environmental Conditions.
The first task in Step 2 is to state the outcomes or changes in the behavioral and environmental causes of the health problem that are expected as a result of the program (Bartholomew Eldridge et al., 2016).

- To state the behavioral outcomes:

1. Review the behaviors identified in the needs assessment and in Phase 3 of the logic model that increase the risk of, or cause, the health problem.
2. Identify key behaviors that if changed to healthier ones, would prevent, reduce, or eliminate the health problem and ultimately improve health and quality of life.
3. Write a statement that contains the healthier behaviors expected as a result of the program. This statement is the behavioral outcome (Bartholomew Eldridge et al., 2016).

For example, in myMoves, a program for people with acquired brain injury, the priority health issues were morbidity and mortality. The needs assessment revealed that reduced physical activity and increased sedentary behavior were their behavioral causes. Therefore, the behavioral outcomes expected from the program were an increase in physical activity and a reduction in sedentary behavior (Jones et al, 2016).

The needs assessment for a program to address vision loss from diabetic retinopathy (damage to the retina from high blood sugar) in young adults found the behavioral cause of the problem was a delay in or failure to have a retinal screening after a diabetes diagnosis. The behavioral outcome expected from the program was an increase in young adults with type 2 diabetes pursing screening for diabetic retinopathy (Lake et al., 2018).

- To state the environmental outcomes:

  1. Review the environmental conditions identified in the needs assessment and in Phase 3 of the logic model that increase the risk of, or cause, the health problem.
  2. Identify key environmental conditions at the different ecological levels— interpersonal, organizational, community, and societal that if changed, would prevent, reduce, or eliminate the health problem and ultimately improve health and quality of life.
  3. Write a statement that contains the healthier environmental conditions expected as a result of the program. These are the expected environmental outcomes (Bartholomew Eldridge et al., 2016).

For example, an entomological (insect) survey was conducted as part of a needs assessment in an eastern Rwandan community prior to developing a program to eliminate malaria. The purpose of the survey was to assess the environmental conditions contributing to the problem, which in this case, was

the mosquito population responsible for transmitting the disease. The results indicated that overall, the mosquito population had increased since the previous survey as did the number of mosquitos found in homes. Based on these environmental causes of the problem, the expected environmental outcome of the program was the prevention of mosquito breeding around homes and mosquito larvae control in the community (Ingabire et al., 2016).

Task 2.2—Identify Performance Objectives for Behavioral and Environmental Outcomes. Performance objectives are statements that describe exactly what the program participants must do, or what must happen in the environment in order for the outcomes to occur. They describe observable actions (Bartholomew Eldridge et al., 2016).

- Performance objectives for behavioral outcomes

The following question serves as a guide for writing performance objectives for the behavioral outcomes.

- What must participants do (what behaviors must they perform) in order for the behavioral outcome to occur?

In the Rwanda malaria elimination program discussed earlier, one of the behavioral outcomes was an increase in the correct and consistent use of insecticide-treated bed netting. In order for this to occur, the program participants had to:

  1. Own bed netting for every bed.
  2. Use the netting correctly every night on every bed (Ingabire et al., 2016).

- Performance objectives for environmental outcomes

In writing performance objectives for the environmental outcome, the following question serves as the guide:

- Who in the environment needs to do what in order for the environmental outcome to happen?

For example, one of the environmental outcomes in the Rwanda malaria elimination program was prevention of mosquito breeding around homes. To accomplish this, homeowners had to:

1. Cover household water collection systems
2. Clear potential mosquito breeding sites (stagnant water sources, overgrown bushes) from around the home (Ingabire et al., 2016).

Task 2.3—Select Changeable Determinants of the Behavioral and Environmental Outcomes. In this task, the focus is on selecting personal and environmental determinants of the performance objectives that are related to the behavioral and environmental outcomes (Bartholomew Eldridge, et al., 2016). The determinants of the performance objectives are factors that enable the participants or environmental agents to do what they have to do, in order to accomplish the expected outcomes.

The behavioral and environmental determinants of the *unhealthy* behavior or the environmental condition identified in the needs assessment are used as a starting point for determining factors that would enable the healthier outcomes to occur. Additional possible determinants of the outcomes are identified through literature reviews, focus groups, or any of the other qualitative or quantitative methods. The aim is to compile a list of possible determinants of the outcomes using the core processes— asking a question, generating answers, and validating the answers.

The preliminary list of determinants is developed from answers to the following questions (Bartholomew Eldridge et al., 2016):

- Why would people engage in the healthier behavior identified in the performance objective?
- Why would an environmental agent make an environmental adjustment (Bartholomew Eldridge et al., 2016)?

To narrow down the list and select the determinants for the basis of the program, each determinant is rated for evidence of its relevance and changeability. Relevance refers to the extent of a determinant's relationship to the behavior described in the performance objective. Changeability refers to the likelihood of the determinant changing as a result of a program (Bartholomew Eldridge et al., 2016).

For example, a performance objective for a program to prevent vision loss from diabetic retinopathy is that—young adults with diabetes are motivated to have a retinal screening (Lake et al., 2018). To identify a determinant of this behavior, the following question is asked: Why would young adults with diabetes have a retinal screening? The answer, they would have a screening because they know it's something they can do to protect their vision (Lake et al., 2018). Therefore, knowledge is a relevant determinant of this performance objective, and it can be changed by a program (Lake et al., 2018).

Ideally, decisions about the relevance and changeability of determinants are based on evidence from the research literature. When the literature doesn't contain enough information to make a judgment, there are three alternatives: (1) collect the data needed to make the decision from the at-risk group, (2) make the decision entirely on a theoretical basis, or (3) use evidence supporting the determinant's relevance or changeability for a behavior similar to the one in the performance objective (Bartholomew Eldridge et al., 2016).

Task 2.4—Construct Matrices of Change Objectives. Change objectives specify the changes needed in the selected determinants in order for the behaviors stated in the performance objectives to happen. These are written as specifically as possible, starting with an action verb followed by the expected result of performing the action. (For a list of action verbs, see Chapter 5, Planning.)

For example, one of the change objectives in the diabetic retinopathy prevention program mentioned previously, is—adopt personal responsibility for retinal screening (Lake et al., 2018). The action is "adopt," the expected result from performing the action (adoption) is—personal responsibility for retinal screening.

The change objectives are presented in a matrix or table format with the performance objective in the far left column and the determinants across the top. The specific change objective is written in the cell on the table where the two intersect (Bartholomew Eldridge et al., 2016).

For example, the needs assessment for a program to address childhood obesity identified three key behavioral determinants: physical activity, diet, and regulation challenges. To address the diet determinant of the health problem, which included unhealthy dietary habits and meal patterns, the following performance objectives were established:

1. Families monitor and reflect on their current dietary habits.
2. Families choose to take part in the program.
3. Families set up to three challenging, realistic goals to improve their dietary habits.
4. Families establish a regular meal pattern that includes at least one family meal each day.
5. Parents develop a weekday meal plan and purchase the food and beverages on the plan.
6. Parents serve appropriate portion sizes to their children.
7. Families choose and try healthier options of unhealthy food and beverages (Stea et al., 2016).

Table 11-1 shows the matrix of change objectives for the following performance objective: families choose and try healthier options of unhealthy food and beverages.

If programs are needed at more than one level of influence, then separate change objectives and matrices are created for each level. For example, in the Keys program, which addresses childhood obesity in home day-care settings by improving diet quality and increasing moderate-rigorous activity, three levels of influence were identified: the day-care provider, the home in which care is provided, and the day-care business itself (Mann et al., 2015). **Table 11-2** shows performance objectives and corresponding change objectives for each level of influence.

To understand the relationship between the behavioral outcomes and the different objectives developed in this step, keep the following in mind:

1. Behavioral outcomes state the behaviors expected as a result of the program.
2. Performance objectives explain what the participant must do (perform) to accomplish the behavioral outcomes.
3. Determinants of performance objectives state the factors that enable participants to perform the behaviors explained in the performance objectives that they must do to accomplish the behavioral outcomes.
4. Change objectives state the changes needed in the determinants of performance objectives that enable participants to perform the behaviors explained in the performance objectives that they must do to accomplish the behavioral outcomes.

Task 2.5—Create Logic Model of Change. The logic model of change developed in this task depicts how the program effects come about. It's developed from left to right and includes the following components: personal and environmental determinants that are the focus of the change

Table 11-1 Sample matrix of change objectives

Performance Objective	Determinants					
	Personal Determinant Change Objectives				Environmental Determinant Change Objectives	
	Knowledge	Awareness	Attitude	Skills	Social influence	Availability
Families choose and try healthier options of unhealthy food and beverages	Families: Distinguish between healthy and unhealthy foods and beverages. Describe problems associated with eating unhealthy snacks and beverages. Identify healthier food and beverage options.	Families: Describe the benefits of increasing their intake of healthier foods and beverages.	Families: Express a positive attitude toward making changes to increase their intake of healthier foods and beverages. Choosing healthier snack and beverage options.	Families can: Explain the health problems related to high consumption of unhealthy foods and beverages. Parents set appropriate limits for their children's consumption of unhealthy food and beverages. Families practice skills for requesting healthy alternatives in different settings. Families taste healthier food and beverage options.	Parents: Praise children for eating healthier. Role model decreased intake of unhealthy food and beverages	Parents: Increase access to healthy snacks and drinks in the home. Decrease presence of unhealthy snacks and beverages in the home.

Adapted from Stea, T. H., Haugen, T., Bernsten, S., Guttormsen, V., Overby, N. C., Haraldstad, K., ... Abildsnes, E. (2016). Using the intervention mapping protocol to develop a family-based intervention for improving lifestyle habits among overweight and obese children: Study protocol for a quasi-experimental trial. *BMC Public Health, 16*(1), 1092. https://doi.org/10.1186/s12889-016-3766-6

Table 11-2 Sample matrices of change objectives for multiple levels of influence

Health problem—Childhood obesity
Behavioral outcome—Improved quality of children's dietary intake while at day care;
increased moderate-vigorous physical activity
Environmental outcomes—Healthy eating habits are role-modeled by day-care providers
A variety of physical activity opportunities are provided for the children

Performance objectives	Change objectives			
	Knowledge	Skills	Self-Efficacy	Attitudes
P.O. 1 Day-care providers limit their intake of foods high in fat, sugar, and salt.	Know the negative effects of a diet high in fat, sugar, and salt. Know common foods that are high in fat, sugar, and salt,	Can read nutritional information on packages and evaluate food quality. Can prepare healthy meal, snack, and beverage alternatives.	Confident in ability to limit high fat, sugar, and salt foods.	Believe limiting fat, sugar, and salt is worthwhile.
P.O. 2 Daily childcare schedule includes a variety of physical activities for the recommended amount of time for children.	Know 120 minutes is the recommended amount of physical activity for children per day.	Can lead children in physical activity twice a day. Can plan outdoor active playtime twice a day.	Confident in ability to help children enjoy physical activity.	Believe physical activity is important for children.
P.O. 3 Day-care business has a contract based on best business practices.	Know the essential components of a contract.	Can create a contract for providing day-care services.		

Adapted from Mann, C. M., Ward, D. S., Vaughn, A., Benjamin Neelon, S. E. B., Long Vidal, J. L., Omar, S., Namenek Brouwek, R. J., & Ostbye, T. (2015). Application of the intervention mapping protocol to develop Keys, a family child care home intervention to prevent early childhood obesity, *BMC Public Health*, *15*, 1227. https://doi.org/10.1186/s12889-015-2573-9

objectives, followed to the right by the behavioral and environmental outcomes, the expected health outcome, and ends on the far right with the quality-of-life improvement the program seeks to accomplish. (See **Figure 11-2**.) **Figure 11-3** is the logic model of change for a diabetic retinopathy prevention program (Lake et al., 2018).

Step 3—Program Design

This step of IM focuses on designing the program. It entails developing a program plan that includes the program themes, components, scope and sequence, theory and evidence-based methods, and practical applications. The plan details how the program will engage different participant groups, the amount of interaction

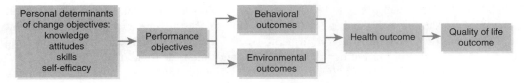

Figure 11-2 Logic model of change components

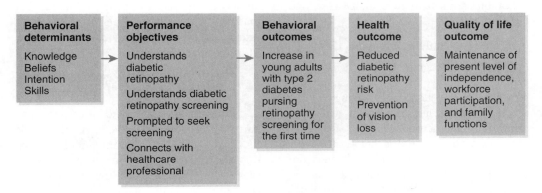

Figure 11-3 Example of logic model of change for a diabetic retinopathy prevention program

Lake, A.J., Browne, J.L., Abraham, C., Tumino, D., Hines, C., Rees, G., Speight, J. (2018). A tailored intervention to promote uptake of retinal screening among young adults with type2 diabetes – an intervention mapping approach. *BMC Health Services Research, 18*(396). https://doi.org/10.1186/s12913-018-3188-5

it will have with each participant group (dose), the scope (extent and duration of the program), and its sequence (the order in which content is presented) (Bartholomew Eldredge et al., 2016).

While each plan differs depending on the program, a few elements are common to them all, including

- Scope and sequence
- Description of each participant group
- Description of how the program interacts with each participant group
- List of materials, staff, and other resources needed for program interaction with participants
- Budgetary and other resource needs

Task 3.1—Generate Ideas, Themes, Components Scope and Sequence. The first task in Step 3 has three parts—generating

ideas for the program, identifying a theme, and developing the components, scope and sequence.

- Part 1—Generating program ideas

The first part of this task focuses on deciding *how* the program will enable the intended audience to accomplish the change objectives, address the health problem, and improve quality of life. To make this decision, the planning committee starts with a list of ideas generated from the following brainstorming, using the core processes, conducting a literature review to identify how others have addressed the same or similar problems, and conducting focus groups with the intended audience to elicit ideas about how to best address the problem and accomplish the change objectives (Bartholomew Eldredge et al., 2016). Once program ideas are compiled and discussed, the planning committee decides on the one it will use as the basis the program. For example, *how* a diabetic retinopathy program for young adults accomplished its intended outcome of preventing vision loss was by developing a brochure tailored to its young adult population (Lake et al., 2018); *how* a childhood obesity prevention program accomplished its intended outcome was by educating providers in childcare and early education settings (Centers for Disease Control and Prevention [CDC], n.d.).

• Part 2—Identifying a program theme

Once the program idea is decided, the planning committee moves on to identifying a program theme, if it chooses. Although a theme is useful in organizing the program, it isn't necessary (Bartholomew Eldredge et al., 2016). Professional associations use themes all the time when planning their annual conference programs. It gives the event structure, a focus. For example, the theme of the American Public Health Association annual conference in 2020 was *Creating the Healthiest Nation: Preventing Violence* (American Public Health Association, n.d.). The National Environmental Health Association's 2020 annual educational conference theme was *The unknown heroes* (National Environmental Health Association, 2019).

A program theme is developed from content related to the program, such as the health problem or the behavioral or environmental change objectives. For example, the theme for a program to prevent occupational skin cancer is *Sun safe worksites,* which is the program's environmental change objective (Walkosz et al., 2018). The theme for the school-based summer safety and environmental health program, *Open the door, get out and explore,* is getting children involved in outdoor activities (San Francisco Unified School District, n.d.).

Themes are also developed from content other than that of the program itself, such as characteristics of the intended audience, the community, or culture. For example, in a quit smoking program for Chinese Americans, the unifying theme was culture. In addition to all protocols and participant materials written in Chinese, the program incorporated critical Chinese social and cultural factors such as Yin–Yang balance and male social status (Wu et al., 2009).

The key to deriving a benefit from using a theme is to make sure it's in sync with the program's behavior change messages. If it is, it can help promote support or adoption of the behavior changes by not only the intended audience, but also secondary audiences, for instance, parents, school personnel, or community members, in general (Bartholomew Eldridge et al., 2016).

• Part 3—Developing program components, scope and sequence

Programs are composed of components, parts, units, or modules (Bartholomew Eldridge et al., 2016). The amount of information the program components cover is the scope. The order in which the information is covered is the sequence.

For example, the diabetic retinopathy prevention program discussed previously, which entails the development and distribution of a tailored brochure, has one component focusing on young adults with type 2 diabetes. The scope of the content covered in the brochure is limited to the individual-level modifiable behavioral determinants identified in the needs assessment. The sequence of the information in the brochure follows a logical order of reading (from the known to the unknown, simple to the more complex) with potentially upsetting or threatening information immediately followed by an empowering or reassuring statement (Lake et al., 2018).

A computer program to promote mothers' acceptance of human papilloma vaccine (HPV) for their daughters has four components. The scope of the content covered in the components includes information about the HPV vaccine, personal values and decision making, getting vaccinated, and frequently asked questions (Pot et al., 2018). The sequence or order in which the related content is covered is shown in **Table 11-3**.

Table 11-3 Scope and sequence of human papilloma virus (HPV) vaccination program

Scope	Sequence
HPV vaccine information	General information HPV and cervical cancer Cervical cancer prevention HPV vaccine side effects Vaccinating young girls HPV/cervical cancer risk HPV vaccination efficacy and safety
HPV vaccination pros and cons	Personal values—decisional balance Values clarification
Practical information	Talking about HPV vaccine Getting vaccinated
Frequently asked questions	Questions about the HPV vaccine Questions about getting vaccinated

Data from Pot, M., Ruiter, R. A. C., Paulussen, T. W. G. M., Heuvelink, A., de Melker, H. E., Vliet, H. J. A., & van Keulen, H. M. (2018). Systematically developing a web-based tailored intervention promoting HPV vaccination acceptability among mothers of invited girls using intervention mapping. *Frontiers in Public Health*, 28. https://doi.org/10.3389/fpubh.2018.00226

Task 3.2 Choose Theory and Evidence-Based Change Methods. This task focuses on methods for changing the determinants of the unhealthy behavior or environmental conditions identified in the needs assessment and in the logic model of the problem developed in Step 1. The aim is to match a theory-based change method with each change objective in the logic model of change developed in Step 2 (Bartholomew Eldridge et al., 2016).

For example, if inability (lack of skill) to check blood sugar levels is a behavioral determinant of poor blood sugar control in diabetics and, if the change objective is the ability (skill) to accurately monitor blood sugar levels, then what behavior change theory explains how new skills are learned? One possibility is the Social Cognitive Theory, specifically the constructs of observational learning and self-efficacy. Observational learning explains that people learn new skills by watching others perform (model) the skill they desire. Self-efficacy explains that people only attempt to do what they believe they can do. Used together, observational learning can increase self-efficacy. Given this, observational learning is used in a diabetes peer-support program focused on improving self-efficacy for diabetes self-management behaviors, which include medication adherence, physical activity, and diet (Cherrington et al., 2012).

To match a change objective with a theory and method:

1. Make a list of the change objectives.
2. Identify the behavioral or environmental determinant for each change objective (knowledge, attitude, skill, etc.).
3. Use the core processes of reviewing the evidence-based literature and behavior change theories (and constructs) to identify evidence-/theory-based change methods for each determinant.
4. Create a chart using the determinants as the headings with the change objective, theory, and method of change under it (Bartholomew Eldridge et al., 2016). See **Table 11-4** for an example.

Table 11-4 Example of change objectives, determinants, theories, and methods

Change objectives	Determinant of change objective
Describe benefits of monitoring blood glucose	Knowledge
Perform glucose monitoring procedure	Skill/ability
Develop glucose monitoring schedule	Skill/ability

Determinant – Knowledge		
Change objective	**Change theory**	**Method**
Describe benefits of monitoring blood glucose	Health belief model— perceived benefits	Present key information during class session in sequence from known to unknown, simple to complex. Provide written material at appropriate reading level to support information presented. Provide time for questions and answers during and after presentation.

Determinant – Skill/ability		
Perform glucose monitoring procedure	Social cognitive theory – Observational learning – Self-efficacy	Demonstrate how to draw blood and use glucose monitoring device. Provide time for supervised practice.
Develop glucose monitoring schedule	Social cognitive theory – Observational learning – Self-efficacy	Demonstrate how to develop a monitoring schedule. Provide time for practice schedule development and feedback.

Data from Song, M., Choi, S., Kim, S., Seo, K., & Lee, S. J. (2015). Intervention mapping protocol for developing theory based diabetes self-management education program. *Research and Theory for Nursing Practice: An International Journal, 29*(2), 94–112. http://dx.doi.org/10.1891/1541-6577.29.2.94

Task 3.3 Select or Design Practical Applications to Deliver Change Methods. Having identified theory- based methods for addressing the determinants of the change objectives in the previous task, the focus of this task is on the practical application of those methods with respect to the context in which the program will take place and the characteristics of the people involved (Bartholomew Eldredge et al., 2016). For example, in the HPV vaccination program mentioned previously, beliefs, attitudes, and risk perception were identified as determinants of the change objectives for the behavioral outcome of increased acceptability of mothers to having their daughters receive HPV vaccine (Pot et al., 2018).

Among the theories and methods used to address these are:

- Theory of Reasoned Action (beliefs and attitudes)—belief selection.
- Social Cognitive Theory (modeling/observational learning)—active learning and modeling.
- Health Belief Model (risk perception)—risk information (Pot et al., 2018).

Table 11-5 shows the practical application of some of the theories and methods used in the HPV prevention program.

Table 11-5 Example of practical application of theories and methods

Behavioral outcome—increased acceptability of mothers to having their daughters receive HPV vaccine

Performance objective—mother makes informed decision to vaccinate daughter

(Selected) Determinants and change objectives	Theory	Methods	Practical Application
Knowledge			
Mother explains that HPV is sexually transmitted. Mother explains that HPV also infects men. Mother explains that HPV is contracted by skin-to-skin contact. Mother explains that condoms are not effective in preventing the spread of HPV. Mother acknowledges that HPV vaccine is 70 percent effective.	Learning theory	Feedback	Provide mothers with basic information about HPV, cervical cancer, and HPV vaccine
Attitude			
Mother assesses the HPV vaccine as positive. Mother acknowledges the health benefits of HPV vaccination.	Trans-theoretical Model Motivational Interviewing	Decisional balance	Provide mothers with a list of vaccine pros and cons to mark as most relevant to her on a scale that reveals her position on HPV vaccination from wanting (positive attitude) to not wanting (negative attitude) her daughter vaccinated.
Beliefs			
Mother recognizes importance of vaccinating daughter before sexual activity begins.	Theory of reasoned action	Belief selection	Mother asked whether she agrees, disagrees, or is neutral to the statement that her daughter is too young for the HPV vaccine. Depending on her response, tailored feedback is provided.
Risk perception			
Mother recognizes daughter's risk of HPV infection and developing cervical cancer if not vaccinated.	Health Belief Model	Risk perception	Mother asked about her perceived risk of her daughter contracting HPV and developing cervical cancer. Depending on her response, tailored feedback is provided, including statistical risk or probability of contracting an HPV infection.

Data from Pot, M., Ruiter, R. A. C., Paulussen, T. W. G. M., Heuvelink, A., de Melker, H. E., Vliet, H. J. A., & van Keulen, H. M. (2018). Systematically developing a web-based tailored intervention promoting HPV vaccination acceptability among mothers of invited girls using intervention mapping. *Frontiers in Public Health*, 28. https://doi.org/10.3389/fpubh.2018.00226

At the end of this third task, the planning committee is responsible for ensuring that each behavioral and environmental outcome has theoretical, evidence-based methods and practical applications in place to address the determinants of the change objectives.

Step 4—Program Production

The information from Step 3 is used in Step 4 to develop the program messages, products (written materials, web postings, billboards, activities, etc.), and protocols. The challenges of this step include creating products that effectively operationalizes the methods and practical applications in order to accomplish the change objectives, and ensuring that the messages' products and protocols are feasible, fit the population, and fit the setting context for which implementation is planned (Bartholomew Eldredge et al., 2016).

If representatives from the intended audience, adopters, and implementers have not been involved in the IM process previously, they are brought in at this point They can provide valuable insight into the intended audience's product preferences, feasibility of delivering products, and goodness of contextual fit (Bartholomew Eldredge et al., 2016).

Task 4.1 Refine Structure and Organization.

This first task of Step 4 entails refining the structure and organization of the program. It focuses on doing a "reality check" of the theme, components, scope and sequence, change methods, and practical applications established in the previous step to make sure what's planned is doable and to adjust what's not (Bartholomew Eldredge et al., 2016).

Two specific issues addressed in this task are

- Reaching the intended audience

What is the feasibility of the intended audience participating in the program how and where it's planned (Bartholomew Eldredge et al., 2016)? This is an issue that representatives of the intended audience on the planning committee can readily address and help with refining, if necessary.

- Budget and time needs

Are the budget estimates and time needs for developing and implementing the program components and products reliable and feasible, given what's available? If not, the program structure, organization, and products will need refinement (Bartholomew Eldredge et al., 2016).

Task 4.2 Prepare Material Design and Production Plans.

This task entails preparing plans to guide the design and production of new program materials (or products) or to refine existing ones to fit programmatic needs (Bartholomew Eldredge et al., 2016). The following questions serve as a guide to determine the goodness of fit of existing materials:

- Would this material enable the intended audience to meet to the change objectives?
- Is this material consistent with the program's change method and practical applications?
- Is this material culturally appropriate and respectful of the relevant cultural aspects of intended audience?
- Is this material compatible with the scope and sequence of the program (Bartholomew Eldredge et al., 2016)?

In addition, existing materials are reviewed to determine their suitability, availability, and readability.

Suitability of existing materials is determined based on content, literacy level, graphics, and layout. Content suitability is determined by answering the following questions:

- Is the purpose of the information evident?
- Does the content focus on the expected behaviors?
- Is the content limited to the scope of the objectives?
- Are the main points of information summarized?

<u>Literacy suitability</u> is determined by answering the following questions:

- Does the reading level match that of the intended audience?
- Is writing in active voice, using simple sentences, common words, and a conversational style?

<u>Graphics suitability</u> is determined by answering the following questions:

- Are cover graphics friendly, attention getting, and representative of the material's purpose?
- Are graphics familiar to the intended audience and age appropriate?
- Do graphics clearly provide key messages?
- Do graphic captions clearly explain the image?

<u>Layout and typography suitability</u> are determined by answering the following questions:

- Is information flow complemented with shading or arrows to guide reader?
- Are graphics next to related text?
- Is paper low gloss with a high-contrast ink color (for example, white paper with black ink, rather than purple paper and brown ink)?
- Is text in sentence case (upper/lower case) with serif font and at least 12 point with no text in all upper case (Bartholomew Eldredge et al., 2016)?

Availability of existing material is determined by answering the following questions:

- Is there access to the quantity needed?
- Can delivery happen within the time frame needed?
- Is the cost within budget (Bartholomew Eldredge et al., 2016)?

Readability of existing material is determined by answering the following questions:

- What is the reading level of the product?
- Is the product's reading level compatible with that of the intended audience (Bartholomew Eldredge et al., 2016)?

Given the uniqueness of each program, it's unlikely that existing materials will exactly meet the criteria for use. At the very least, however, they provide a basis for developing materials that do.

The aim is to have materials that are culturally appropriate, consistent with the program objectives, change methods, and practical applications (Bartholomew Eldredge et al., 2016). To do this, aspects of the culture related to health and health behavior are reflected in the program materials. For example, family relationships, communication styles, acceptable emotional expression, individual vs. community orientation, spirituality/religiosity, beliefs/myths, and time orientation (Deshpande et al.,2009).

Strategies for accomplishing this include

- Ensuring materials are visually appealing and comfortable for the intended audience (Kreuter et al., 2003).

This is achieved by incorporating characteristics common to the culture such as images, language, and familiar faces (Bartholomew Eldredge et al., 2016) and by avoiding characteristics, such as a color that can have unintended meanings. For example, in Chinese culture, the color yellow is associated with pornography, in Middle Eastern cultures orange is associated with mourning, and in most South American cultures green is associated with death (Briggs, 2016).

- Reminding the intended audience of the significance of the health problem in their cultural group (Kreuter et al., 2003).

For example, African American infants are more than twice as likely to die from sudden infant death than are non-Hispanic whites (U.S. Department of Health and Human Services—Office of Minority Health [USDHHS—OMH], 2019); Hispanic/Latino Americans have a greater than 50 percent chance of developing diabetes compared to a 40 percent chance overall for the U.S. adult population, a greater likelihood of developing it at a younger age, and greater rates of complications, including kidney failure and vision loss (CDC, 2019a).

- Preparing materials in the language spoken by the intended audience (Kreuter et al., 2003).

To increase the accuracy of translated materials into the language of the intended audience (also called the target language):

o   Use a professional translator

It's best to use a professional translator rather than relying on a native speaker on the planning committee to translate material or using an online "machine translation" tool. Translating information from one language to another is more than just replacing words, it's also knowing dialects, idioms, expressions, grammar and sentence structure, words without direct translation or with multiple meanings (Common challenges of translation, 2019).

Following are two tips for hiring a professional translator:

TIP 1 Ask for credentials –
A bachelors' degree and American Translators Association (ATA) certification are indications of competence (American Translators Association, 2019).

TIP 2 Ask for examples of previous work – Review translations from English into the target language that were translated back into English to ensure writing ability, knowledge of health terminology, and understanding of the intended audience's culture (Zarcadoolas & Blanco, 2000).

o   Translate the material back into English

Once the material is translated into the target language, it should be translated back into English to compare the two versions and make sure the information in the translation is correct. This process can take a few rounds before an accurate translation is produced (Bartholomew Eldredge et al., 2016).

A good example of a public health translation failure occurred in 2018 during an outbreak of measles in ultra-Orthodox Jewish communities in New York State. In an effort to contain the outbreak, the New York State Department of Health developed, printed, and distributed more than 45,000 door hangers in Yiddish with information about measles and the need for vaccination. The door hangers were filled with errors, barely comprehensible, and practically indecipherable. Measles was spelled three different ways, the word used for "runny nose" doesn't exist in Yiddish, and some of the information just didn't make sense such as—the rash is allowed to take 4–2 days after the fever raises (Cohen, 2019). Here are some translation errors from global companies that didn't work out very well for them:

> Coors translated its "Turn it loose" slogan into Spanish and missed the fact that "*turn it loose*" in Spanish is slang for "*having diarrhea.*"

> The American Dairy Association's "got milk?" campaign translated into Spanish as—"*Are you lactating?*"

> Mercedes-Benz marketed a car in China under the brand name "Bensi," which in Chinese means "*rush to die.*"

> Ford didn't do much better when it introduced its "Pinto" brand in Brazil. Unfortunately, "pinto" in Brazilian-Portuguese means "*tiny male genitals*" (James, 2014).

Using a professional translator doesn't guarantee an accurate translation 100 percent of the time. But, having materials translated into the target language and then translated back into English again with an online translation tool *and* a native speaker of the target language is likely to result in more accurate materials.

- Involving representatives from the intended audience (Kreuter et al., 2003).

Getting input from the intended audience to ensure the program is culturally appropriate is invaluable. To do this, include representatives from the intended audience/cultural group on the planning committee, hire program staff from the cultural group, or train people from the cultural group as lay or community health workers (Kreuter et al., 2003).

Lay health workers are often used to reach Hispanic communities and migrant and seasonal farm workers in rural communities along the United States–Mexico border. Because these health workers are themselves members of the community, they share the cultural, social, and economic characteristics of the intended audience. They are trained to provide a range of services such as patient advocacy, mentoring, education, and translation. For example, in one program they provide culturally appropriate diabetes education in rural communities. In another, they provide information on cervical cancer and HPV vaccine to migrant farmworker women (Rural Health Information Hub [RHIhub], 2019).

The planning committee conveys its intentions for program materials to either a subcommittee or consultant through a *design document*. (See **Table 11-6**.) This document includes the following three sections (Bartholomew Eldredge et al., 2016):

1. A prospectus—

This describes the intended audience, main message of the material, intended impact of the material, length of the material (if applicable), method of user interaction with the material, and budget or cost of the material.

2. Change matrices from Step 2—

These highlight each set of change objectives and how each set of change objectives relate to each product.

3. Detail design documents—

These documents contain the materials, change objectives the materials address grouped by determinant, method of use and practical application, and message content.

Task 4.3 Draft Program Messages and Materials. In this task program messages and materials are drafted. These products enable the use of the methods chosen by the planning committee in Step 3 to address the change objectives (Bartholomew Eldredge et al., 2016).

Table 11-6 Detailed design document for a heart attack intervention

Product/ material/ activity	Change objectives by determinant	Methods/ applications	Message
Brochure	**Knowledge** Lists heart attack symptoms Describes whom to call—911	Information transfer	Every second counts Don't wait to RACE R—recognize symptoms A—acknowledge emergency C—call 911 E—eat an aspirin
	Skill Recognizes heart attack symptoms Demonstrates giving person instructions to chew and swallow aspirin (unless contraindicated)	Observational learning/modeling	

Data from Bartholomew Eldredge, L. K., Markham, C. M., Ruiter, R. A. C., Fernandez, M. E., Kok, G., & Parcel, G. S. (2016). *Planning health promotion programs: An intervention mapping approach* (4th ed.). San Francisco: Jossey-Bass; Morgenstern, L. B., Bartholomew, L. K., Grotta, J. C., Staub, L., King, M., & Chan, W. (2003). Sustained benefit of a community and professional intervention to increase acute stroke therapy. *Archives of Internal Medicine, 163*(18), 2198–2202; Morgenstern, L. B., Staub, L., Chan, W., Wein, T. H., Bartholomew, L. K., King, M., . . . Grotta, J. C. (2002). Improving delivery of acute stroke therapy: The TLL Temple Foundation Stroke Project. *Stroke, 33*(1), 160–166.

- Messages

Program messages are based on the information collected in Steps 1–3 and are meant to help the intended audience accomplish the change objectives. They are written to promote thought and application of the information rather than memorization. Following are guidelines for writing messages:

- Limit the number of concepts introduced in each message to the most important that support the change objectives.
- Start with information known to the intended audience before presenting new information.
- Present information in a logical sequence following the order in which the reader will use it.
- Use active voice.
- Write at the reading level of the intended audience.
- Avoid medical terminology, abbreviations or terms above the intended audience's reading level without also providing the more commonly used term. For example, if using myocardial infarct (MI) indicate that it's a heart attack, hypertension is high blood pressure.
- Use one- and two-syllable words and short sentences.
- Use subheadings to break up information.
- Use graphics that match the messages.
- Make each item on a list a complete sentence rather than using an introductory sentence.

For example, use this—

Do not skip brushing your teeth before bed.

Do not drink sugary beverages.

Rather than this—

Do not:

skip brushing your teeth before bed.

drink sugary beverages (Bartholomew Eldredge et al., 2016).

- Print materials

Regardless of whether a subcommittee or a consultant is responsible for the actual design and production of the printed program materials, the following are taken into consideration:

Design elements, which include tables, graphs, charts, graphics, lists, and instructions. The more "elements," the more complicated the material. It's best to keep the design simple.

Organizational standards, which are the graphic requirements of the organization producing the material, such as logos, paper color, etc.

Review and approval process, which are the procedures for getting planning committee input and acceptance of the final product.

Distribution method, which is the process that will be used for sharing the material.

Costs and constraints, which are the estimated costs and needed resource availability (Bartholomew Eldredge et al., 2016).

Task 4.4—Pretest, Pilot Test, and Revise. Although time consuming, pretesting program materials and messages and piloting the program before implementation is time well spent. These undertakings identify problems and uncover unforeseen challenges that might impact program implementation or effectiveness. Because they are conducted before the program is fully implemented, there is time to make corrections.

- Pretesting

Pretesting is a way to try out the program messages and materials with representatives of the intended audience to determine if they find them attractive, understandable, relevant, acceptable, persuasive, or in need of adjustment

Table 11-7 Product pretest questions

Product characteristic	Questions
Attractiveness Does the product get the attention of the intended audience?	What was the first thing you noticed about this product*? What do you like or find pleasant about this product? What do you dislike or find unpleasant about this product?
Comprehensibility Does the intended audience understand the information correctly?	What is the product all about? Who do you think the product is written for? What words, sentences, or pictures are hard to understand? What is the product asking you to do?
Relevance Does the intended audience find the information important or significant?	What people do you think should read this product? How are you different or the same as these people?
Acceptability Does the intended audience find the information culturally and socially acceptable?	Did you find anything in this product? Is there anything in this product someone in your community might find offensive or inappropriate?
Persuasiveness Does the intended audience find the product convincing?	How likely are you to do what the product is asking you to do? Why do you think you should or shouldn't do what the product is asking you to do?
Completeness Does the intended audience find the product in need of improvement?	What information would you like added to this product? What other changes would you suggest?

* Product refers to program messages, brochures, booklets, and any other print or online materials.
Data from Johns Hopkins University Center for Communication. (2016). Social and behavior change communication (SBCC) for emergency preparedness implementation kit: Pretest messages and materials. Retrieved December 30, 2019, from https://sbccimplementationkits.org/sbcc-in-emergencies/pretest-messages-and-materials/

(Bartholomew Eldredge et al., 2016; Johns Hopkins University Center for Communication Programs [JHU-CCP], 2016). Focus groups and interviews are good ways to elicit this information (Bartholomew Eldredge et al., 2016). See **Table 11-7** for sample questions to guide pretesting.

- Pilot testing

Pilot testing is a way to try out the program methods, products, and procedures with a small group of people (pilot group) from the intended audience before it's implemented with the entire audience. It's done to uncover problems that could impact program implementation and or effectiveness. When these issues are identified before the program is fully implemented, there is still time to make corrections or adjustments.

Following are tips for pilot testing:

TIP 1 Follow the implementation plan exactly in order to identify problems.

TIP 2 Have a plan in place for collecting feedback from the pilot group.

TIP 3 Have a plan in place for collecting feedback from the program presenters.

TIP 4 Track the outcome (success/failure) of activities.

TIP 5 Record which aspects of the program need adjustment (U.S. Department of Health and Human Services, Office of Adolescent Health [USDHSS-OAH], n.d.).

Step 5— Plan Program Implementation

A program's successful outcome depends not only on its content, but also on its implementation. This is especially true for evidence-based programs. Unsuccessful programs, those that fail to deliver what they were intended to deliver, often result from poor implementation rather than poor design. (See Chapter 6—Implementing.)

Task 5.1—Identify Who Will Do What.

The focus of this task is to identify—

- Who will adopt the program?
  - Which agency or organization will make the program available to the intended audience?
  - Which agencies and organizations with a history of or the potential for reaching the intended audience and sufficient resources are preferable? ?
- Who will implement the program?
  - Who at the agency or organization will deliver the program components to the intended audience (Bartholomew Eldredge et al., 2016)?
  - Does the organization have adequate personnel to implement the program and time for training?
- Who will maintain the program?
  - Who (agency, organization, or people) will ensure the program continues (Bartholomew Eldredge et al., 2016)?

If the planning committee identified "who will do what" before this point in the planning process, then the focus of this task is on confirmation rather than identification.

Task 5.2 State Outcomes and Performance Objectives for Program Use. In this task, the planning committee focuses on the following:

1. Determining who must do what in order to achieve the program outcomes with fidelity.
2. Identifying the program use outcomes.

Program use outcomes are similar to the program objectives developed in Step 2, but instead of stating expected behavioral and environmental outcomes, they state the expected outcomes for the program to accomplish adoption, implementation, and maintenance.

- Program adoption

Program adoption refers to an agency or organization's decision to use the program and become the program adopter (Bartholomew Eldredge et al., 2016).

Adoption outcomes specify:

who [the name of the agency or organization]

is adopting what [the name of the program]

as indicated by [the evidence or document indicating adoption] (Bartholomew Eldredge et al., 2016)

For example:

The Any City agency is adopting the ABC early childhood program as indicated by the signed Memorandum of Understanding.

Adoption performance objectives answer the following question:

- What must a potential program adopter do to adopt the program?

For example, adopters will review the program description, agree to participate in the program, agree to conduct an evaluation, sign a Memorandum of Understanding, gain support for the program from stakeholders (Bartholomew Eldridge et al., 2016).

- Program Implementation

Program implementation refers to an agency or organization's use of the program.

Implementation outcomes specify:

who [the agency, organization, or individual]

will implement what [the innovative program]

including use of [program components]

For example:

The Any City Health Clinic director will implement the mobile oral health screening program including use of the appointment tracking system, follow-up assessments, and phone consultations (Bartholomew Eldridge et al., 2016).

Implementation performance objectives answer the following question:

– What must the agency/organization/staff do in order to implement the program?

For example:

To implement the program, the clinic director will:

– provide regular updates to the board, designate time for staff training, and approve
– increased mobile screening.

To implement the program, the coordinator will:

– arrange for community health workers to participate in the program,
– arrange for community health worker training,
– arrange for increased screening hours, - set screening goals- monitor barriers to implementation.

• Maintenance

Maintenance refers to the sustainability or continuation of a program over time and its integration into the routines of the organizations (Bartholomew Eldridge et al., 2016).

Maintenance outcomes specify:

– Who [the agency, organization, or individual],
– Will maintain what [the program or its components].

– As indicated by [how the program is integrated into the organization].

For example:

The clinic director will maintain the XZY program as part of the standard clinic practice for every patient at the end of the initial funding period.

Maintenance performance objectives answer the question:

– What must the organization/agency/staff do to integrate the program into its routines?

For example, the clinic director will:

– discuss continuation of the program after initial funding with decision makers.
– approve steps to integrate program components into regular clinic routines.
– add program tasks to normal clinic routines (Bartholomew Eldridge et al., 2016).

In preparation for constructing the matrices of change objectives for adoption, implementation, and maintenance in the next task, keep the following in mind:

– Adoption performance objectives specify what an organization must do to adopt (use) the program.
– Implementation performance objectives specify what an organization must do to implement the program.
– Maintenance performance objectives specify what an organization must do to integrate the program into its routines.

Task 5.3—Construct Matrices of Change Objectives for Program Adoption, Implementation, and Maintenance.
The matrices of change objectives are composed of the performance objectives for adoption, implementation, and maintenance, and determinants of the performance objectives such as: program awareness, familiarity with elements of the program, opinions about the

program, perceived benefits of using the program, skills needed for implementation, and resource needs. Determinants of performance objectives are identified by the planning committee through the same brainstorming process used in Step 2 to identify determinants of the health behaviors and environmental conditions (Bartholomew Eldredge et al., 2016).

The following questions guide their identification.

- Why would an agency decide to adopt or use the program?
- Why would an adopter do what is necessary to implement the program?
- Why would an adopter do what is necessary to make sure the program is maintained over time? (Bartholomew Eldridge et al., 2016)

Once the planning committee identifies all the possible determinants of the performance objectives, each determinant is assessed to ascertain the strength of its association with program adoption and implementation and the likelihood of it changing with program implementation (Bartholomew Eldredge et al., 2016). The determinants found to be most associated with program adoption and implementation and likely to change are used to create the matrices of change objectives. These matrices are created using the same process used in Step 2 for creating the matrices of change objectives for behavioral and environmental outcomes (Bartholomew Eldredge et al., 2016).

Task 5.4—Design Implementation Methods, Delineate Scope and Sequence, and Produce Materials. This task begins with designing the program methods and practical applications. It entails the following:

- Brainstorming change methods and practical applications for each of the change objectives listed in the matrices of change objectives.

- Compiling a provisional list of change methods and practical applications.
- Reviewing the literature to confirm or modify the methods and practical applications on the provisional list.
- Compiling a final list of change methods and practical applications.
- Linking the practical applications and change methods to theoretical methods (Bartholomew Eldredge et al., 2016).

In delineating the scope and sequence of implementation, the planning committee takes the following into consideration:

- Awareness and adoption of the program by the intended audience.
- Training, capacity development, and ongoing technical support for the staff.
- Transitioning from implementation to maintenance by the implementing agency (Bartholomew Eldredge et al., 2016).

In producing materials for the program, the planning committee focuses on:

- Promoting program awareness
- Assisting implementation (an implementation manual)
- Supporting implementer training (Bartholomew Eldredge et al., 2016).

Step 6— Plan Evaluation

Outcome and impact evaluation answers questions about program efficacy and effectiveness. Did the program work in the "real world"? Did the program accomplish its behavioral, environmental, and implementation outcomes?

Process evaluation provides answers to questions about program implementation. Why was the program delivered the way it was (Bartholomew Eldredge et al., 2016)?

Planning for evaluation takes into consideration that programs aim to change future behavior. Consequently, program effects are not evident immediately. Change needs time to occur, especially if the change is on a community level (Bartholomew Eldredge et al., 2016).

What this means is that evaluations done in the short term are not appropriate for determining if behavior change occurred. Rather, short-term evaluation focuses on changes in behavioral or environmental determinants such as knowledge, skills, and self-efficacy (Bartholomew Eldredge et al., 2016).

Because program outcomes and impact are affected by the processes used to implement the program, process evaluation is also done. The key components of process evaluation, context, reach, dose, fidelity, and implementation are discussed in detail in Chapter 7, Evaluating.

Task 6.1 Write Evaluation Questions.

Developing evaluation questions is the first task in this final step. To begin writing these questions, the evaluator or evaluation subcommittee committee starts with the logic models developed in Steps 1 and 2. These present the causes of the health problem and how the program intends to change health, quality of life, and the behavioral and environmental causes of the problem. The goals developed for these are the basis for the evaluation questions.

For example:

- To what extent did the quality-of-life problem change during the program time frame?
- To what extent did the health problem change during the program time frame?
- What changes occurred in the behavioral and environmental conditions (Bartholomew Eldredge et al., 2016)?

Evaluation questions also generate data to determine the program's effect on performance and change objectives. To glean this data, questions are written based on the determinants of the change objectives (Bartholomew Eldredge et al., 2016). For example, if knowledge is a determinant of a change objective for a fall prevention program, then the evaluation question is—Did participants of the Fall Prevention program increase their knowledge of fall risk reduction strategies?

Task 6.2 Develop Measures and Indicators.

In this task, the planning committee focuses on developing indicators and measures to evaluate the program's effects (outcome and impact) and planning and implementation processes. An *indicator* is a measurable characteristic, for example, life expectancy, disease incidence, use of healthcare services, socioeconomics (CDC, 2015). A *measure* is the means by which an indicator is quantified or categorized, usually by applying numbers to the indicator. For example, number of minutes walked each day is a measure for the indicator—participation in physical activity (Bartholomew Eldredge et al., 2016). For the indicator of increased childhood vaccination rates, one measure is the number of children entering school fully vaccinated.

To begin developing these, the matrices of change objectives created in Step 2 are used. The determinants in the matrices are the indictors for evaluation. The change objectives linked to each of the determinants are the basis for their measurement (Bartholomew Eldridge et al., 2016).

After the health indicators are selected, a protocol for measuring each is developed (Bartholomew Eldridge et al., 2016). For example, if the indicator is blood pressure within normal limits, and the measure is a blood pressure reading, the protocol is the daily recording of the blood pressure reading.

Task 6.3 Specify Evaluation Design.

Evaluation designs are of two types, qualitative and quantitative. *Qualitative* methods collect descriptive data, data that are nonnumerical. These methods are frequently used for process evaluation. They include focus groups, interviews, and observation (CDC, 2010).

Quantitative methods include surveys, reports, checklists, attendance logs, self-administered questionnaires, project archives, and community profiles (Linnan & Steckler, 2002). They produce data that are numerical and answer *what* and *where* questions. (See Chapter 7, Evaluating, for a more detailed discussion of evaluation designs.)

Task 6.4 Complete Evaluation Plan.

The evaluation plan is a comprehensive document that includes the following:

- Process evaluation questions.

- Effect (outcome and impact) evaluation questions.
- Outcome indicators and measures.
- Evaluation design and timing of measures.
- Protocol for carrying out the evaluation.
- Required resources.
- Stakeholder reporting procedure (Bartholomew Eldredge et al., 2016).

Table 11-8 is an example of an IM evaluation plan.

Table 11-8 Sample IM plan for outcome and process evaluation of a binge drinking program for college students

Determinant	Evaluation question	Indicator	Measure	Timing
Outcome				
Knowledge of detrimental effects of binge drinking	Did the program increase student knowledge about the potential detrimental effects of binge drinking?	Knowledge of the potential detrimental effects binge drinking	Items on survey instrument	Baseline beginning of fall semester freshman year and spring semester follow-up
Self-efficacy to decline participation in drinking games	Did the program increase student ability to decline participation in drinking games?	Ability to decline participation in drinking games	Self-efficacy scale on survey instrument	Baseline beginning of fall semester freshman year and spring semester follow-up
Process evaluation plan				
Reach	How many freshmen participated in the program?	Number of students attending program sessions	Session attendance records	First semester freshman year
Dose	How many program sessions did each student attend?	Number of students attending each program session	Session attendance records	First semester freshman year
Fidelity	How many counselors attended training?	Number of counselors at training session	Training session attendance records	August, prior to the beginning of the academic year
	Did counselors implement the program components as written?	Number of program components completed as written	Implementation logs Session observations	End of fall semester

Data from Bartholomew Eldredge, L. K., Markham, C. M., Ruiter, R. A. C., Fernandez, M. E., Kok, G., & Parcel, G. S. (2016). *Planning health promotion programs: An intervention mapping approach* (4th ed.). San Francisco: Jossey-Bass.

Chapter Summary

Intervention mapping consists of six core processes and six consecutive planning steps that entail the development of objective matrices in each step, which serves as the foundation for the following step.

Planning in Practice Chapter Activity

When a child gets sick in a community with limited access to healthcare professionals, and the parents/caregivers don't access the health care that is available fast enough, the consequences can be deadly. Read the article below, and answer the questions that follow to learn how one country addressed this problem.

Article: *Development of a theory and evidence-based program to promote community treatment of fevers in children under five in a rural district in southern Ghana: An intervention mapping approach* (Abbey, Bartholomew, Chinbuah, Gyapong, Gyapong, & van den Borne, 2017)

Article link: https://bmcpublichealth.biomedcentral.com/articles/10.1186/s12889-016-3957-1

(Note: Download PDF)

Article Questions

1. What is the goal of this program?
2. Why was this program needed?
3. What factors did the authors identify as contributing to the problem in developing countries?
4. What were the reasons given for the factors that contribute to the problem?
5. How was needs assessment data collected in Step 1?
6. What was done to verify the accuracy of the primary qualitative data collected in Step 1?
7. How were the data collected in Step 1 used to inform the tasks completed in Step 2?
8. Which core process was used in Step 2? Support your response with examples from the article.
9. What were the matrices of change objectives based on?
10. For what decisions did the matrices of change objectives serve as the basis?
11. How were the matrices created in Step 2, used in Step 3?
12. According to the logic model of the problem, what is the main health problem the program is addressing, and what are the contributing factors and their underlying causes?
13. What theory informed the creation of the program activities? Support your answer with an example.
14. What was done to ensure the program messages were acceptable to the intended audience?
15. What parental/caregiver performance objective addresses the root cause of the problem, and what attitudinal change is expected to remedy the situation?
16. Whose behavior did the program components influence, and by what methods?
17. Which determinant is addressed in all the program components, and which theory-based method is used to affect change in all of them?
18. In Step 5 of the IM process, who implemented the program?
19. How were community members recruited to participate in the program?

20. What was the format for the community program, and how were local customs respected?

21. What did the community health worker component of the program consist of, and how were local customs respected?

22. How was the primary outcome of the program evaluated in Step 6, and what were the results?

23. How were the attrition and retention rates of the community health workers evaluated?

24. How was community health worker compliance with fever management guidelines evaluated?

25. How were community utilization and other factors associated with community health workers evaluated?

References

American Public Health Association. (n.d.). Annual meeting theme. Retrieved December 6, 2019, from https://www.apha.org/events-and-meetings/annual/why-attend/annual-meeting-theme

American Translators Association. (2019). Certification. Retrieved December 21, 2019, from https://www.atanet.org/certification/

Baranowski, T., Cerin, E., & Baranowski, J. (2009). Steps in the design, development and formative evaluation of obesity prevention-related behavior change trials. *International Journal of Behavioral Nutrition & Physical Activity*, 6(1), 6. https://dx.doi.org/10.1186%2F1479-5868-6-6

Bartholomew, L. K., Parcel, G. S., & Kok, G. (1998). Intervention mapping: A process for designing theory- and evidence-based health education programs. *Health Education & Behavior*, 25, 545–563. https://doi.org/10.1177/109019819802500502

Bartholomew Eldredge, L. K., Markham, C. M., Ruiter, R. A. C., Fernandez, M. E., Kok, G., & Parcel, G. S. (2016). *Planning health promotion programs: An intervention mapping approach* (4th ed.). San Francisco: Jossey-Bass.

Briggs, O. (2016). What colors mean in other cultures. Retrieved December 17, 2019, from https://www.smartertravel.com/what-colors-mean-in-other-cultures/

Buunk, A., & Van Vugt, M. (2013) *Applying social psychology*. Thousand Oaks, CA: Sage Publications.

Centers for Disease Control and Prevention0([CDC). (n.d.). Early childcare and education obesity prevention program. Retrieved December 5, 2019, from https://www.cdc.gov/obesity/strategies/ece-obesity-prevention-program.html

Centers for Disease Control and Prevention (CDC). (2010). Evaluation. Retrieved January 17, 2020, from https://www.cdc.gov/healthcommunication/cdcynergy/Evaluation.html

Centers for Disease Control and Prevention, National Center for Health Statistics. (2015). Health indicators warehouse. Retrieved January 16, 2020, from https://www.cdc.gov/nchs/ppt/nchs2015/Pendley_Monday_BrooksideAB_C1.pdf

Centers for Disease Control and Prevention. (2019a). Hispanic/Latino Americans and type 2 diabetes. Retrieved December 18, 2019, from https://www.cdc.gov/diabetes/library/features/hispanic-diabetes.html

Cherrington, A., Martin, M. Y., Hayes, M., Halanych, J. H., Andreae, S. J., Safford, M., Wright, M. A., & Appel, S. J. (2012). Intervention mapping as a guide for the development of a diabetes peer support intervention in rural Alabama. *Preventing Chronic Disease, 9*(E36). http://dx.doi.org/10.5888/pcd9.110053

Cohen, E. (2019). Trying to convince ultra-Orthodox Jews to vaccinate, New York messes up the Yiddish. Retrieved December 19, 2019 from https://www.cnn.com/2019/05/22/health/ny-mangled-measles-messaging/index.html

Common challenges of translation. (2019). Retrieved December 21, 2019, from Smartling—https://www.smartling.com/resources/101/common-challenges-of-translation/

Deshpande, A. D., Sanders Thompson, A. L., Vaughn, K. P., & Kreuter, M. W. (2009). The use of sociocultural constructs in cancer screening research among African Americans. *Cancer Control*, 16(13), 256–265. https://dx.doi.org/10.1177%2F107327480901600308

Fernandez, M. E., Hoor, G. A., van Lieshout, S., Rodriguez, S. A., Beidas, R. S., Parcel, G., Ruiter, R. A., Markham, C. M., & Kok, G. (2019). Implementation mapping: Using intervention mapping to develop implementation strategies. *Frontiers in Public Health, 7, 158.* https://doi.org/10.3389/fpubh.2019.00158

Ingabire, C. M., Hakizimana, E., Kateera, F., Rulisa, A., Van Den Borne, B., Nieuwold, I., Muvunyi, C., … Alaii, J. (2016). Using an intervention mapping approach for planning, implementing and assessing a community-led project towards malaria elimination in the eastern province of Rwanda. *Malaria Journal, 15, 594.* https://doi.org/10.1186/s12936-016-1645-3

James, G. (2014). 20 epic fails in global branding. Retrieved December 21, 2019, from https://www.inc.com/geoffrey-james/the-20-worst-brand-translations-of-all-time.html

Johns Hopkins University Center for Communication. (2016). Social and behavior change communication (SBCC) for emergency preparedness implementation kit: Pretest messages and materials. Retrieved December 30, 2019, from https://sbccimplementationkits.org/sbcc-in-emergencies/pretest-messages-and-materials/

Jones, T. M., Dear, B. F., Hush, J. M., Titov, N., & Dean, C. M. (2016). Application of intervention mapping to the development of a complex physical therapist intervention. *Physical Therapy, 96*(12). *1994–2004.* https://doi.org/10.2522/ptj.20150387

Kok, G., Peters, L. W. H., & Ruiter, R. A. (2017). Planning theory- and evidence-based interventions: A conceptual review of the intervention mapping protocol. *Psicologia: Reflexão e Crítica, 30*(19). Retrieved October 27, 2019, from https://link.springer.com/article/10.1186/s41155-017-0072-x

Kreuter, M. W., Lukwago, S. N., Bucholz, R. D., Clark, E. M., & Sanders Thompson, V. (2003). Achieving cultural appropriateness in health promotion programs: Targeted and tailored approaches. *Health Education and Behavior, 30*(2), *133–146.* https://doi.org/10.1177/1090198102251021

Lake, A. J., Browne, J. L., Abraham, C., Tumino, D., Hines, C., Rees, G., & Speight, J. (2018). A tailored intervention to promote uptake of retinal screening among young adults with type 2 diabetes—an intervention mapping approach. *BMC Health Services Research, 18*(396). https://doi.org/10.1186/s12913-018-3188-5

Linnan, L., Steckler, A. (2002). Process evaluation for public health interventions and research: An overview. In: Steckler, A., Linnan, L. (Eds.), *Process Evaluation for Public Health Interventions and Research* (pp. 1–23). San Francisco: Jossey-Bass.

Mann, C. M., Ward, D. S., Vaughn, A., Benjamin Neelon, S. E., Long Vidal, J. L., Omar, S., Namenek Brouwek, R. J., & Ostbye, T. (2015). Application of the intervention mapping protocol to develop Keys, a family childcare home intervention to prevent childhood obesity. *BMC Public Health, 15, 1227.* https://doi.org/10.1186/s12889-015-2573-9

National Environmental Health Association. (2019). NEHA 2020 Annual educational conference (ACE) & exhibition. Retrieved December 6, 2019, from https://www.neha.org/news-events/aec-annual-educational-conference-0

Pot, M., Ruiter, R. A. C., Paulussen, T. W. G. M., Heuvelink, A., de Melker, H. E., an Vliet, H. J. A., & van Keulen, H. M. (2018). Systematically developing a web-based tailored intervention promoting HPV vaccination acceptability among mothers of invited girls using intervention mapping. *Frontiers in Public Health, 6, 226.* https://doi.org/10.3389/fpubh.2018.00226

Rural Health Information Hub [RHIhub]. (2019). Promotora de salud/Lay health worker model. Retrieved December 23, 2019, from https://www.ruralhealthinfo.org/toolkits/community-health-workers/2/layhealth

San Francisco Unified School District. (n.d.). Monthly health themes. Retrieved December 5, 2019, from https://www.healthiersf.org/News/HealthAwarenessMonths/index.php#may

Stea, T. H., Haugen, T., Bernsten, S., Guttormsen, V., Øverby, N. C., Haraldstad, K., ... Ablidsnes, E. (2016). Using the intervention mapping protocol to develop a family-based intervention for improving lifestyle habits among overweight and obese children: Study protocol for quasi-experimental trial. *BMC Public Health, 16.* https://doi.org/10.1186/s12889-016-3766-6

Tufel-Shone, N. I., Siyjua, T., Watahomigie, H. J., & Irwin, S. (2006). Community-based participatory research: Conducting a formative assessment of factors that influence youth wellness in the Hualapai community. *American Journal of Public Health, 96*(9), *1623–1628.* https://dx.doi.org/10.2105%2FAJPH.2004.054254

U.S. Department of Health and Human Services, Office of Minority Health [USDHHS-OMH]. (2019). Infant mortality and African Americans. Retrieved December 17, 2019, from https://minorityhealth.hhs.gov/omh/browse.aspx?lvl=4&lvlid=23

U.S. Department of Health and Service, Office of Adolescent Health [USDHHS-OAH]. (n.d.). Tips and recommendations for successfully piloting testing your program. Retrieved January 2, 2020, from https://search.hhs.gov/searchblox/hhs/index.html?query=tips%20on%20pilot%20testing&page=1&pagesize=10&sort=relevance&sortdir=desc&HHS=Search&adsCname=HHS&adsDisplay=true&cname=hhsgov_only&default=AND&tune=true&tune.0=10&tune.1=8&tune.2=2&tune.3=5&tune.4=365&tune.5=30

Walkosz, B. J., Buller, D., Buller, M., Wallis, A., Meenan, R., Cutter, G. ... Scott, M. (2018). Sun safe workplaces: Effect of an occupational skin cancer prevention program on employee sun safety practices. *Journal of Occupational and Environmental Medicine, 60*(11). https://dx.doi.org/10.1097%2FJOM.0000000000001427

Wu, D., Ma, G. X., Zhou, K. Zhou, D., Liu, A., & Poon, A. N. (2009). The effect of a culturally tailored smoking cessation for Chinese American smokers. *Nicotine Tobacco Research, 11*(12), *1448–1457.* https://dx.doi.org/10.1093%2Fntr%2Fntp159

Zarcadoolas, C., & Blanco, M. (2000). Lost in translation: Each word accurate yet ... Retrieved December 21, 2019, from https://www.managedcaremag.com/archives/2000/8/lost-translation-each-word-accurate-yet

Frameworks for Specific Issues and Methods

STUDENT LEARNING OBJECTIVES

After reading this chapter, the student will be able to:

- Describe how frameworks for specific issues and methodologies differ from other frameworks.
- Use an issue- or method-specific framework to plan a hypothetical program.

Introduction

Although for the most part, any of the planning frameworks will work with any health issue, some frameworks are designed for particular health issues or a specific type of program methodology. Following are summaries of three of these, the Strategic Prevention Framework for substance abuse issues, Protocol for Assessing Community Excellence in Environmental Health for environmental health issues, and Making Health Communication Programs Work, for health communication programs.

Strategic Prevention Framework (SPF)

The Strategic Prevention Framework [SPF], developed by the National Institutes of Health—Substance Abuse and Mental Health Services Administration (SAMHSA), is specific to substance misuse issues in the community. The SPF is guided by two principles—cultural competence and sustainability—which are integrated into the framework's five steps summarized here (SAMHSA, 2019). (See **Figure 12-1** and **Table 12-1**.)

A detailed explanation of the framework is available at https://www.samhsa.gov/sites/default/files/20190620-samhsa-strategic-prevention-framework-guide.pdf.

Step 1—Assess Substance Misuse Problem. This initial step in the SPF focuses on gaining an understanding of the community's substance misuse prevention needs. Data from a variety of sources (see Chapter 4, Assessing Needs) are used to identify and prioritize misuse problems (for example,

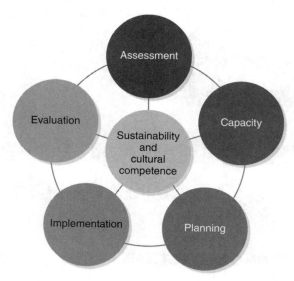

Figure 12-1 Strategic prevention framework

U.S. Department of Health and Human Service. Substance Abuse and Mental Health Services Administration [SAMHSA]. (2019). A Guide to SAMHSA's Strategic Prevention Framework. Rockville, MD: Center for Substance Abuse Prevention. Substance Abuse and Mental Health Services Administration. Retrieved from https//:www.samhsa.gov/sites/default/files/20190620-samhsa-strategic-prevention-framework-guide.pdf

Table 12-1 Strategic prevention framework steps and tasks

Steps	Tasks
Step 1—Assess substance misuse problem	Assess misuse and related problems Prioritize problems and behaviors Assess risk and protective factors
Step 2—Build capacity for addressing needs	Involve diverse stakeholders Create a diverse prevention team Increase community awareness
Step 3—Develop prevention program plan	Prioritize factors associated with the misuse Identify evidence-based programs Combine evidence-based programs Develop a logic model
Step 4—Implement prevention program plan	Balance fidelity with the need for adaptation Adhere to core program components Establish supports for implementation Monitor the program
Step 5—Evaluate prevention program	Conduct process and outcome evaluations Make recommendations to improve program Share results

Data from Substance Abuse and Mental Health Services Administration (SAMHSA). (2019). A Guide to SAMHSA's Strategic Prevention Framework. Rockville, MD: Center for Substance Abuse Prevention. Substance Abuse and Mental Health Services Administration.

overdoses, alcohol poisoning) and their related behaviors (for example, prescription drug misuse, underage drinking), and risk and protective factors.

- Assess misuse problems and related behaviors

The following questions guide this assessment:

- What are the substance misuse problems and related behaviors in the community?
- How often are these problems happening, and which are happening most often?
- Where are these problems happening (at large home parties, in vacant lots)?
- Who is misusing substances and engaging in related problem behaviors (males, females, teens, certain cultural group members)?
- What resources are available for establishing and maintaining a substance misuse prevention program?
- How ready, motivated, and willing is the community to commit resources to substance misuse prevention?

- Prioritize problems and behaviors

If the previous assessment uncovers multiple misuse problems and behaviors, they are prioritized to determine the most significant. The criteria used for prioritizing should result in an unbiased view of each problem and behavior, its impact on the community, and its potential for change. The following are sample criteria for prioritizing:

- Magnitude—How extensive the problem and behavior are in the community.
- Severity—How large of an impact the problem and behavior are having on the people affected or the community as a whole.
- Trends—How the problem is evolving.
- Changeability—How likely it is to modify the problem and behavior.

(See Chapter 4, Assessing Needs, for more information about prioritizing.)

- Assess risk and protective factors

Risk and protective factors influence the chances of a person engaging in behaviors related to a misuse problem. Risk factors increase the chances of a person developing the misuse problem, such as peer pressure and impulsivity. Protective factors decrease the chances of a person developing the misuse problem, such as academic achievement and family stability.

Consequently, effective misuse prevention programs focus on reducing risk factors and increasing protective factors.

Step 2—Build Capacity for Addressing Substance Misuse Prevention Needs.
Building capacity entails ensuring the community is ready for a prevention effort and willing to commit resources. To support capacity building:

- Involve diverse stakeholders in the prevention initiative, including community residents, healthcare and treatment providers, community leaders, law enforcement, faith communities, academia, youth, and organizations.
- Create a diverse prevention team (planning committee) composed of stakeholders.
- Increase community awareness by meeting with community opinion leaders, hosting events, and writing articles for the local newspapers, church bulletins, neighborhood newsletters, and social media to share information about the substance misuse problems, conducting focus groups to get community input about the problems.

Step 3—Develop Substance Misuse Prevention Plan.
Developing a substance misuse prevention program entails involving diverse stakeholders, making decisions based on data, and evidence of effectiveness. To ensure the plan addresses the misuse issue (problem and related behaviors):

1. Prioritize the factors associated with the misuse issue that were identified in the needs assessment.
2. Identify evidence-based, contextually appropriate programs (in the literature) for addressing each of the priority factors associated with the misuse issue.
3. Combine evidence-based programs for a broad approach to addressing the misuse issue.
4. Develop a logic model with short-term and long-term outcomes. (See Chapter 5, Planning.)

Step 4—Implement Substance Misuse Prevention Program Plan. Putting the prevention program plan into action requires attention to the following:

• Balancing fidelity to the original plan with the need for adaptation,
• Adhering to core program components,
• Establishing supports for implementation and successful outcomes such as having stakeholder leadership and support, the most qualified person to deliver the program, trained staff, a comprehensive action plan with all tasks, deadlines, and responsible parties,
• Monitoring and evaluating the program.

(For more information on program implementation, see Chapter 6, Implementing.)

Step 5—Evaluate Substance Misuse Prevention Program. Evaluation is done to facilitate data-informed decision making and improve program effectiveness. It entails:

conducting process and outcome evaluations,

making recommendations for program improvement,

sharing results. (See Chapter 7, Evaluating.)

Evaluation results are used for:

– Documenting and describing substance misuse prevention activities in the community.
– Providing information about the prevention program to stakeholders and funders.
– Documenting the outcomes of the program on substance misuse and its related behaviors.
– Improving the prevention program.
– Determining which components of the prevention program work and which don't.
– Building support for substance misuse prevention programing in the community.
– Increasing the knowledge base of which substance misuse programs work and which don't.

Protocol for Assessing Community Excellence in Environmental Health (PACE-EH)

The Protocol for Assessing Community Excellence in Environmental Health (PACE-EH) was developed jointly in 1995 by the Centers for Disease Control's National Center for Environmental Health (CDC-NCEH) and the National Association for County and City Health Officials (NACCHO). It provides guidance on conducting community environmental health assessments, including how to identify the local environmental health issues, determine priority environmental health issues for action, identify populations most at risk of the priority environmental health issues, and address the identified environmental health issue (NACCHO, 2000)

PACE-EH entails 13 tasks and corresponding actions summarized from the *Protocol for Assessing Community Excellence in Environmental Health: A Guidebook for Local Health Officials* (NACCHO, 2000), available at: https://www.cdc.gov/nceh/ehs/ceha/pace_eh.htm.

Task 1—Determine Community Capacity to Undertake the Environmental Assessment. Community capacity refers to the resources (human, organizational, and social) in a community that, when combined, can improve its ability to solve problems or maintain well-being (Chaskin, 2001).

Following are the corresponding actions for completing this task.

- Determine resources *needed* to conduct the environmental health assessment.

Resources needed to conduct the assessment include money, personnel skills and capacities, for example, data collection and analysis, public relations and marketing, access to technical support.

- Determine resources *available* to conduct the environmental health assessment at the local public health agency and in the community.

  Available resources are contingent upon:

  - the local public health agency's data collection and analysis capabilities;
  - staff availability, relationships, and collaborations with stakeholders, other agencies, and organizations, the community's profile and asset map. (See Chapter 9, MAPP, for more information on asset mapping.)

- Determine the collaborative capacities of the agency and community.

Collaborative capacity takes into consideration community conflicts, mistrust issues, success rate of previous collaborative endeavors, and the availability of credible and committed leaders and a willingness of the agency overseeing the assessment to share its decision-making power.

- Determine the level of support for an environmental health assessment.

All the information gathered previously in this task is taken into consideration in determining if the level of support is enough to implement the assessment

Task 2—Define the Community and Its Characteristics. How the community is defined influences its assessment activities, for example, selecting the environmental health issues, deciding on the extent of community member involvement in the assessment process, choosing community partners for the assessment, identifying collaborative opportunities, determining available resources, and creating the plan to address the environmental health issues.

Following are the corresponding actions for completing this task:

- Define the community.

A community is often defined by a geographic boundary—a neighborhood, a section of a town or city, a school district, or a voting district. Other ways to define a community are by a common characteristic of the people, such as profession, religion, ethnicity, age, or by a common interest such as a hobby.

- Describe the community.

The community description includes information about who the community members are, their concerns, level of civic engagement, key leaders, and how they function as a group and make decisions. It is based on demographics data, health status, socioeconomic status and education level, in addition to language, culture, and religion.

- Refine the community definition

How the community is defined is essential for identifying people from the community to serve on the environmental health assessment team (assessment team) conducting the assessment. Once the initial assessment team is assembled (in Task 3), the community definition is reviewed in light of the assessment team's composition and refined to better reflect the perspectives of the community members, if needed.

Task 3—Assemble an Environmental Health Assessment Team. The assessment team is responsible for conducting the environmental health assessment and should represent a broad cross section of the defined community, including members from organizations, businesses, and politics.

Following are the corresponding actions for completing this task:

- Clarify assessment team member expectations.

It's essential that the roles, responsibilities, and rights of team members are clearly explained and provided to potential members at the time they are invited and before they accept the invitation to serve on the team.

- Invite people to design and implement the assessment.

Potential members of the assessment team include representatives from the following community entities: healthcare providers/facilities; educational institutions including schools, colleges, and universities; news media outlets; local government; trade/professional groups; businesses; labor groups; faith groups; voluntary and nonprofit organizations; neighborhood associations; first responders (fire, emergency medical services); law enforcement; environmental organizations and associations; and cooperative extension services.

- Establish governing and decision-making structure and rules.

The organizational or administrative structure frames how the assessment team will work. For example:

- If there is a chairperson, what are this person's responsibilities?
- Will certain tasks become the responsibility of subcommittees?
- Will all members of the team have an equal voice in decision making with decisions made by consensus or majority vote?

- What rules are members expected to follow regarding active participation, speaking time limits, listening to and respecting other's opinions, fact versus fiction, constructive criticism, positive confrontation?

Task 4—Define Goals, Objectives, and Assessment Scope. All members of the assessment team work together to identify the goals, objectives, and scope of the environmental health assessment.

Following are the corresponding actions for completing this task:

- Establish assessment goals and objectives. (See Chapter 5, Planning.)
- Develop a shared environmental health assessment vision. (See Chapter 9, MAPP.)
- Determine the scope of the environmental health assessment.

It's important for the team to decide which issues are acceptable for an "environmental health assessment" and which are not. For example, will the environmental health assessment only address the human health effects from environmental sources, or the health of the environment, or the health of the community in general?

- Define key terms.

Establish agreed-upon definitions for key terms pertaining to the assessment to prevent potential disagreement among assessment team members about their meaning.

Task 5—List the Environmental Health Issues. This task focuses on identifying the environmental health issues of concern to the community and determining their prevalence.

Following are the corresponding actions for completing this task:

- Choose methods for data gathering. (See Chapter 4, Assessing Needs.)
- Collect data on community environmental health issues. (See Chapter 4, Assessing Needs.)

- Compile a manageable list of the community's environmental health issues.

Condense the entire list of issues identified by the community to a manageable list of those that meet a set of criteria agreed upon by the assessment team. For example, the criteria for remaining on the list might include that the issue is within the scope of the assessment, related to human health, of local concern, of concern to a significant majority of the community, or supported by other information from the community for inclusion.

Task 6—Analyze the List of Environmental Health Issues. The environmental health issues from Task 5 are analyzed to identify the set of interrelated factors promoting each of them. This task is completed using the Analyzing Framework (see **Figure 12-2**) to identify the following:

Contributing factors—These are the policies (activities and practices) and personal behaviors that affect the environmental issue or put people at potential risk of its effects.

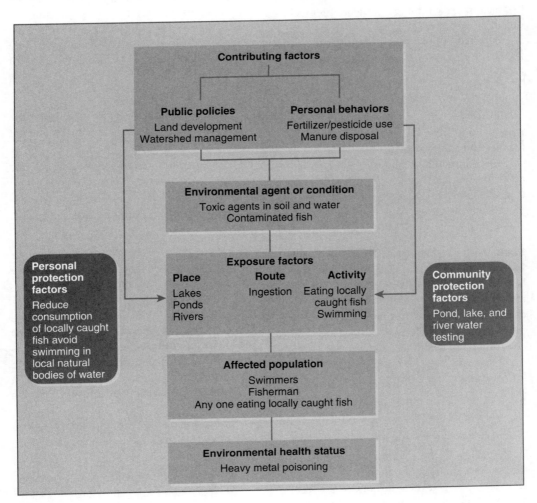

Figure 12-2 PACE-EH analyzing framework example

Data from Centers for Disease Control and Prevention (CDC). (2000). *Protocol for assessing community excellence in environmental health: A guidebook for local health officials.* Washington: CDC/NACCHO.

Environmental conditions and health links—These are possible connections between hazardous chemicals, biological agents, radiation, and other physical conditions (for example, dust, water pollution) and environmental health, human health, or quality of life.

Exposure factors—These are the places where exposure to the environmental agent or condition occurs (for example, work, school, outdoors), the route or how exposure occurs (for example, ingestion, inhalation, absorption), and the activities that lead to exposure (for example, swimming, on the job, remodeling an older home).

Affected populations—These are the people at risk of exposure to the hazardous environmental agent or condition.

Protection factors—These are the personal behaviors and community actions that can modify or prevent the environmental health issue or contribute to the maintenance of environmental health quality.

Environmental health status—This is an acute or chronic health condition or quality-of-life issue with a suspected or known link to an environmental cause.

Task 7—Develop Quantitative Indicators. In the previous task, the connections between the various factors related to the environmental issues are identified in descriptive or qualitative terms. In this task, quantitative indicators are developed for measuring the environmental health issue.

Following are the corresponding actions for completing this task:

- Create a list of potential quantitative indicators

Identify ways to quantify or measure the factors related to the environmental issue using the results of the Task 6 analysis as the basis. For example, quantitative indicators of a concern about watershed contamination might include:

- the rate of pesticide and fertilizer use.
- the number of people who fish in local waters.
- the number of people who eat fish caught in local waters.
- the rate of heavy metal poisoning among the affected populations.

- Identify key quantitative indicators from the list of potential indicators

The list of potential quantitative indicators is revised to contain only *key* indicators, those that effectively describe the most important elements related to the environmental health issue. This is done by assessing each indicator against a set of criteria developed by the assessment team. For example:

- Simplicity—Does the indicator measure only one factor?

- Understandability—Does the indicator make sense with the environmental issue?

- Acceptability—Is the indicator in line with community characteristics and concerns?

- Measurability—Is the indicator quantifiable?

- Defensibility—Does the indicator establish the relationship between the environmental issue and health?

Task 8—Select Standards to Compare Indicators Against. The focus of Task 8 is to identify the standards or benchmarks for each key quantitative indicator identified in Task 7 for use as a comparison to measure progress against.

Following are the corresponding actions for completing this task:

- Identify local, state, and national data/ goals for environmental health that may serve as standards to measure progress in addressing the community issue.

- Agree upon the use of indicators with local data (for example, the number of people who eat fish caught in local waters) that can serve as a starting point or benchmark for determining progress over time.

Task 9—Create Profiles for Environmental Health Issues.
The focus of Task 9 is on creating a profile or written report for each environmental health issue in preparation for ranking them in Task 10.

Following are the corresponding actions for completing this task:

- Select the profile components and format. For example, each profile might include:
  - a description of the issue.
  - a summary of the local conditions related to the issue.
  - the standards and their data sources from Task 8.
  - the community indicators from the Analyzing Framework in Task 7.
  - the Analyzing Framework results from Task 7.

(See **Figure 12-3**.)

Environmental Health Issue Profile

Issue: _____

Issue description:

Local conditions summary:

Standards and data sources:

Analyzing framework indicators:

Assessment team analysis results:

Figure 12-3 Sample environmental health issue profile format

Data from Centers for Disease Control and Prevention (CDC). (2000). *Protocol for assessing community excellence in environmental health: A guidebook for local health officials.* Washington: CDC/NACCHO.

• Collect the same information for each issue

The same information at the same level of detail is collected for each component of each issue's profile in preparation for ranking and prioritizing the issues in the next task.

Task 10—Rank the Environmental Health Issues. In this task, the assessment team uses the profiles completed in Task 9 to determine the relative importance of each environmental health issue when compared against all the others.

Following are the corresponding actions for completing this task:

• Determine the purpose of ranking the issues

The following questions are a guide for discussing and coming to agreement on the purpose of ranking the issues:

– What outcomes are expected from the ranking?
– What uses are there for the results?

• Decide on the ranking criteria

Having set criteria for comparing each issue against the others provides assurance that the ranking process is fair and valid. Examples of ranking criteria include the following:

– The number of people in the community likely at risk of negative health consequences from exposure to the issue.
– The locations where risk of exposure is greatest (the workplace, schools, or homes).
– The populations within the community most at risk (older adults, teens, or those with chronic lung disease).
– The severity of the health effects of the issue (high mortality rate, irreversible harm, negative impact on ecosystem).
– The state of the issue or its health effects (improving, stabilizing or worsening).

• Select a ranking method

A suggested method of ranking is to generate quantitative data by developing a

worksheet that contains the ranking criteria for which numerical values (criteria scores) are assigned. A worksheet is completed by each assessment team member for each issue. A ranking score is computed for each issue by adding the criteria scores. (See **Table 12-2.**)

To generate qualitative ranking data, assessment team members complete the worksheets, review the ranking scores, and make a judgment as to their level of concern—high, moderate, or low.

• Rank the issues

Based on the ranking score, the level of concern, or both, the issues are compared and put into order from those with the highest score and/or of highest concern to lowest. Those with the highest scores and of highest concern are prioritized in Task 11.

Task 11—Prioritize Environmental Health Issues. Prioritizing takes into account the obstacles and opportunities presented by the legal, economic, social, scientific, and political circumstances of the community.

Following are the corresponding actions for completing this task:

• Determine criteria for setting priorities

The criteria for prioritizing the health issues are more subjective than those for ranking and depend on the assessment team's understanding of the community. For example, prioritizing criteria might include political support for addressing the issue, legal constraints of addressing the issue, or community demand for addressing the issue.

• Select a prioritizing method

One way to prioritize the issues is to develop a worksheet similar to the ranking worksheet used in the previous task, to assess the issues against the priority criteria. For example, is there high, moderate, or low political support for the issue, community demand

Table 12-2 Sample environmental health issue ranking worksheet

Environmental Health Issue: _____

Instructions: Circle the number in the Response Value column that corresponds to your answer. To compute the criteria score, total the circled response values.

Criteria—The number of people in the community affected by the environmental health issue. (Select one)	Response value
Less than 25% of the community	1
25–50% of the community	2
50–75% of the community	3
75–100% of the community	4
Criteria score	

Criteria—The location where people are most affected by the environmental health issue. (Select all that apply)	Response value
Home	1
School	1
Child day care centers	1
Adult day care or senior centers	1
Workplace	1
Outdoors	1
Criteria score	

Criteria—The populations most affected by the environmental health issue. (Select all that apply)	Response Value
Children	1
Teens	1
Adults	1
People with chronic respiratory diseases	1
Criteria score	

Criteria—Human health effects of the environmental health issue. (Select all that apply)	Response Value
High mortality rate	1
High disability rate	1
Irreversible harm to those affected	1
Criteria score	

(continues)

Table 12-2 Sample environmental health issue ranking worksheet *(continued)*

Criteria—Status of the environmental health issue.	Response value
Improving	1
Stable	2
Increasing	3
Criteria score	

Instructions:
To compute the environmental health issue ranking score, insert the criteria scores and total.

Criteria	Criteria Score
The number of people in the community affected by the environmental health issue.	
The location where people are most affected by the environmental health issue.	
The populations most affected by the environmental health issue.	
Human health effects of the environmental health issue.	
Status of the environmental health issue.	
Ranking score	

Data from Centers for Disease Control and Prevention (CDC). (2000). *Protocol for assessing community excellence in environmental health: A guidebook for local health officials.* Washington: CDC/NACCHO.

for addressing the issue, or risk of legal implications. (See **Table 12-3**.) (For other methods of prioritizing, see Chapter 4, Assessing Needs.)

- Determine the priorities

The purpose of prioritizing is to determine which issues are of greatest importance to the community and feasible to address. One way to accomplish this is by identifying the three issues with the highest priority scores.

Task 12—Develop an Action Plan. The focus of this task is developing plans to address the priority issues identified in Task 11.

Following are the corresponding actions for completing this task:

- Develop goals and SMART objectives. (See Chapter 5, Planning.)
- Review the contributing factors identified in Task 6 in the Analyzing Framework.
- Identify potential evidence-based programs for implementation. (See Chapter 5, Planning, and Chapter 6, Implementing.)
- Assess each potential evidence-based program against the PEARL test (see Chapter 5, Planning, and Chapter 9, MAPP), and select the most appropriate for implementation.
- Identify potential barriers to implementation using the information collected in

---

Table 12-3 Sample environmental health issue priority-setting worksheet

Environmental Health Issue: _____

Instructions: Assess the extent to which the environmental health issues meets the priority criteria using the following scale:

1 = doesn't meet the criteria

2 = somewhat meets the criteria

3 = meets the criteria

To compute the priority score, add the values in the criteria score column.

Priority criteria	Criteria score
Political support for addressing the issue	
Community demand for addressing the issue.	
Availability of effective evidence-based interventions for addressing the issue	
Priority score	

Data from Centers for Disease Control and Prevention (CDC). (2000). *Protocol for assessing community excellence in environmental health: A guidebook for local health officials.* Washington: CDC/NACCHO.

Task 2 about the community characteristics and Task 9 about constraints and barriers.

- Determine resource needs and availability to implement the selected programs.
- Determine community assets applicable to the issue using the community asset map created in Task 1.
- Identify potential implementation partners using the information about community capacity gathered in Task 1.
- Provide training to those with responsibility for program implementation.
- Develop a timeline. (See Chapter 5, Planning.)

Task 13—Evaluate Progress. Evaluation measures the degree to which the program is meeting its objectives, achieving its expected outcomes within the allotted time frames.

Following are the corresponding actions for completing this task:

- Determine the evaluation questions. (See Chapter 7, Evaluating.)
- Evaluate success of the assessment process.

The indicators identified in the Analyzing Framework in Task 6 are used as the criteria to evaluate the success of the assessment process.

- Plan for ongoing assessment activities

The PACE-EH is a process for tracking key environmental health indicators over time. The knowledge gained from completing the initial assessment is used to plan ongoing assessment activities. See **Table 12-4** for the framework tasks and actions.

Table 12-4 Protocol for Assessing Community Excellence in Environmental Health (PACE-EH) tasks and actions

Tasks	Actions
Task 1—Determine community capacity to undertake the environmental assessment.	– Determine resource needs. – Determine resources available. – Determine the collaborative capacities. – Determine the level of support.
Task 2—Define the community and its characteristics.	– Define the community. – Describe the community. – Refine the community definition.
Task 3—Assemble environmental health assessment team.	– Clarify assessment team member expectations. – Invite people to design and implement assessment. – Establish governing and decision-making structure and rules.
Task 4—Define goals, objectives, and assessment scope.	– Establish assessment goals and objectives. – Develop shared environmental health assessment vision. – Determine the scope of environmental health assessment. – Define key terms.
Task 5—List the environmental health issues.	– Choose methods for data gathering. – Collect data on community environmental health issues. – Compile list of the community environmental health issues.

Task 6—Analyze list of environmental health issues.	– Use the Analyzing Framework to identify:
	    – Contributing factors
	    – Environmental conditions and links
	    – Exposure factors
	    – Populations affected
	    – Protection factors
	    – Environmental health status

Task 7—Develop quantitative indicators.	– Create list of potential quantitative indicators. – Identify key quantitative indicators potential indicators list.
Task 8—Select standards to compare indicators against.	– Identify environmental health data/goals for measuring progress. – Agree upon use of indicators.
Task 9—Create profiles for environmental health issues.	– Select profile components and format. – Collect the same information for each issue.
Task 10—Rank environmental health issues.	– Determine purpose of ranking the issues. – Decide on ranking criteria. – Select ranking method. – Rank issues.

(continues)

Table 12-4 **Protocol for Assessing Community Excellence in Environmental Health (PACE-EH) tasks and actions** *(continued)*

Tasks	Actions
Task 11—Prioritize environmental health issues.	– Determine criteria for setting priorities. – Select prioritizing method. – Determine priorities.
Task 12—Develop action plan.	– Develop goals and SMART objectives. – Review contributing factors identified in the Analyzing Framework. – Identify potential evidence-based programs for implementation. – Assess potential evidence-based programs using PEARL test. – Identify potential implementation barriers. – Determine resource needs and availability. – Determine community assets. – Identify potential implementation partners. – Train those responsible for implementation. – Develop a timeline.
Task 13—Evaluate progress.	– Determine evaluation questions. – Evaluate assessment process. – Plan ongoing assessment activities.

Data from Centers for Disease Control and Prevention (CDC). (2000). *Protocol for assessing community excellence in environmental health: A guidebook for local health officials.* Washington: CDC/NACCHO.

Making Health Communication Programs Work

This framework, originally developed in 1989 by the Office of Communication of the National Cancer Institute, is an approach for planning health communication programs (National Cancer Institute [NCI], 2004). These programs use communication channels to change the knowledge, attitudes, and behaviors of the intended audience (Rural Health Information Hub [RHIhub], 2020) and inform and influence individual and community decisions that improve health (NCI, 2004). Communication channels include broadcast media (radio, television), print media (newspapers, brochures, flyers), social media (Facebook, Twitter, YouTube), and the Internet.

The four stages of the framework: planning and strategy development; developing and pretesting concepts, messages, and materials; implementing the program; and assessing effectiveness, serve as *guidelines* rather than hard and fast procedures to follow because they may not apply in every situation (NCI, 2004). They are depicted in **Figure 12-4** and summarized here from the National Cancer Institute's *Making Health Communication Programs Work* ("the pink book") (NCI, 2004), available at: https://pubs.cancer.gov/ncipl/detail.aspx?prodid=T068.

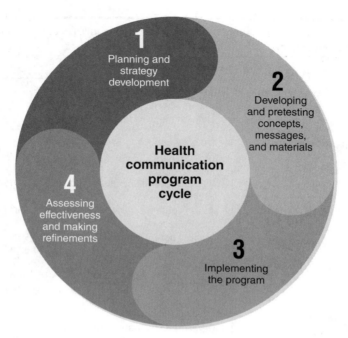

Figure 12-4 The health communication framework

Stage 1—Develop Plan and Strategy. The first stage of the health communication planning process guides the design of a program plan. It entails the following steps.

- Step 1-1 Assess the health problem and identify solution components.

This initial step involves collecting data to describe the health problem, the people affected, the changes needed, and the components of a solution (goal) to affect the changes. (See Chapter 4, Assessing Needs, for more information about data collection.) The role health communication might play in the solution is also assessed to determine if it alone can accomplish the needed changes or if the changes involve policy (laws, regulations) or technologies (new products, drugs, services, or treatments).

- Step 1-2 Define communication objectives

The communication objectives should meet the criteria for SMART objectives, contain the intended outcomes of the communication program, and suggest the message and content needed to achieve them. (For more information about writing objectives, see Chapter 5, Planning.)

- Step 1-3 Define intended audiences

This step focuses on pinpointing the specific intended audience of the communication program from within the larger population. This is done by segmenting or separating the population into subgroups based on characteristics related to the health problem targeted for change. Segmenting enables the development of messages, materials, and activities relevant to the intended audience, as well as identification of the best communication channels for reaching them.

The following are characteristics typically used for segmenting:

Behavior—health choices, lifestyle practices, information seeking, readiness to change.

Culture—language preferences and English proficiency, religion, ethnicity, family composition, and lifestyle habits.

Demographics—age, gender, occupation, income, education, level, and residence and work situations.

Health history—health risk exposure, personal or family health history.

Psychographics—attitudes, perspective on life and health, self-esteem, beliefs, values.

To select the intended audience from among the segments, the following questions are asked for each segment:

- What is a realistic and reasonable communication objective (behavior change) if this segment is the intended audience? That is, what behavior change can this audience realistically make?
- Will accomplishing this communication objective (behavior change) contribute to attaining the program goal? That is, are there enough people in this segment for a change in their behavior to make a worthwhile contribution to attaining the goal?
- To what extent would this segment benefit from communication about the behavior change? That is, how many people in this segment are *not* already engaged in the desired behavior?
- To what extent can available resources and channels of communication reach this segment and affect change? That is, with what is available, how likely is it to reach this segment and change their behavior?

Once the intended audience is selected, further information is often needed before objectives are set. The following questions are offered as a guide for gathering this additional data:

- What does the intended audience already know about the health issue?
- What are the intended audience's beliefs, attitudes, and barriers to change relative to the health issue?
- How ready is the intended audience to make a change?

- What social, cultural, and economic factors are likely to impact program development and implementation?
- What time, locations, communication channels, and learning styles are best for reaching the intended audience?

- Step 1-4 Explore ways to best reach intended audience

The focus of this step is to determine the most effective, efficient settings, channels, and activities to reach the intended audience.

Settings include

- Places where the program can reach the audience. For example, at home, in the car, on mass transit, at school, work, or a healthcare provider's office.
- Places where the audience can act upon the message.
- Places where they will find the message most credible.
- Times when the audience is most attentive.

Communication channels and activities include:

- Interpersonal communication channels— such as those between physician and patient, clergy and parishioner, coach and player, family members, and friends. They are effective for changing attitudes, skills, and behavioral intent through counseling, instruction, and informal discussion activities.
- Group communication channels—such as those between people with a common interest or characteristic gathered together in one place such as a classroom, lunch at a worksite, a club meeting. These channels allow for easy access to the intended audience with messages tailored to their common characteristic disseminated instruction and informal discussion activities.
- Organization/community channels— such as advocacy groups, coalitions, and nonprofits. Using these channels enables the dissemination of the program message through newsletters, bulletins, and

activities such as events, meetings, and worksite campaigns.

- Mass media channels, such as radio, television, magazines, direct mail, and newspapers, are known for their effectiveness in raising awareness about a health issue, increasing knowledge, changing attitudes, and motivating intended audiences to seek services and information. They entail letters to the editor, op/ed pieces, ads, feature stories, and talk shows.
- Interactive media channels—such as websites, email, and social media enable dissemination of highly tailored messages to the intended audience.

- Step 1-5 Identify possible program partners

The process of identifying suitable partners begins with making a list of entities that can bring resources, expertise, or credibility to the program and can fill a role that supports its success. Once completed, a partnering plan is developed that includes the following:

- Program title.
- Communication objectives.
- Intended audiences.
- Potential partner organizations, agencies, or individuals.
- Potential partner roles and responsibilities.
- Benefits to potential partners of partnering.
- Process for approaching and engaging potential partners.

- Step 1-6 Develop a strategy, evaluation plans, and a timeline

Results from the previous step are used to develop a communication strategy and plan and evaluation plans in this step. A communication strategy, also called a creative brief, is a guiding principle for all program products and activities. The communication strategy contains all the information needed to communicate with the intended audience, including:

- a definition of the intended audience.
- a description of the actions (changes) specified in the objectives that the intended audience is expected to take.

- a list of barriers or obstacles to taking action.
- an explanation of how the intended audience will benefit from taking action.
- the settings, channels, and activities that will reach the audience.
- the tone, look, and feel of the messages and materials.

The communication plan is developed taking the following into consideration:

- That the evaluation design is appropriate for the communication activity it will evaluate.
- That the evaluation time frame is compatible with the implementation time frame.
- That the level of evidence expected is acceptable for reporting and decision-making purposes.
- That the evaluation is measuring the extent of change that occurred against the expected change specified in the communication objectives.

The communication plan contains the individual plans developed for specific elements of the program. It includes the communication strategy, partnering, message and materials development and testing, implementation, outcome evaluation, and task completion (timeline).

The outcome evaluation plan guides the process for determining the extent to which the communication objectives were met. (For more information about outcome evaluation, see Chapter 7, Evaluating.)

Evaluating a communication program presents some unique challenges not typically seen with other types of programs. For example, it's difficult, if not impossible, to separate out the effects of a communication activity because behavior change does not usually result from one activity.

Communication programs take place in real-world settings where there are other influences on the intended audience, including other organizations and programs addressing the same problem, making it difficult to attribute any change to a specific program.

Communication objectives are sometimes not measurable because the change in behavior occurs in too few people and falls within a typical margin of error.

The timeline for developing the communication and evaluation plans includes every possible task necessary to accomplish these endeavors. This is a flexible document that is updated regularly to manage the program and track its progress. (See Chapter 5, Planning, for more detailed information on developing timelines.)

Stage 2—Develop and Pretest Concepts, Messages, and Materials. Developing messages and materials is key to a health communication program. Creating and pretesting messages early in the program planning process enables confirmation of their effectiveness in reaching the intended audience and reduces the likelihood of going through the entire program using an ineffective message.

Message, material, and concept development are based on the communication strategy from the previous stage and the following.

• Step 2-1 Review existing materials

Existing materials are reviewed to determine if they are usable or if it's necessary to create new materials.

• Step 2-2 Develop and test message concepts

Message concepts are preliminary message ideas, suggestions, or ways of presenting the program information to the intended audience. Developing at least two concepts allows for a discussion of which one is most likely to work as *the* program message.

• Step 2-3 Decide on materials to develop

Making a decision about materials to develop is based on:

– the nature of the message (its complexity, style, sensitivity).
– the function of message (bring awareness, increase knowledge, teach a skill).
– the activities and channels decided in Step 1.
– the budget and other resources.

• Step 2-4 Develop messages and materials

The aim in developing messages and materials is for the audience to understand, accept, and use them. To accomplish this, materials and messages are assessed against the following criteria:

– Accuracy—Is the message conveying accurate information?
– Consistency—Are all messages and activities consistent with each other and the communications strategy?
– Clarity—Are the messages and materials written clearly, simply, and at a level appropriate for the intended audience?
– Relevancy—Are the messages and materials of value to the intended audience, and what incentives beyond health benefits might encourage them to change their behavior?
– Credibility—Are there spokespersons or organizations seen as credible by the audience that are associated with the message and practice the behavior recommended in the messages and materials?
– Appeal—Are the materials of high quality, and do they draw the attention of the intended audience?

• Step 2-5 Pretest messages and materials

Messages and materials are pretested to find out if the intended audience understands them, identifies with them, and finds any topic confusing, sensitive, or controversial. Pretesting entails the following:

– Determining the objectives of the pretest.
– Selecting the pretesting methods (interviews, focus groups, questionnaires, observations).
– Securing moderators, and facilities.
– Recruiting and screening reviewers.
– Conducting pretest.
– Analyzing pretest results.
– Revising messages and materials, as needed.

- Step 2-6 Plan for production, distribution and promotion of materials, and process evaluation.

In this step, the quantity of materials needed and a schedule for producing them are determined by taking the following into account:

- The distribution channels and number of materials needed for dissemination through each.
- The plans for promoting the use of the materials.
- The plans for monitoring material usage (process evaluation).

Stage 3—Implement the Program.
Prior to initiating any implementation activities, ensure sufficient quantities of materials are ready and staff are trained.

Putting the plan into action entails the following:

- Step 3-1 Prepare for program launch and implementation.

There are several ways to start implementing a program. (See Chapter 6, Implementing.) One way used with communication programs is to launch (start) with a kickoff, an event that introduces the program to the public. To enhance the effectiveness of a kickoff:

1. Inform the media of the event in a timely manner to improve chances of getting coverage.
2. Launch events in multiple locations on the same day to increase their newsworthiness.
3. Create media kits to facilitate accurate reporting.
4. Invite spokespersons who support the program and attract media attention.
5. Tie it into a community event or other newsworthy happening, such as the Great American Smoke Out or National Wear Red Day.

- Step 3-2 Hold a press conference.

A press conference is an event the press (journalists, reporters) are invited to where information about the program is shared with them and their questions are answered. The following are suggestions for increasing press attendance at a press conference:

- Alert press about the press conference at least 3–4 days in advance.
- Invite local press rather than press from national news outlets.
- Have those whose names carry clout in the community speak about the program.
- Limit the press conference to 15 minutes.
- Have media kits available (press conference agenda, press release, statistics on the health issue, speaker biographies, copies of charts/graphs and program materials or reports, name and contact information of someone who can answer questions and verify information about the program).

- Step 3-3 Maintain media relations.

Getting media coverage at the launch is one thing, maintaining coverage throughout the program is another. To ensure coverage continues:

- Create a list of key media contacts, and nurture relationships with them.
- Identify and train three people with authority in the program to act as media spokespersons.
- Track media coverage to identify and correct misstatements and errors.
- Offer an expert opinion to news media contacts when something happens that is related to the program or the issue the program addresses.

- Step 3-4 Manage implementation.

Managing ongoing program implementation entails the following:

- Monitoring staff, activities, and budget.
- Solving problems that arise.

- Conducting process evaluations.
- Assessing audience response to activities and materials.
- Revising plans as needed.

• Step 3-5 Maintain partnerships.

Maintaining good relationships with partners and keeping them involved takes work.

To support the maintenance of partnerships:

- Contact partners regularly to find out about their progress.
- Credit partners in news releases and other program publicity and materials.
- Inform partners of program evaluation results, both positive and negative.
- Provide partners with new program materials and program-related information

Stage 4—Assess Effectiveness. In this stage, the outcome evaluation plan developed in Stage 1 is used to determine what changes, if any, occurred in knowledge, attitude, or behavior as a result of the program.

To determine how effective the program is

• Step 4-1 Review and revise outcome evaluation plan.

Review the evaluation plan developed in Stage 1 to make sure it will produce the data needed to determine if the program met the outcome objectives by asking the following questions:

- What are the communication objectives?
- What is the intended audience expected to think, feel, or do after the program compared to before, and what methods can measure these changes?
- How is change expected to occur?
- Is the change expected to occur quickly or take time, and what must happen (change) along the way before the outcome behavior change can occur?
- How long is the program expected to last?

- Given the program time frame, what changes are reasonable to expect? What changes are reasonable to expect from year to year over the life of the program?
- Which outcome evaluation methods can measure the size of the change expected to occur?
- Which data collection methods and statistical analysis are likely to capture change in a small percent of the population that normally would fall within the margin of error?
- Which component of the outcome evaluation plan best fits the organization's priorities?
- How do the results of the evaluation contribute to the organization's mission and priorities?
- Are the contributions sufficient to ensure availability of the resources needed to evaluate the program activities?

• Step 4-2 Conduct outcome evaluation.

See Chapter 7, Evaluating.

• Step 4-3 Refine the health communication program.

The evaluation results from the previous step are used to determine if there are aspects of the program that need revision, removal, or reinforcement, or if the program in its entirety should or should not continue.

To make these determinations, the following are examined.

Goals and objectives

- Have the goals and objectives changed? If so, do they need revision or removal?
- Is the program meeting the objectives? If not, what are the barriers? Would revising them overcome the barriers?
- Does the program meet enough of the objectives to justify its continuation?

Information needs

- Is there new health information available that would reinforce the program message?

- Are there activities and strategies that need revision or reinforcement?

Success implications

- Which objectives were met, and by which activities?
- Should use of successful activities continue?
- Is it possible to expand successful activities to other audiences or situations?

Activity costs

- What are the costs and results of different program aspects?

- Are some activities as effective as others, but less costly?

Accountability

- Is there evidence of program effectiveness?
- Were program results shared with the organization leadership, partners, and other stakeholders?
- Do the results indicate a need for new activities that require additional partners?

See **Table 12-5** for a synopsis of the stages and steps of Making Health Communication Programs Work.

Table 12-5 Making Health Communication Programs Work Stages and Steps

Stage	Steps
Stage 1—Develop plan and strategy.	1-1 Assess health problem and identify solution components. 1-2 Define communication objectives. 1-3 Define intended audiences. 1-4 Explore ways to reach intended audience. 1-5 Identify possible program partners. 1-6 Develop strategy, evaluation plans, and timeline.
Stage 2—Develop and pretest concepts, messages, and materials.	2-1 Review existing materials. 2-2 Develop and test message concepts. 2-3 Decide on materials to develop. 2-4 Develop messages and materials. 2-5 Pretest messages and materials. 2-6 Plan for production, distribution, and promotion of materials and process evaluation.
Stage 3—Implement the program.	3-1 Prepare for program launch and implementation. 3-2 Hold a press conference. 3-3 Maintain media relations. 3-4 Manage implementation. 3-5 Maintain partnerships.
Stage 4 - Assess effectiveness.	4-1 Review and revise outcome evaluation plan. 4-2 Conduct outcome evaluation. 4-3 Refine the health communication program.

Data from National Cancer Institute (NCI). (2004). *Making health communication programs work: A planner's guide, pink book.* Washington, DC: U.S. Department of Health and Human Services, National Institutes of Health.

Chapter Summary

Issue and method-specific frameworks provide distinct guidance for developing programs that are consistent with their focus.

Planning in Practice Chapter Activity

Access the following article through your college or university library:

Shrosphire, A. M., Brent-Hotchkiss, R., & Andrews, U. K. (2013). Mass media campaign impacts influenza vaccine obtainment of university students. *Journal of American College Health*, 61(8), 435–443. https://doi.org/10.10 80/07448481.2013.830619

Read the article, and then answer the following questions.

Article Questions

1. Why was this program needed?
2. What beliefs are associated with getting vaccinated?
3. What beliefs are barriers to vaccination?
4. What specific barrier was identified for college students?
5. What health behavior theory is used to explain behaviors associated with flu vaccination?
   (This information is not in the article.)
6. What mass media methods were used in this program?
7. What was the timeline of the mass media campaign?
8. How was the campaign implemented, that is, what was actually done?
9. Was the mass media campaign effective, and how was this determined?
10. If you were to implement this program on your campus, what would you do differently, and why?
11. If this program was for a COVID-19 vaccination program, how might it differ?

References

Chaskin, R. J. (2001). Building community capacity: A definitional framework and case studies from a comprehensive community initiative. *Urban Affairs Review*, 36(3), 291–323. https://doi-org.ezproxy.wpunj.edu/1 0.1177%2F10780870122184876

National Association for County and City Health Officials (NACCHO). (2000). Protocol for assessing community excellence in environmental health (PACE-EH). Washington, DC: NACCHO. Retrieved January 24, 2020, from https://www.cdc.gov/nceh/ehs/ceha/pace_eh.htm

National Cancer Institute (NCI). (2004). *Making health communication programs work: A planner's guide, pink book*. Washington, DC: U.S. Department of Health and Human Services, National Institutes of Health.

Retrieved February 4, 2020, from https://pubs.cancer.gov/ncipl/detail.aspx?prodid=T068

Rural Health Information Hub (RHIhub). (2020). Health communication. Retrieved February 5, 2020, from https://www.ruralhealthinfo.org/toolkits/health-promotion/2/strategies/health-communication

Substance Abuse and Mental Health Services Administration (SAMHSA). (2019). *A guide to SAMHSA's strategic prevention framework*. Rockville, MD: Center for Substance Abuse Prevention. Substance Abuse and Mental Health Services Administration. Retrieved June 25, 2020, from https://www.samhsa.gov/sites/default/files/20190620-samhsa-strategic-prevention-framework-guide.pdf

Choosing a Planning Framework

STUDENT LEARNING OBJECTIVES

After reading this chapter the student will be able to:

- Recognize the generic stages of program planning in frameworks.
- Select a suitable framework for a given program.

Introduction

While there is no one perfect planning framework, some work better than others with certain populations, health issues, cultures, and organizations. Some are more detailed than others or have more steps or stages. Some differ by the types of data (quantitative, qualitative, primary, secondary) sources and indicators used, the extent of community involvement, the length of time the process takes, and whether they are broad and comprehensive or focused on one particular issue (Centers for Disease Control and Prevention [CDC], 2015).

Regardless of their differences, all planning frameworks address the four generic stages of program planning—assessing, planning, implementing, and evaluating. See **Table 13-1** for a comparison of these stages in select planning frameworks.

Guidelines for Choosing a Framework

With the plethora of planning frameworks available, choosing which to use for a given program can be challenging. To ease this process, the following should be taken into consideration:

- Planning committee expertise
  - Do planning committee members or stakeholders have experience and expertise with a particular planning framework?

- Framework effectiveness
  - Is there one framework with proven effectiveness in prior programs for the same intended audience?
  - Is there one framework with proven effectiveness in prior programs addressing the same health issue?

Table 13-1 Comparison of select planning frameworks

Generic steps for program planning	PRECEDE-PROCEDE	Mobilizing for Action Through Planning and Partnership (MAPP)	Mobilize, Assess, Plan, Implement, Track (MAP-IT)	Intervention Mapping (IM)
		Phase 1—Organize for success and partnership development	Step 1—Mobilize coalition	
		Phase 2—Visioning		
Step 1— Assess health needs	Phase 1—Social assessment	Phase 3—Four assessments Community health status assessment	Step 2—Assess	Step 1—Create logic model of the problem
	Phase 2—Epidemiological assessment	Community themes and strength assessment		
		Local public health system assessment		
		Forces of change assessment		
		Phase 4—Identify strategic issues		
Step 2— Plan goals, objectives, and intervention activities	Phase 3—Educational and ecological assessment	Phase 5—Formulate goals and strategies	Step 3—Plan	Step 2—Develop objectives outcomes, and logic model of change
	Phase 4—Administrative, organizational, and policy assessment			Step 3—Program design
				Step 4—Program production
Step 3—Implement plan	Phase 5—Implementation	Phase 6—Action cycle	Step 4—Implement	Step 5—Program implementation plan
Step 4—Evaluate process, impact, and outcomes	Phase 6—Process evaluation	Phase 4—Step 4.6 Conduct process evaluation	Step 5—Track outcomes	Step 6—Evaluation plan
	Phase 7—Impact evaluation	Phase 5—Step 5.7 Conduct process evaluation		
	Phase 8—Outcome evaluation	Phase 6—Step 6.7 Conduct process and outcome evaluations		

- Time availability
  - How much time is available for planning?
  - Which frameworks are compatible with the time available for planning?
  - Are there less time-consuming frameworks?
- Resource needs and availability
  - What resources are available for planning in terms of staffing, equipment/technology, and funding?
  - Which frameworks are compatible with the available resources?
- Expected audience involvement
  - How much involvement in the planning process is expected from representatives of the intended audience?
  - Which frameworks are compatible with the expected level of intended audience involvement?
- Funder requirements
  - Does the funding agency have a preferred or required planning framework?
- Framework fluidity
  - Is the framework fluid or sequential in nature with one stage building upon the previous one (Edelstein, 2018)?
- Framework flexibility
  - Is the framework flexible or adaptable (Edelstein, 2018)? Does it allow

for adjustment to meet the needs of the planning committee and program stakeholders?
- Framework functionality
  - Is the framework functional? Does it focus on improving health rather than producing a program plan (Edelstein, 2018)?

Working through the guidelines can help avoid using a framework that doesn't work as well as it should or could. For example, when intervention mapping was used to develop a smoking cessation program, time and resource (funding) restrictions made it impossible to complete all the tasks required (Dalum, Schaalma, & Kok, 2012). Although intervention mapping was found helpful in planning a program to address weight gain during pregnancy, it was time consuming and unwieldy when used to address a health issue as complex as gestational weight management (Merkx, Ausems, DeVries, & Nieuwenhuize, 2017).

PRECEDE-PROCEED was used for a peer-to-peer online suicide prevention program because of its known effectiveness as a guide for planning health promotion programs. However, because it's a broad framework that doesn't provide specific guidance for prioritizing factors associated with the behavior being changed, it resulted in very diffuse peer counselor training (Bridges, Sharma, Lee, Bennett, Buxbaum, & Resse-Smith, 2018).

Chapter Summary

Because each framework provides guidance for completing the generic stages of program planning in its own unique way, the one used should be carefully chosen to ensure its unique aspects help, rather than hinder, program development.

Planning in Practice Chapter Activity

The CDC has tips for college health and safety at:https://www.cdc.gov/family/college/index.htm

Read the tips for each of the eight health issues.

Choose one tip/issue to use as the basis of a hypothetical program for your campus, then answer the following questions.

Article Questions

1. Which health issue did you choose, and why?
2. If you were planning a program to address this health issue, who would you have on your planning committee, and why?
3. Which of the planning frameworks would you use to develop your program, and why?

References

Bridges, L. S., Sharma, M., Lee, J. H. S., Bennett, R., Buxbaum, S. G., & Resse-Smith, J. (2018). Using the PRECEDE-PROCEED model for an online peer-to-peer suicide prevention and awareness for depression (SPAD) intervention among African American college students: Experimental study. *Health Promotion Perspective*, 8(1),15–24. doi: https://dx.doi.org/10.15171%2Fhpp.2018.02

Centers for Disease Control and Prevention (CDC). (2015). Assessment & planning models, frameworks & tools. Retrieved June 21, 2020, from https://www.cdc.gov/publichealthgateway/cha/assessment.html#two

Dalum, P., Schaalma, H., & Kok, G. (2012). The development of an adolescent smoking cessation intervention—an Intervention Mapping approach to planning. *Health Education Research*, 27(1), 172–181. https://doi.org/10.1093/her/cyr044

Edelstein, S. (Ed). (2018). *Nutrition in public health* (4th ed.). Burlington, MA: Jones & Bartlett Learning.

Merkx, A., Ausems, M., DeVries, R., & Niewenbhuize, M. J. (2017). Come on! Using intervention mapping to help healthy pregnant women achieve healthy weight gain. *Public Health Nutrition*, 20(9), 1666–1680. doi: https://doi.org/10.1017/s1368980017000271

Index

Note: Page numbers followed by *f* or *t* indicate materials in figures or tables respectively.